The Cognitive Revolution in Psychology

The Cognitive Revolution in Psychology

Bernard J. Baars

University of California, San Francisco

The Guilford Press
New York   London

Library of Congress Cataloging in Publication Data
Baars, Bernard J.
    The cognitive revolution in psychology.

    Bibliography: p.
    Includes index.
    1. Cognition.   2. Behaviorism (Psychology)
3. Psychology—Methodology.   I. Title.   [DNLM: 1. Cognition.   2. Psychology—trends.   BF 408 B111c]
BF311.B225   1986   150.19   84-25311
ISBN 0-89862-656-0

To my parents

—for their love and patience

Preface

In recent years the scientific approach to psychology has changed fundamentally, in ways that many consider revolutionary. This book aims to clarify the quiet revolution in thinking that has taken scientific psychology from a strong behaviorist viewpoint to a "cognitive" one. Toward this end, 17 psychologists on both sides of this revolutionary shift are interviewed, each explaining the issues from a personal perspective.

Behaviorism is defended by such major contributors to that approach as B. F. Skinner, Howard Rachlin, Howard H. Kendler, Irving R. Maltzman, and Alan O. Ross. The shift toward a cognitive point of view is discussed by George A. Miller, Noam Chomsky, Ulric Neisser, Donald A. Norman, George Mandler, Jerrold A. Fodor, James J. Jenkins, Walter Weimer, Marvin Levine, Michael A. Wapner, Ernest R. Hilgard, and Herbert A. Simon. Chapters 3, 5, 6, and 7 present the 17 interviews; Chapters 1, 2, and 4 attempt to place behaviorism and cognitive psychology in historical context. The final chapter raises some questions of interpretation: Has the century-long attempt to use the scientific method in psychology lived up to its promise? Have the means of application been appropriate? Does scientific psychology tend to denigrate human nature? If so, with what justification? Although there can be no final agreement on these interpretive issues, they are nonetheless worth raising.

This book is aimed at three possible audiences. First, professional psychologists may be curious to know how the cognitive shift was understood by some of its major protagonists. Those readers interested in the history, philosophy, and sociology of the human sciences will find the interviews a source of insight on a revolutionary change in our scientific conception of human beings. Third, and most important, this book is addressed to students who are within a few years of becoming professional psychologists — graduate students and advanced undergraduates. They are the ones most likely to feel torn between the competing perspectives of their teachers, and they may benefit most from a clear presentation of the circumstances that led to the present state of psychology.

Inevitably, the telling of history is shaped by one's point of view. The psychologists interviewed in this book take a number of different perspectives, and in the historical chapters I attempt a coherent sketch of the major events that have led to contemporary psychology. Because the standard history of psychology, E. G. Boring's *History of Experimental Psychology* (1950), was written from a very specific and strongly held point of view (see Blumenthal, 1975, 1977b), my own attempt to sketch out the events that have shaped contemporary thinking may strike some readers as "revisionist history." Undoubtedly, the narrative of my historical chapters reflects the views of a contemporary cognitive psychologist; however, I have attempted to be sensitive to other points of view, and I am not uncritical of cognitive psychology itself. Still, there is no historiography without perspective, and any perspective both reveals and conceals the actual stream of events. Thus, although the historical chapters represent many years of thinking about the issues, I do not claim them to be the last word on the cognitive shift in psychology.

A cognitive metatheory now dominates most scientific work in psychology, yet there are still a number of viable behavioristic research programs. Does the predominance of the cognitive approach invalidate contemporary behavioristic research? The claim made here is not that "behaviorism is false," but that, in point of historical fact, it has fallen from favor among the majority of active workers in the field. Behaviorists may deplore this development as a deviation from the right way to do scientific psychology, but they do not dispute that the cognitive shift *is* a fact. Indeed, insofar as it represents the philosophical position of "physicalistic monism" — one of the perennial positions on the mind–body problem — behaviorism can probably never be *proven* false. Nor does it make much sense to say that behaviorism "lost" in the cognitive revolution, any more than it would to say that Newtonian physics "lost" to relativity theory in the early decades of this century. Einstein's contribution is inconceivable without the background of Newtonian physics, and the cognitive metatheory can be understood only against the background of behaviorism.

Some of the central tenets of behaviorism are at this point so taken for granted that they have simply become part of standard experimental psychology. All modern psychologists restrict their *evidence* to observable behavior, attempt to specify stimuli and responses with the greatest possible precision, are skeptical of theories that resist empirical testing, and refuse to consider unsupported subjective reports as scientific evidence. In these ways, we are all behaviorists.

At the core of the disagreement between cognitive and behavioristic psychology is the role of theory. This book defines "cognitive psychology" in the first instance as a metatheory — an approach to scientific psychology — that encourages psychologists to infer unobservable constructs on the basis of observable phenomena. Classical behaviorism historically resisted this kind of theoretical inference (see Chapters 1 and 2); but more recent work by behaviorists suggests a greater reliance on theoretical constructs. Thus, in this critical respect, the differences between behaviorists and their cognitive colleagues may well disappear in a few decades.

On the other hand, most of the natural sciences are characterized by the perennial debate between experimenters and theoreticians — between those who are comfortable with theoretical entities such as "genes" and "electrons" and those who must see and touch the phenomena to be sure they are real. In this sense, the dynamic tension between the behavioral and cognitive points of view may well continue in the future, though it may be *called* something else. It may begin to resemble the perennial debate between experimental and theoretical scientists in the natural sciences.

This book owes a great deal to a number of people. The interview participants graciously gave of their time and effort. Others helped with the very large clerical effort involved, especially Ms. Connie Fremont, whose epic battles with computer terminals and text editors were awesome to behold, and certainly indispensable. Magdalena Palmer volunteered her time and energy to organize a sizeable bibliography. Mark Mattson, Michael T. Motley, and Kenneth Giroux gave helpful comments on several chapters, and Professors Aaron Carton, Marvin Levine, and Leonard Krasner provided important historical insights. Professor Lyn Abramson (now of the University of Wisconsin) joined me in interviewing Alan O. Ross (Chapter 3). Comments and reviews by Arthur Blumenthal, Arthur Reber, Howard Gardner, and Donald G. MacKay were most helpful. I also wish to thank my editor, Seymour Weingarten, for his patience and confidence, and for incisive editorial comments. My father, Louis J. Baars, helped design the book jacket. The finishing touches were put on this book while I was Visiting Scientist at the Program for the Study of Conscious and Unconscious Processes, Langley Porter Psychiatric Institute, supported by the John D. and Catherine T. MacArthur Foundation and directed by Mardi J. Horowitz. They are hereby gratefully acknowledged.

Contents

The Cognitive Revolution in Psychology

Introduction: Scientific Psychology in Search of a Framework

For at least 50 years, until very recently, scientific psychology was dominated by a philosophy of science known as behaviorism. Behaviorism is, in many ways, a radical position. Many behaviorists denied the legitimacy of ideas such as consciousness, thinking, feelings, motives, plans, purposes, images, knowledge, or the self. Much of the everyday vocabulary we take for granted in describing human behavior and experience was rejected as unscientific. Thus the most prestigious form of psychology, taught in all major colleges and universities, utterly rejected the major psychological concepts of Western thought. The reasons for this radical rejection of everyday ideas are complex; they involve not only the historical circumstances under which experimental psychology came about and was maintained, especially in the United States, but also the philosophical issue of the mind–body problem, and the nature of science. All of these reasons will be touched on in the course of this book. Over the past several decades, however, a significant shift has taken place in the research community, away from behaviorism and toward a "cognitive" or "information-processing" position. Fewer scholars at major universities now call themselves behaviorists in the traditional sense. In fact, "behaviorism" is often referred to in the past tense, and many commonsense notions of human experience and action are again gaining wide currency in the scientific literature. This shift has been referred to as "the cognitive revolution in psychology" (*e.g.*, Dember, 1974; Joynson, 1970; Weimer & Palermo, 1973; Palermo, 1971), and this book presents the thoughts of some of the most prominent psychologists who figured on both sides of this conceptual revolution.

The changes that have occurred in the last 20 years or so can be interpreted from different vantage points, and will undoubtedly be the source of many disagreements. But no one doubts that something has happened, and that it is fundamental. Sociologists and philosophers of science may differ on how best to characterize the "cognitive revolution," but for working scientists in psychology, the effects of the shift have been concrete and practical: Topics and phenomena that were rejected as "unscientific" are again the subject of lively thinking and experimentation, and much of the 19th-century psychology of Wilhelm Wundt, William James, and others has become relevant again. And conversely, research topics that constituted the very core of the scientific approach to psychology a few decades ago are now dormant, and often considered to be contrived or irrelevant. Along with this, the "reference experiments" that seemed to provide analogues for all other problems have changed. Experiments in animal associationism, such as the work of Pavlov, Watson, and Skinner, seem less relevant now to many psychologists. Reputations have fallen, and reputations have been made. A number of workers who were trained under the older viewpoint are sympathetic to the cognitive revolution, yet seem unable to disengage from the older point of view. The editorial control of journals has shifted, and new journals have sprung up. Along with this have come the new buzz-words — "cognitive," "information processing," "structure," "organization," "psycholinguistics," and so on. The human cost has sometimes been considerable.

Human experimental psychology has been the major focus of the cognitive revolution, but other areas of psychology are beginning to feel the impact. Animal psychology has long been the stronghold of a behaviorism, but recent work indicates the beginnings of a shift there, too (*e.g.*, Hulse, Fowler, & Honig, 1978). Developmental psychology has been similarly affected. And even clinical work with emotionally disturbed people, which has gained the most practical benefits from behavioral ideas and findings, may be shifting in a more cognitive direction (*e.g.*, Mahoney & Arnkoff, 1978; Beck, Rush, Shaw, & Emery, 1979).

Why should anyone outside the field really care about these specialized debates between scholars? Are they not, in fact, very far removed from our everyday concerns? The cognitive revolution warrants general interest for several reasons:

1. *The experimental psychology community has made a profound effort to apply scientific methods to the study of human beings.* At times the operative conception of "scientific method" may have been naïve or based on excessive borrowing from the physical sciences. Nevertheless, both behaviorism

and cognitive psychology represents efforts to be as objective as mere humans can be about ourselves, and neither can be understood apart from this devotion to an idealistic conception of science. Both the behavioristic and cognitive paradigms represent cases of "scientism" in modern life, certainly one of the dominant themes of this century. If the turning away from the behavioristic approach represents a case of "scientism gone wrong," it should concern all of us as a demonstrated limit of what is perhaps the deepest faith of the 20th century.

2. *The cognitive revolution may represent a living example of a "scientific revolution."* Historians and sociologists of science are currently much concerned with the nature of scientific revolutions — radical shifts in the viewpoints of whole research communities (Kuhn, 1962). The best-known examples of such shifts are associated with the great names in the history of science: the Copernican revolution, the Einsteinian revolution, the Darwinian, and so on. It has been argued that the cognitive shift is not at all like these classical revolutions; yet the basic phenomenon — a relatively sudden turnabout in the perspective of a community of scientists — is very similar. Most important, it is happening today, and the majority of the participants in this remarkable event in the life of a scientific community are still alive to give us their impressions.

3. *Because their work carries the status of science, experimental psychologists are highly influential.* Experimentalists have tremendous long-term influence not only over the lives of college students, but also over practicing psychologists, educators, social workers, and others in the "helping professions." Today's research ideas are likely to show up elsewhere — not tomorrow, for there is a considerable time lag before ideas become widely known — but within the next 5 or 10 years. On most college campuses psychology is the most popular subject. But because of the time lag between research and teaching, many undergraduate students even today are taught the behavioristic perspective on human psychology as if it were still dominant in the thinking of researchers.

4. *The scientific approach may yet succeed in understanding human nature.* Probably most scientific psychologists would agree that our understanding is quite limited. But nothing is more fascinating to most of us than the study of humanity itself, and this book may, in a sense, be treated as a progress report on the historic *quest for scientific certainty* in our understanding of human beings and the human puzzle. Even those who view science with suspicion have reason to care about the course of experimental psychology: We have enough experience today with the benefits and drawbacks of successful science to know that the more widely

a scientific approach is understood, the less likely it is to be misused. If war is too important to be left to the generals, then certainly scientific psychology is too important to be left to the psychologists.

In spite of what some popular figures have said about scientific psychology, we in the field are not about to manipulate masses of people against their will. Indeed, current research findings might be held to suggest the impressive capability of people to *resist* manipulation. This book tends, if anything, to emphasize the limits of our current understanding of human beings, and the researchers whose words are recorded herein are very frank about those limits.

In yet a different way, I hope that these interviews reveal the human dimension of psychologists as they devote their professional lives to extending our knowledge about ourselves. Certainly there are failures, and doubts, and some of the less praiseworthy aspects of humanity have their role here as elsewhere. Overall, experimental psychologists are dedicated to a compulsion that all of us share to some degree: the pursuit of knowledge, the attempted satisfaction of a fathomless curiosity about mankind. They have tried to pursue this ideal in a highly disciplined way, refusing to claim anything unless they could prove their claim in the most rigorous way. Sometimes this great cautiousness makes psychologists appear silly, as when they seem to explain laboriously, or even to deny, some utterly commonplace fact. But it must be understood that scientific standards of evidence are much more demanding than those we use in everyday life — in fact, it may be this self-disciplined approach that has ultimately led to the power of the scientific approach in so many areas of life.

The Cognitive Revolution as a Change in the Metatheory of Psychology

Roughly in the decade from 1955 to 1965 a quiet revolution in thought took place among many research psychologists. The dominant metatheory of the previous 50 years was discarded or changed fundamentally, and a new point of view began to take shape. A "metatheory" in science is a viewpoint about how one goes about doing the science, and because psychology is a young and, in many ways, uncertain discipline, its metatheories are even more important than its theories. The theories that psychologists propose to explain their observations are usually quite limited and prone to change, but the metatheory defines the field itself, often for many decades. Psychologists may disagree about any particular topic, but if they share the same metatheory, they will be able to agree on what constitutes evidence for or against their claims. On the other hand, if they cannot define their standards of evidence or their views about the proper domain for psychology, scientific work and communication become nearly impossible.

Thus, it is of major importance that the behavioristic metatheory, which defined the scientific approach to psychology from about 1913 to about 1960, has undergone a fundamental change, a change so profound that most active researchers began to refer to the new point of view with a new name: usually, "cognitive psychology" or "information-processing psychology."

This new metatheory has not yet spread to all areas of psychological research, but everywhere, there is a strong trend in a cognitive direction. Behavioristic influence does remain strong, however, in those areas where it has apparently been very fruitful, especially in animal research and clinical psychology. And because history seldom fits our categories very neatly, it may be that the behavioral influence in these areas will continue to be strong for some time.

Some Ambiguities

Practically all of the words used to describe the events I am outlining have several meanings. "Behaviorism" is a fairly good label for the scientific metatheory that dominated psychology between 1913 and 1960, but a closer look shows that there are many varieties of behaviorism: operant conditioners (Skinnerian), S-R behaviorists, Hullian behaviorists, functionalists, reflex behaviorists, and even "cognitive behaviorists" (*e.g.*, Tolman, 1932). Furthermore, the word "cognitive" is ambiguous: Although it may denote "conscious, intellectual functions," this is *not* the primary sense in which modern cognitive psychologists use it (see Chapter 2). The term "cognitive psychology" is also used to specify a field within human experimental psychology that applies an information-processing metaphor to human functioning. This book uses the term in an even broader sense: It treats cognitive psychology as a new metatheory for psychology — a new approach to the subject matter of scientific psychology — and, thus, as an alternative to behaviorism. This book attempts to use all such labels as consistently as possible, but the reader should be sensitive to possible ambiguities.

Even the word "science" is ambiguous. In one sense, it refers to an established body of fact, integrated by an elegant and powerful theory, but it is also used to characterize a specific *approach* to the establishment of fact, an approach using precise measurement and observation, rigorous reasoning about the observations, and a preference for experimental manipulation of phenomena. Psychology is *not* a science in the first sense, because it lacks an overarching theory. But the psychological research community has worked very hard, at times brilliantly, to develop a *scientific approach* to human conduct and experience. In this second sense, psychology has been scientific for at least 100 years. It has been remarkably difficult to understand human beings in a scientific way, and what progress has been made has been hard won. Yet we have progressed, despite the problems.

Three Metatheories for Psychology

Some fundamental themes will be found throughout this book. One is that three metatheoretical viewpoints have dominated experimental psychology so far, usually called *introspectionism, behaviorism*, and *cognitive* psychology. Each specifies a domain for psychology, a set of techniques for investigating that domain, and a research program to integrate the findings into the body of human knowledge and practice.

Introspectionism claims that the special domain of psychology is conscious human experience. No other science deals directly with human experience as such, and it is the job of psychologists to discover ways to investigate the contents of consciousness. Introspectionism in this sense is usually attributed to Wilhelm Wundt (1832–1920), the major experimental psychologist of the 19th century. But recently it has become clear that Wundt's view is very much broader than introspectionism proper, though he did use "systematic self-observation" to analyze "simple" mental contents. This basic misinterpretation of Wundt's psychology is apparently due to Edward B. Titchener (1867–1927), who was considered the foremost exponent of Wundtian psychology in America (Blumenthal, 1980). It is actually Titchener who best represents the kind of introspectionism against which the behaviorists revolted near the beginning of this century.

Thus, the word "introspectionism" is problematic. Strictly speaking, it is best suited to the work of Titchener, who used the term to describe his own technique of analytic self-observation. Other 19th-century psychologists did not use the term to describe their own work, nor did Wundt. On the other hand, there was general agreement among academic psychologists in the 19th century that the primary *mission* of psychology was to investigate conscious experience.

We could therefore refer to 19th-century academic psychology as "consciousness psychology" — or even as "mentalism." Throughout this book when I use the term "introspectionism," I will use it in the sense of "the consciousness psychology" of the 19th century to include any psychologists who defined psychology primarily as the quest for conscious experience.

Behaviorism came to dominate experimental psychology in America following the work of John B. Watson (1878–1958). From about 1913 on, American experimental psychologists began to outnumber all other psychologists in the world, and because behaviorism dominated American psychology, the bulk of the world's experimental psychology was behavioristic. Although Gestalt psychology, psychoanalysis, and Piagetian psychology flourished in Europe, these significant movements had only marginal impact on behavioristic thought in the United States. Behaviorism utterly rejected the idea that psychology was the study of the contents of consciousness, claiming instead that psychology was the science of observable *behavior*. Indeed, radical behaviorists such as John B. Watson and B. F. Skinner generally denied the scientific validity of conscious experience altogether. During the behavioristic period, psychology grew enormously in the sophistication of its research methods and in the use of experimental design and statistics, but the theories that grew out of behaviorism were easily shown to be weak. In general, behaviorists tended to be antitheoretical, though they were, and are, excellent experimentalists.

Notice that introspectionism and behaviorism both had a definition about the proper domain of psychological science. Introspectionists thought psychology was about the contents of consciousness. Behaviorists decided that it was about behavior, the physical, observable movements organisms make in space.

Cognitive psychologists also have a claim about the domain of a scientific psychology — essentially, it is that psychologists observe behavior in order to make inferences about underlying factors that can explain the behavior. They agree with behaviorists that the data of psychology must be public, but the purpose of gathering this data is to generate theories about unobservable constructs, such as "purposes" and "ideas," which can summarize, predict, and explain the data. In particular, cognitive psychologists often talk about the *representations* that organisms can have of themselves and of their world, and about the transformations that these representations undergo. "Transforming representations" is sometimes called *information processing*. Using this kind of theoretical metaphor, cognitive psychologists can interpret commonsense psychological terms in a rather straightforward way. Thought, language, knowledge, meaning, purpose, imagery, motives, even consciousness and emotion — all the commonsense vocabulary inherited from our culture becomes scientifically useful again. Indeed, it becomes clear that meta-theoretically, our everyday psychology *is* cognitive, since common sense is constantly making inferences about events that underlie the observable world.

Introspectionism, behaviorism, and cognitive psychology are fundamentally different ways of approaching the study of human beings. In a larger sense, they also tell us something about the cultural conditions of science — why was it that different metatheories caught the imagination of psychologists at different times and places? Even more interesting is the fact that each of these positions also represents a traditional stance on the most basic *philosophical* issue in psychology — usually known as the "mind–body" problem.

The Mind–Body Problem

This fundamental issue runs throughout Western philosophy, going back at least to Plato and Aristotle, and forward via Descartes to today's philosophical journals (*e.g.*, Rieber, 1980). And although psychologists today rarely debate the mind–body question, it is easy to show that 19th-century psychology and behaviorism, at least, were explicitly defined in its terms.

For several thousand years the mind–body problem has been discussed in terms of the "fundamental substance of reality": Is reality basically physical or mental? Apparently irrefutable arguments can be mounted either way, but common sense is unlikely to choose either extreme physicalism or mentalism. Commonsense psychology has, indeed, two separate sets of words to talk about physical and mental states. We speak of physical objects and mental ideas in the same breath. Commonsense psychology is *dualistic*, a position first stated explicitly by René Descartes (1596–1650), who argued that consciousness and the physical world exist in two fundamentally different realms of reality. But dualism has its own problems: How does the realm of subjective experience relate to reality "out there"? This problem preoccupied early psychologists. For example, Gustav Fechner, the 19-century founder of experimental psychophysics, was deeply concerned with proving that all physical events are at bottom mental. Psychophysics is today the oldest continuing research tradition in experimental psychology, and of course the very name "psycho-physics" is a reference to the mind–body problem (Greek: *psyche* = mind, soul, or breath; *physis* = body or nature).

When psychology proclaimed itself an independent discipline about

100 years ago, many psychologists wanted their profession to be purely scientific and empirical, and therefore unconcerned with philosophical issues. Over time, professional psychologists lost track of the philosophical underpinnings. This antiphilosophical attitude still prevails today. But is it, in fact, a valid stance? The first metatheory for psychology, the consciousness psychology of the 19th century, defined psychology as the study of conscious contents. To these psychologists, mind was real. The second metatheory, behaviorism, defined psychology as the study of physical movements of organisms. To the behaviorists, mind was an illusion; only the physical world was real. The third metatheory, cognitive psychology, would appear to define psychology as the study of internal processes, conscious or not, which may be inferred by an outside observer on the basis of an organism's behavior. To cognitive psychologists, then, mind is an *inferred* entity, but the history of science shows that inferred constructs gradually begin to take on reality as people become used to them. It is easy to see that the definitions of psychology promulgated by our three metatheories correspond rather neatly to the traditional points of view on the mind–body question: 19th-century psychologists tended to be either mentalists or dualists; behaviorists were clearly physicalists. And most cognitive psychologists are probably "dual-aspect physicalists," at least implicitly, tending to believe that reality is ultimately physical, and that subjective experience is merely a different perspective on the physical world.

It is one of those wonderful historical ironies that, even as psychologists were claiming to be purely scientific, going beyond philosophy to look only at the facts, they found themselves trapped in the oldest philosophical argument of all.

The core issues in this book arise out of the peculiar, and indeed unique, nature of the scientific enterprise in psychology. Unlike any other scientist, a psychologist is an instance of his or her own subject matter. In the last century this was thought to be a great advantage, in that psychologists had unique access to the inner workings of the mind. In the first half of the 20th century, the fact that psychologists are people who study people was held to be a serious scientific *dis*advantage, and private experience was often dismissed as scientifically useless, or even nonexistent. Contemporary psychology has by no means solved this problem, but it may be learning to live with it. Private experience is well and good, but we cannot expect to persuade someone else of our own experience unless we can find some common evidence for it in our shared reality. And science, so the claim goes, is concerned exclusively with evidence and reasoning that can be *publicly shared*.

Whether this is the ultimate resolution of the issue we cannot know, but it seems unlikely that the problem will ever wholly disappear. Philosophers have tried to resolve it for several thousand years, and for scientific psychologists — relative newcomers to the field — a degree of modesty may be well advised. This book will not help to solve the mind–body issue, either, but it may throw some light on the encounter of Western scientists with something new — themselves — and on how this encounter has led to some unexpected problems.

Scientific Revolutions and the Importance of Shared Frameworks

In 1962, the physicist and historian of science Thomas Kuhn published a seminal monograph on the nature of scientific development, entitled *The Structure of Scientific Revolutions* (see also Kuhn, 1970). In this book he argued, contrary to the conventional wisdom, that scientific communities develop not only by slow increments of new knowledge, but also by occasional sudden and dramatic shifts in perspective. Kuhn calls these sudden major changes "paradigm shifts" or "scientific revolutions," and he calls the viewpoint of the scientific community between such revolutions a "paradigm." Paradigm shifts, he claims, take place not only in the great scientific revolutions associated with Copernicus, Newton, Einstein, and Darwin, but also in small scientific groups in a less spectacular, but nonetheless remarkable way: A whole group of scientists will appear to change suddenly, almost in unison, within a short period of time. Those who do not change with the group generally lose their standing as active participants in the group. This kind of paradigm shift is often preceded by a period of crisis, a time when the previous paradigm seems to run into trouble.

Although it has been difficult for Kuhn and others to specify precisely what constitutes a paradigm and what does not, however, Kuhn's description of the paradigm shift elicits an immediate sense of recognition in the mind of the working scientist. Every scientist recognizes that there is a shared framework within which problems are defined and which can, on occasion, go through a rapid consensual change.

Whether or not experimental psychology has a paradigm is a controversial question (Palermo, 1971; Briskman, 1972; Warren, 1972; Mackenzie, 1972; Weimer & Palermo, 1973). The controversy is due, in part, to the fact that the word "paradigm" is generally used rather loosely, but also to the fact that contemporary psychology is viewed differently by different observers. The slippery nature of the world "paradigm" will help to introduce another theme of this book—that scientific terms in general *are meaningful only when understood in a historical context*.

Masterman (1970) has pointed out that Kuhn's famous book used the word "paradigm" in no fewer than 22 different senses (Kuhn, 1970, p. 174). Yet in the minds of many readers, Kuhn seemed to be making a genuine and distinctive point. How can these facts be reconciled? Actually, there is no problem. Kuhn's claims must be seen against the background of his predecessors, especially the influential views of his great teacher Karl Popper. Popper believed that science should function as an essentially rational enterprise, wherein differences between scientists are debated and decided essentially on the merits of the available evidence. Kuhn pointed out that very often scientists with different points of view literally cannot talk to each other, because they base their reasoning on different assumptions and perforce interpret their facts in incompatible ways. *As an objection to Popper's position*, Kuhn's viewpoint is quite meaningful. *Within* Kuhn's viewpoint, however, a large number of ambiguities remain unresolved.

This kind of problem of interpretation is very common in science. It suggests that a scientific issue is meaningful only in its historical context. For example, the once hotly debated issues regarding the "latent learning" controversy of the 1940s are simply meaningless in today's psychological community. Today's issues are similarly *undefinable* within the framework of classical behaviorism.

The terms employed in this book, then—"science," "revolution," "cognitive," "behavioristic," and so on—are sometimes problematic. Some of the psychologists interviewed in this book doubt whether current experimental psychology can even be considered fully scientific in Kuhn's terms, and question whether a paradigm in any of Kuhn's senses obtains in the psychological community. As we shall see, experimental psychology has many, but not all, properties of science as defined by Kuhn. At this point we are confronted by a question of terminological nicety— are the differences between experimental psychology and Kuhn's definition of science great enough to justify using a completely different set of terms for the properties involved? Using the standard words emphasizes commonalities and threatens to obscure differences. Using different terms has the reverse effect, and begins to exhaust the available vocabulary.

Given that our current scientific approach to psychology may be "preparadigmatic," I avoid the word "paradigm" as much as possible in this book, using instead words such as "framework," "perspective," and "exemplar." What is important is to describe the actual views and practices of the experimental psychology community without undue clumsiness.

Shared Frameworks in Science:
A Source of Insight and Blindness

It is often said that the role of a theory is to summarize current results and predict new ones. That description is somewhat narrow. One very important role of theory is to define the nature of the world for a community of scientists. It is impossible to view the world without some theory, although one may shift between different theories for different domains. Consider a simple example. Suppose some people are collecting small objects on a beach, and putting them into different bags according to color and size. All small white objects go into one bag, all large brown ones into another, and so on. This seems to be a reasonable mode of classification — for instance, it would allow the collectors to predict facts about the number of objects per bag. They could also set up experiments, which would result in their knowing that a bagful of small objects weighs less than a bagful of large ones.

Suppose then that someone begins to notice that the objects on the beach are of different sorts: Some are shells, others are rocks and pebbles. This new classification can be just as well-defined in terms of observable properties; moreover, it gives new meaning to the experimental results found earlier: Bags of small objects weigh less than bags of large ones, because there are more shells among the smaller objects, and shells weigh less per volume than the larger rocks. The new theory cuts across the old one. It may render irrelevant some properties that were considered important before, such as the fact that white shells and brown shells belonged together as small objects. Conversely, it has created new distinctions where there were none before, such as the fact that small white shells and small white pebbles are now considered different.

Because of this new classification, the beach people can ask questions that were difficult to articulate in the older theory. What is the origin of shells? Is it different from the origin of pebbles? When you break a shell of any color, the inside looks white — does that mean that all shells are made of the same substance inside? What about the insides of rocks? And so on.

Thus, even a simple theory about objects at the beach will affect the way a community does many things. The new classification has reduced the complexity of searching for objects. It cuts across other reasonable theories, and thus calls attention to some aspects of the phenomena involved, while obscuring others. Both theories make predictions, and it is not obvious which theory is the better one. If the beach people are interested exclusively in the weight of a bag of objects, they may decide that the first theory is good enough for them. If they are ambitiously speculating about the origins of things, the second classification is preferable. If someone who views the world in terms of the first theory meets someone who knows only the assumptions of the second, *he will not be able to understand many of the questions that are obvious to the other person.* This is also true of scientific frameworks. Kuhn (1970) notes that the world views of scientists adhering to competing paradigms are partly *incommensurable.*

In the first place, the proponents of competing paradigms will often disagree about the list of problems that any candidate for paradigm must solve. Their standards or their definitions of science are not the same. More is involved, however, than incommensurability of standards. Since new paradigms are born from old ones, they ordinarily incorporate much of the vocabulary and apparatus, both conceptual and manipulative, that the traditional paradigm had previously employed. But they seldom employ these borrowed elements in quite the traditional way. Within the new paradigm, old terms, concepts, and experiments fall into new relationships with each other. . . . The layman who scoffed at Einstein's theory of relativity because space could not be "curved"— it was not that sort of thing—was not simply wrong or mistaken. . . . What had previously been meant by space was necessarily flat, homogeneous, isotropic, and unaffected by the presence of matter. If it had not been, Newtonian physics would not have worked. *To make the transition to Einstein's universe, the whole conceptual web whose strands are space, time, matter, force, and so on, had to be shifted and laid down again on nature whole.* (pp. 148–149, italics added)

[Thus] debates over theory-choice cannot be cast in a form that fully resembles logical or mathematical proof. . . . That debate is about premises, and its recourse is to persuasion as a prelude to the possibility of proof. . . . There is no neutral algorithm for theory-choice, no systematic procedure which, properly applied, must lead each individual in the group to the same decision. (pp. 199–200)

And in the same vein, but more pessimistically, Max Planck has written that " . . . a new scientific theory does not triumph by convincing its opponents and making them see the light, but rather because its opponents eventually die, and a new generation grows up that is familiar with it" (quoted in Kuhn, 1970, p. 150).

Thus, new paradigms or frameworks are not accepted by some entirely formal proof procedure, but rather by a process of persuasion that can involve many ingredients. Nor does it follow that the losing side in a scientific revolution is necessarily wrong—merely that it loses. Those individuals who fundamentally disagree with the new direction are likely to be increasingly viewed as outsiders to the shared concerns of the community.

The Adolescence of Psychology

Another theme of this book can be stated as an analogy. There is an interesting parallel between the development of scientific psychology and adolescence. Adolescents are often unsure of themselves; consequently, they emphasize differences between themselves and others. Conversely, they also tend to idolize their favorite role models. These points can be made as well about experimental psychology in its first 100 years. It is young, as sciences go, and has often been unsure of itself. Among its older brothers, the established natural sciences, it was obliged to carve out its own domain. Because physiology preceded the establishment of psychology, psychologists often claimed that their science had no direct connection with the physiology of the nervous system. In order to separate itself from philosophy (which at one time included psychology), psychologists emphasized the fact that they were *empirical*, whereas philosophers spent their time in "armchair speculation." Psychologists often brashly established such differences in order to delimit a legitimate domain for their discipline, one that permitted a scientific approach not already claimed by the older sciences.

Psychologists also had a special problem in the fact that there already exists a reasonably effective psychology of everyday life, which employs a rich and apparently meaningful vocabulary. Thus every brand of scientific psychology must not only create a place for itself somehow among the formal scientific disciplines, but must also separate itself from commonsense psychology. This obligation has created its own characteristic difficulties. Just as adolescents sometimes indulge in uncritical imitation of heroes and heroines, psychologists initially tended to idolize certain sciences, especially physics, the first and perhaps the most beautiful of the sciences. This general, uncritical adoration of anything scientific has been called "scientism" (Koch, 1959; Koestler, 1967), and it was sometimes indulged to an embarrassing extent. Nevertheless, the adoration of established science yielded some clearly useful methods, so that maybe it was worthwhile. The trouble was perhaps, that there were no good "role models" in the human sciences, and many of the growing pains of experimental psychology have resulted from the fact that it had to find its own way. Other human sciences such as sociology, linguistics, and political science have experienced similar growing pains (*e.g.*, Andreski, 1972).

The Scientific Community as an Ecosystem

Another useful theme metaphor for this book may be borrowed from biology, namely, the notion of the scientific community as an *ecosystem*. Science, at least in the West, is always the product of a *community* of thinkers with shared interests and shared criteria for acceptable evidence. Such a community requires methods of internal communication and publication; it requires the intellectual resources, time to think, the opportunity to discuss issues, money for equipment and trained assistance, and so on. All these requirements tend to encourage professionalization, and there is only a finite number of "niches" available — spaces in the professional ecosystem for individuals whose demands for time, support, social status, and the like can be satisfied. Furthermore, the psychological ecosystem competes for resources with other research communities. Indeed, scientific psychology found its primary home in Germany in the 19th century and in the United States in the 20th largely because the resources needed were available in these countries, and the claims for legitimacy made by psychologists were likely to be believed. All this meant that psychology became professionalized. This is somewhat peculiar, since even today we are not sure if psychology warrants characterization as a "science" in the strong sense of that word. One indication of this professionalization is that we credit psychology with a birthdate: The first psychological laboratory was opened in Leipzig in 1879 by Wilhelm Wundt. Note that this is an *institutional* birthdate; very good experimental work had been done earlier, by Helmholtz and Fechner, for example, but not in a psychological research institution. It is unusual in the history of a science to be able to pinpoint beginnings with such specificity — who knows when physics or astronomy began? With the Babylonians? With Archimedes or Aristarchus? In fact, the beginnings of the established sciences are indeterminable because the early scientists did not know they were doing science. The very distinction we make between "empirical science" and other scholarly fields is modern, and one could not self-consciously begin a science without this conception. Thus empirical psychology, like medicine, became a profession before it found a sound scientific basis.

Professionalization has well-known penalties. In a professional science, scientists cannot be satisfied with an office, a laboratory, and a salary. They must continually justify their existence in terms of some unique contribution to the field. If the scientist's work is like someone else's, no one will read it, and he or she will ultimately lose the position. But if the scientist does things so differently from everyone else that the work cannot be understood, no one will read it either, and again, one will lose one's professional position. In order to survive, scientists must have their own "conceptual niches." In practice, every scientist can label his or her colleagues: "Oh yes, Jane Jones does x in physical chemistry, which differs completely from John Jones, who does y in chemical physics." But what happens if the scientific community is not certain of its own domain? Then it becomes impossible for an individual scientist to establish a reliable niche in a recognized field, or to make a recognizable contribution.

The history of psychology is clearly the search for a valid domain. The metatheory for experimental psychology may well change when a set of particular conceptual niches has been exhausted and the older metatheory simply provides no more ideas to keep the community going. In the absence of valid content, a professional group will often engage in empty jargon and mystification, attempting to justify its existence. The history of medicine provides many telling examples of this kind of coping device (Zilboorg, 1941). In the case of psychology, it would appear that psychologists have repeatedly rejected the psychology of common sense in an effort to prove that scientific psychology is necessary. But commonsense psychology seems to serve most people rather well.

One major penalty of professionalization is the danger of *fixedness* (Duncker, 1945). If a community becomes established before it is sure of its proper content, the development of new points of view, which are necessary to the progress of science, is inevitably retarded. In medicine, for example, there was a great deal of resistance to the ideas of Pasteur because the medical community was committed to other modes of therapy, which were, in fact, less effective. Indeed, it is said that prior to about 1910, the majority of drugs used by physicians were either ineffective or actually harmful (Shapiro, 1960). Fixedness is probably universal — one can demonstrate it in any kind of problem-solving situation (Duncker, 1945; Levine & Fingerman, 1974; Luchins, 1942). It is especially harmful when it involves a *denial* of possibility. Scientists are typically quite good when they *assert* some fact in their field, but they have a rather bad record when it comes to denying the possibility of some hypothesis. Almost every great advance in the history of science was initially debunked by some highly respected scientist.

The Framework Dilemma

This point leads to a final theme of this book, which I will call the "framework dilemma," as follows. In order to think about any subject, we need to establish a framework — some set of assumptions that reduces to manageable proportions the number of ways to view the subject. The framework of 19th-century consciousness psychology assumed that trained observers could observe their own, internal processes. Behavioristic framework assumptions include associationism, peripheralism, experimentalism, and the like (see Chapter 2). Frameworks are absolutely necessary, but they may also be false or misleading. This is a true dilemma — there really is no way to avoid using frameworks, because one cannot deal with the multiplicity of possibilities without some simplifying assumptions. Nor is there any way to avoid the possibility of being led astray by the framework. (It *is* useful to be tolerant and willing to listen to other points of view, to encourage competing perspectives, and to minimize the number of assumptions if possible.)

A framework, as the word is used here, is very similar to a "paradigm," but, as I suggested earlier, there is a great deal of debate about the meaning of the word paradigm," which seems fruitless to repeat here. Furthermore, we can define the idea of a framework psychologically as a set of assumptions that guide the scientist in thought, action, and communication by *reducing the number of possibilities that can be imagined*. While scientists are thinking about a specific problem or talking about it to one another, these assumptions are typically not focally conscious. They become focal and explicit only when a scientist is dealing with *outsiders* to the community, such as students, or other scientists who maintain different framework assumptions. Some of the assumptions a scientist makes are merely metaphors, and "machine metaphors" are especially important in the history of psychology. Other assumptions are heuristic, having to do with the intangibles of a successful research strategy. Because they are often not consciously examined, some of the working assumptions scientists maintain may be surprisingly naïve. But good scientists are very thoughtful, and do, in the course of their careers, spend a great deal of time examining assumptions. The interviews in this book ask psychologists to make explicit some of the assumptions on which they have based their whole professional lives.

Among these framework assumptions are the "metaphysical foundations of science" (Burtt, 1955), such as the assumption of determinism. One does not test determinism in a laboratory. It is only a convenient way of thinking about the world, and insofar as a science is successful, we learn more about how one specific factor determines another. Occasionally one will hear a psychologist say that we now *know* that human behavior is *determined*. Such a statement is highly questionable — it is merely part of the metaphysical framework of science. We assume it, we do not test it.

2

Behaviorism: The Rise of an Objectivist Psychology

In the year of our Lord 1432, there arose a grievous quarrel among the brethren over the number of teeth in the mouth of a horse. For thirteen days the disputation raged without ceasing. All the ancient books and chronicles were fetched out, and a wonderful and ponderous erudition, such as was never before heard of in this region, was made manifest. At the beginning of the fourteenth day, a youthful friar of goodly bearing asked his learned superiors for permission to add a word, and straightway, to the wonderment of the disputants, whose deep wisdom he sore vexed, he beseeched them to unbend in a manner coarse and unheard-of, and to look in the open mouth of a horse and find answer to their questionings. At this, their dignity being grievously hurt, they waxed exceedingly wroth and joining in a mighty uproar, they flew upon him and smote his hip and thigh, and cast him out forthwith. For, said they, surely Satan hath tempted this bold neophyte to declare unholy and unheard-of ways of finding truth contrary to all the teachings of the fathers. After many days of grievous strife the dove of peace sat on the assembly, and they as one man, declaring the problem to be an ever-lasting mystery because of a grievous dearth of historical and theological evidence thereof, so ordered the same writ down.

— Francis Bacon (quoted in Meese, 1934)

If we take in our hand any volume — of divinity or school metaphysics, for instance — let us ask, *Does it contain any abstract reasoning concerning quantity or number?* No. *Does it contain any experimental reasoning concerning matters of fact and existence?* No. Commit it then to the flames, for it can contain nothing but sophistry and illusion.

— David Hume (1748/1962, p. 163)

Behaviorism is a natural outcome of a trend in Western thought that is at least four centuries old: a trend toward empirical testing of hypotheses, and away from a reliance on scripture and authority; toward physicalism, and away from a reliance on mental events; toward a faith in science, and away from religious faith. Francis Bacon (1561–1626), who wrote the satirical story of the theologians' dispute quoted above, was one of the first notable figures in this trend. And several centuries later, David Hume (1711–1776) carried it to its logical conclusion: All "metaphysical" thought was to be discarded unless it could be tested empirically. By the end of the 19th century this view was sweeping philosophical thinking in the form of positivism and later, logical positivism (Ayer, 1946). Behaviorism is really an extension of this view to psychology. As far as behaviorists were concerned, any hypotheses that did not lead to physically quantifiable, measurable behavior were to be discarded. In Hume's fiery metaphor, they were determined to "Commit it then to the flames, for it can contain nothing but sophistry and illusion." Thus behaviorism was a major attempt to extend scientific physicalism to its apparent logical conclusion, to show that even the human mind could be reduced to the basic physics of the 19th century. In this chapter we will look at the rise of behaviorism, starting with its physicalistic antecedents.

The attempt to create a scientific psychology — to study human conduct and experience objectively — is a most peculiar enterprise from the outset. There would seem to be a basic dilemma in any effort to study human beings "as if from the outside." Human beings always seem to take an insider's viewpoint on ourselves, our society, and our world. We make assumptions that become so much a part of us that we take them as given and unquestionable. Being scientific means taking a distance from ordinary human conduct, taking an outsider's point of view to study "the facts" minutely while holding in abeyance what we think we already know.

Further, each of us has a great many experiences that would be hard to prove to others. Someone may have a stomach ache, or be color blind. Someone may have wonderful feelings listening to music, or take a particular point of view toward the world. How would anyone convince another rational person that these experiences are "real"? This puzzle (which is really a variant of the philosophical mind–body problem) is at the bottom of the three great phases of experimental psychology during the last 100 years. As noted in the introduction, these great phases can be roughly characterized by the labels *introspectionism, behaviorism, and cognitive psychology*, and each copes with the mind–body distinction somewhat differently.

Most 19th-century psychologists claimed that the main role of scientific psychology was to study the contents of consciousness — a radical *insiders'* viewpoint. In his popular introduction to experimental psychology, Wundt (1912/1973) wrote:

If psychologists are asked, what the business of psychology is, they generally make some such answer as follows, if they belong to the empirical school: that this science has to investigate the facts of consciousness, its combinations and relations, so that it may ultimately discover the laws which govern these relations and combinations. (p. 3)

And Wundt was quite sure that these laws of mental life were fundamentally different from physical laws. He was not a dualist — he asserted repeatedly that only one reality underlies the two perspectives of mind and body (Blumenthal, 1979) — but to Wundt, the unique character of psychology is that it permits us to understand its subject matter in its own terms, from the "inside."

Behaviorists utterly denied this view, claiming that the only proper study of psychology was *external* manifestations — that is, human behavior. Everything of interest would ultimately reduce to physical movements in space, the "insider's" point of view would be shown to be illusory.

Modern cognitivists, curiously enough, tend to ignore the philosophical ramifications of the mind–body question, taking no explicit position on it. They simply run what they think are interesting studies and pursue the theoretical implications of their results. But one might infer from their practices a position as follows: To each of us our individual consciousness is directly in evidence, but to the rest of the world it must be inferred from our words and actions (Mandler & Kessen, 1959). Hence, if we make a claim about our experience, and intend to use this claim as scientific evidence, it behooves us to find a publically observable correlate of that claim. Given some ingenuity, this can be done in a surprising number of cases. Thus, the picture of the human mind that emerges from the cognitive approach is based on evidence that is observable to anyone. It leads to theories that do not so much violate common sense as go beyond it in certain ways (*e.g.*, Neisser, 1967; Newell & Simon, 1972; Norman, 1976).

As we go from 19th-century psychology to behaviorism to cognitive psychology, we can detect in each metatheory a point of view on the mind–body problem, but also a *decreasing* concern with making this point of view explicit. 19th-century psychologists were openly concerned with the mind–body controversy. Behaviorists were initially concerned with it, but subsequently simply assumed that physicalism was the only possible scientific position, so that the issue was no longer discussed. And many cognitive psychologists today would be surprised to find that their work relates at all to the mind–body question.

The fact that empirical psychologists have all but lost sight of the vexing philosophical issues is probably a sign of their increasing confidence in the subject matter of psychology. This pragmatic strategy does not *solve* the mind–body problem. It simply circumvents it, confident that an interesting set of issues can be dealt with without becoming embroiled in empty controversy. But cognitive psychologists may be drawn in spite of themselves to consider some surprising philosophical implications of their position. For example, Bakan (1980) and Szilard (1929/1964) have suggested that the formal concept of "information" raises the same problems that have long been associated with "mind." And, of course, "information" is a fundamental idea in physics and biology, as well as increasingly in psychology (see also Bateson, 1979).

To understand the conditions in which behaviorism rose and flourished for a half century, it is well to recall the place of science in the outlook of late 19th- and early 20th-century America. Along with much of the Western world, Americans shared the view that "science" and "Progress" were inseparable, and that each scientific advance forced a concomitant retreat in the religious view of life. Copernicus represented an advance in scientific knowledge over Ptolemaeus, but in return, the world ceased to be geocentric and instead became heliocentric. With Newton, the entire solar system became an arbitrary locus in unbounded space. And with Darwin, humanity lost its special place in the biological world. Darwin's theory led to the epic battle of 19th-century science against religion, and in the eyes of most observers, science won. Indeed, religion was increasingly viewed as the preeminent opponent of scientific advancement (read: Progress)—from Galileo's trial by the Inquisition to the Scopes Monkey Trial in Tennessee. By the end of the 19th century, the last refuge of religion appeared to be the soul, which had become identified by many with human consciousness. So it was that just as a scientific approach to psychology was about to be born, the most basic cultural and philosophical struggle was going on about the very issues that the new psychology would have to investigate.

As theological claims began to retreat, a genuine scientific ideology was taking shape, a faith often held with truly religious fervor. It may be no accident that many of the most fervent advocates of a scientific psychology were brought up in religious homes (*e.g.*, Watson, Pavlov, and Skinner). In biology, the scientific and antireligious trends appeared in the form of Darwinism and its offshoots, especially in the *antivitalist* movement. Vitalism was a philosophy holding that there is some unique essence that animates living things and separates them from the inanimate world; this vital essence could never be reduced to mere physics (*e.g.*, Bergson, 1907/1926; McDougall, 1923). Antivitalism attempted to disprove vitalism's argument, and in the process seemed to take on the characteristic ideological quality of an opposing religious view. Against the philosophy of vitalism the great physiologist Claude Bernard wrote in 1865:

I propose to prove that the science of vital phenomena must have the same foundations as the science of the phenomena of inorganic bodies, and that there is no difference in this respect between the principles of biological science and those of physico-chemical science. (quoted in Miller, 1962, p. 193)

According to Miller (1962), "in Germany, the science of physiology was controlled by four men: Herman Ludwig von Helmholtz, Emil Du Bois-Reymond, Ernst Brücke, and Carl Ludwig." These four formed a private club in Berlin whose members were pledged to destroy vitalism, a pledge that one of them phrased so:

No other forces than the common physical–chemical ones are active within the organisms. In those cases which cannot be explained by these forces or their action by means of a physical–mathematical method or assume new forces equal in dignity to the chemical–physical forces inherent in matter, reducible to the force of attraction and repulsion. (Jones, 1953)

"And it was in this intellectual atmosphere," Miller points out,

that the pioneer psychologists were educated. Freud was Brücke's student; Pavlov studied under Ludwig; Wundt was Du Bois-Reymond's student and Helmholtz's assistant. With physiology reduced to chemistry and physics, the next step was to reduce psychology to physiology . . . Freud to the end of his life talked about the mind in hydraulic, mechanical, electrical, and other physical metaphors. Pavlov would never concede that his physiological interpretation of conditioning experiments was merely an elaborate figure of speech. And even Wundt, who tried to break with the positivistic tradition, founded his new psychology by writing a text, not on psychology, but on physiological psychology. (p. 194)

Thus the believers in scientism actively advocated a *program* not merely of research, but of ideological physicalism. They confidently expected all of human knowledge to yield to the assault of the scientific method that had proved so successful in physics, astronomy, and major areas of biology and chemistry. And they further assumed that the successful natural sciences were not vulnerable to fundamental change (a false assumption, as Einstein and others were about to show the world).

What about the human sciences? In the second half of the 19th century, ambitious attempts were made to found new scientific approaches to psychology, sociology, and political science in a deliberate and self-conscious way. In the last chapter I pointed out how peculiar it is that scientific psychology has an official birthdate. One cannot establish a science deliberately without first *having* the conception of what a science is, and in the latter half of the 19th century, science was understood as an empirical, precise, theoretically explicit sort of enterprise, which must, in order to succeed, be free of the fetters imposed by metaphysical philosophy and theology. None of the natural sciences were deliberately founded — they grew organically, over thousands of years, with no sense that scientific work was somehow different from philosophy or theology. Indeed, until the middle of the 19th century, physics was called "natural philosophy." Newton considered his *Principia* to be of minor interest compared with his commentary on the Book of Job. Only about 100 years ago did empirical science became a separate entity, and only then do we see the rise of a scientific ideology, pledged to do battle the metaphysical ghosts of the past.

Psychological thought had its own version of vitalism. Sentient beings were said to differ fundamentally from physical objects because they were conscious and purposeful. Some philosophers and psychologists interpreted this perceived difference in explicitly spiritual terms (*e.g.*, Bergson, 1907/1926; McDougall, 1923). Others, such as Wundt, believed that psychology could function as a science, but that it would have to proceed in a way fundamentally different from the physical sciences. Thus Wundt cautioned that given the conscious and volitional character of human perception, thought, and action, "Attempts to subsume mental processes under the types of laws found in the physical sciences (including physiology) will never be successful." Wundt believed that human perception, thought, and action were essentially directed toward goals, whereas physical activity occurred as the result of prior causes (Wundt, 1873, quoted in Blumenthal, 1979, p. 549). The idea that psychology is unique and different from physical science thus came down to two issues: consciousness and purpose.

To some partisans of physicalistic science, the arguments supporting the existence of consciousness and purpose posed a threat to the scientific world view: First, if consciousness involved some nonphysical form of reality, then physicalism was incomplete. Second, if the laws of psychological functioning involved goal-directed activity, then everything could not be reduced to physical causality. It is against these two views — mentalism and *teleology* (after the Greek *telos*, meaning end or goal) — that behaviorism ultimately defined its program.

In pursuit of this program, it became necessary for advocates of scientific physicalism to deny two commonsense ideas about people — that they are conscious and that they have goals. How were physicalists going to deal with consciousness? T. H. Huxley, the famous spokesman for Darwinism, proposed that consciousness might have some sort of existence, but no function:

Consciousness . . . would appear to be related to the mechanism of the body . . . simply as a [side] product of its working, and to be completely without any power of modifying that working, as the [sound of] a steam whistle which accompanies the work of a locomotive . . . is without influence upon its machinery. (quoted in James, 1890/1983, p. 135)

This position, that consciousness exists, but without power to affect the world, is usually known as *epiphenomenalism*. Other physicalists seemed to deny the existence of consciousness altogether. Chief among these, of course, were the radical behaviorists, notably Watson and Skinner. Indeed, Skinner has defined radical behaviorism in these terms:

It is . . . possible to be a Behaviorist and recognize the existence of conscious events. . . . We may set up a distinction between a public and a private world, the first a communicable one . . . and the latter forever reserved from scientific treatment. If psychology is to be a science (i.e. a public science) its concepts must be defined as if they did not refer to a private world. . . . But I preferred the position of *radical behaviorism* in which the existence of subjective entities is denied. (1978, p. 117)

Even the radicals at times held different positions on the issue of consciousness (*e.g.*, Skinner, 1979). But the overall *effect* of their views was to discredit consciousness as a respectable topic of research and theory. Behaviorists who were inclined to take the issue seriously were forced into a highly defensive stance. And if one must be defensive about even mentioning a topic, it becomes effectively impossible to explore it in depth. Thus, the effect of the radical arguments was to put the entire topic of personal experience outside the pale of respectable psychology. Only in the last few years have experimental psychologists begun to take another serious look at consciousness (Posner, 1973; Mandler, 1984; Baars, 1983a). This is only one illustration of the massive impact that the 19th-century physicalistic philosophy of science has had, even on today's scientific research in psychology.

Physicalists also denied the existence of *human purpose*. The concept of purpose has a curious philosophical background. Aristotle, the most influential thinker in Western history, defined four kinds of "causality," and his distinctions have remained the basis for our own. Among the four was "efficient causality," the kind of "billiard ball" causality for which we, in the English language, reserve the word "cause" itself. But Aristotle also defined a "final cause," or *telos* — the purpose for which a thing is made. The connection between the efficient cause and the final cause has always seemed deeply puzzling. If something happens to a billiard ball, we can attribute that event to *preceding* events. But purpose seems to involve an "effect" of a *future state*. It would appear to run counter to the direction of ordinary causal time. Some of the antiphysicalists thought that this was a devastating argument in their favor: How could goals and purposes ever be reduced to mere physical causality?

The response of many physicalists was to deny the existence of purposes altogether. Although this seemed to fly in the face of everyday reality, physicalists were wont to point out that at least one kind of human activity was *not* purposeful: namely, the physiological reflexes. One merely taps the tendon on the knee, and the foot swings out, just as one merely strikes a billiard ball with a cue, and the ball will roll. One does not give the knee a goal, or ask it to move. Of course, only a tiny percentage of normal activity is reflexive in this sense. But could this example of physical causality be extended to explain psychological cause as well?

In the mid-19th century the Russian physiologist I. M. Sechenov (1829–1905) proposed that it could. He wrote in his doctoral dissertation of 1860 that " . . . all movements bearing in physiology the name voluntary are in a strict sense reflexive" (quoted in Razran, 1965, p. 354). Furthermore,

If a conscious psychical act is not accompanied by any external manifestations, it still remains a reflex. . . . A thought is two-thirds of a psychical reflex . . . only the end of the reflex, i.e., movement, is completely absent. . . . Association is effected through a continuous series of reflexes in which the end of a preceding reflex coincides in time with the beginning of a subsequent [one]." (quoted in Razran, 1965, p. 354).

Sechenov anticipated the behaviorism of the 20th century even more in his emphasis on the physiological, and even just muscular, nature of psychological events. In this connection he claimed in 1863 that

No conceivable demarcation will be found between obvious somatic, i.e., bodily, nervous acts and unmistakable psychic phenomena . . . A child laughing at the sight of a toy, a young girl trembling at the first thought of love, Garibaldi smiling when he was driven from his country because his love for it was too great, Newton discovering and writing down the laws of the universe — everywhere, the final act is a muscular movement. (quoted in Razran, 1965, p. 354)

Sechenov was much admired by I. P. Pavlov (1849–1936) who half a century later gave further legitimacy to this point of view. Pavlov showed how *new* events in the environment could come to evoke standard reflexes, such as salivation, leg flexion, or pupillary contraction. Such "psychic reflexes" were supposed to explain, at least in principle, how normal actions — which are complex, voluntary, and apparently purposeful — could be reduced to the causality of reflexes and billiard balls.

The denial of purpose has been central to behaviorism as well. More accurately, perhaps, one of the behaviorism's primary tasks has been to show that apparently purposive behavior can be explained in terms of ordinary physical causality. Some behaviorists — for example, Edward

Tolman—were content to assert simply that behavior was fundamentally purposive, and that somehow, eventually, the causal chain would be puzzled out. In the meantime it seemed wise to accept purpose as a fact. Others, such as Skinner, denied the *concept* of goals or purposes, but developed alternative ways of analyzing the observations that lead us to think that goals and purposes are real. Indeed, Skinner (1974) wrote that "Operant behavior is the very field of purpose and intention" (p. 61). And, finally, Clark Hull, the major theoretician of the behavioristic period, devoted great effort to proving that goal-directed behavior could be explained causally; he postulated that a chain of tiny internal stimuli and responses, acquired by learning, extends backward to the beginning of an action by a process of generalization. We will look at behaviorism's efforts to resolve the problem of teleology in more detail below.

To a generation brought up with computers, the foregoing arguments may seem curious. In a real sense, even a simple thermostat is a goal-directed machine. One begins by setting a desirable temperature, and by a continual process of adjustment the thermostat causes the heating system to turn on and off, thereby narrowing the difference between the preset goal and the room temperature. This kind of cybernetic feedback loop is so commonplace today that one does not bother about specifying the *particular* mechanisms that cause the temperature to approach the goal. Such mechanisms are presumably causal in the sense of classic efficient causality, but the technical end of the process does not concern us—we tend simply to use the vocabulary of goals in describing the activity of the thermostat. Computers are large conglomerations of cybernetic feedback loops, and it has become common to speak of a computer "attempting to reach" some solution to a preset problem, especially if it can do so with a high degree of flexibility. There is no implication that the ability to function in terms of goals makes the computer somehow nonphysical.

But this point did not always seem so obvious. Gregory Bateson, one of the first to apply cybernetic ideas in psychology and anthropology, has described his own development as follows:

In the 1930's I was already familiar with the idea of "runaway" (a positive feedback loop). . . . But at that time, I had no idea that there might be circuits of causation which might be self-corrective (i.e., negative feedback loops). Many self-corrective systems were also already known. That is, individual cases were known, but the *principle* remained unknown . . . Discoveries and rediscoveries of the principle include Lamarck's transformism (1809), James Watt's invention of the governor for the steam engine (late 18th century), Alfred Russel Wallace's perception of natural selection (1856), Clerk Maxwell's mathematical analysis of the steam engine with a governor (1868), Claude Bernard's *milieu interne*, Hegelian and Marxian analyses of social process, Walter Cannon's *Wisdom of the Body* (1932). . . . Finally, the famous paper in *Philosophy of Science* by Rosenblueth, Wiener and Bigelow (1943) proposed that the self-corrective circuit and its many variants provided possibilities for modeling the adaptive actions of organisms. The central problem of Greek philosophy—the problem of purpose, unsolved for 2,500 years—came within range of rigorous analysis. (1979, p. 117)

Thus it was only in 1943 that the cybernetic principles were stated in a general and precise form (Wiener, 1961). This made it possible to be scientific and physicalistic, and still acknowledge the existence of goals and purposes. This idea has become so commonplace today that the fight both for and against "teleology" is difficult for us to understand. But the struggle against teleology motivated a great deal of behavioristic thought.

To be a scientist at the end of the 19th century was to be on the side of progress and against superstition. It meant believing that Newtonian physics described the fundamental nature of reality, and that any other knowledge of reality should ultimately be reduced to it. The resulting need to explain psychological phenomena in terms familiar in physics implied, for many people at least, that any obstacles to extending physicalism to the world of consciousness and volition were to be denied. Indeed, the very existence of conscious experience and purpose was denied. It is one of those great ironies that a scientific devotion to empirical fact led scientific physicalists to deny facts that can be observed and tested in everyday life. It is important to be reminded, in this regard, that behaviorists and other physicalists saw themselves as an idealistic vanguard, struggling against superstition and its hold on the human mind. If it was necessary to deny some apparent phenomenon such as purpose, this was perhaps a temporary price to pay in order to establish a truly scientific study of humanity.

The denial of consciousness and purpose always had a curiously paradoxical air about it. The commonsense view of human psychology is so strong and perhaps so fundamentally true, that physicalists found themselves asserting in their actions precisely what they were denying in words—attempting, as it were, to make their opponents *conscious* of the fact that *consciousness* does not exist; having *as a goal* the extension of a scientific philosophy that denies the existence of goals. All varieties of scientism in psychology have this air of paradox, and behaviorism does so to an extraordinary degree: Many behaviorists believed that beliefs are not believable, that thought is unthinkable, that one can have a theory of human beings who cannot have theories, and so on. This paradoxical quality did not go unnoticed by behaviorists themselves, but it was usually ascribed to a temporary need to use the commonsense language until a more adequate description became available (Bergman & Spence, 1941).

By the end of the 19th century, then, the stage was set for a thoroughgoing physicalistic psychology. But in fact, experimental psychology was officially founded, not by physicalists, but by scholars who believed in the reality of consciousness, purpose, and all the other ideas of commonsense psychology. "Introspectionism" is the name which the next, behavioristic generation, gave to the psychology of the 19th century often in an effort to discredit it. From a modern point of view, much of this work is again seen as interesting and useful. It is important to understand the thinking of those psychologists who used "self-observation" as well as objective measures, not only for its own sake, but because behaviorism *defined itself against what it thought 19th-century psychology was*. It is quite impossible to understand behaviorism without understanding what came before it.

The 19th-Century Background

If the major cultural trends over four centuries have been in the direction of physicalism, it seems surprising that experimental psychology began with a program for the investigation of conscious experience. But in the 19th century the belief in the independent reality of mental events was associated with some of the great names in German philosophy, such as Hegel, Kant, and Schopenhauer; and it was in Germany that experimental psychology first began. Further, some of the pioneers in experimental psychology, such as Fechner and Wundt, were apparently drawn to psychology precisely because of its potential to prove the inadequacies of physicalism. Early psychologists were well versed in philosophy, and it is only toward the end of the 19th century that the science-oriented philosophy of positivism began to dominate thought on the European continent (Danziger, 1979).

The first empirical work of importance begins early in the 19th century with the work of Gustav Fechner (1801–1887), a physicist and nature mystic, who founded the field of psychophysics. Psychophysics is today the oldest continuing research tradition in experimental psychology, and it still aims to determine with precision the relationship between physical dimensions and their experiential concomitants. Even the basic law of modern psychophysics is not dramatically different from

Fechner's law — whereas Fechner claimed that physical quantities relate to experience by a logarithmic function, most modern psychophysicists favor a power function. What *is* different about modern psychophysics is its perceived mission. "Psycho-physics" means, of course, "mind–body," and for Fechner the mission of psychophysical research was to show that physical quantity can be reduced to conscious experience. Most modern psychophysicists probably believe the reverse — that conscious experiences are determined by physical energies. In point of fact, psychophysical research demonstrates neither presumption; it merely investigates the functional relationship between experience and physical energy, without showing which is more basic. It is an irony of history that modern psychophysics has reinterpreted Fechner as though he had demonstrated the physical basis of experience, but it is not surprising in view of the overall trend toward physicalism.

The story of Wilhelm Wundt (1832–1920), founder of the first experimental psychology laboratory, reveals a similar conversion over time of the real man into a caricature of the 19th-century psychologist. Wundt, too, began from a philosophical point of view that was not physicalistic, and thus was very much at odds with the cultural trends (Danziger, 1979; Wundt, 1912/1973). But recent historical research indicates that Wundt's point of view was seriously misunderstood by the major 20th-century historian of experimental psychology, E. G. Boring. Because of Boring's great reputation, his description of Wundt in his monumental *History of Experimental Psychology* (1929/1950) was not questioned until recently. Apparently, however, Boring took his conception of Wundt from his own teacher, Edward B. Titchener, and it now appears that Titchener constructed Wundt in his own image (Blumenthal, 1979). Thus Wundt has been represented as a believer in trained introspection as the sole tool of psychological investigation. This process involved a subjective analysis by trained observers of the contents of experience. At the time, some psychologists believed that such analysis would yield the "elements" of mental life, and that these elements would be comparable to the elements of chemistry. The theory was that by some principles of association it would be possible to synthesize such mental elements, thus reconstructing ordinary experience. For most of this century experimental psychologists have understood the founder of experimental psychology in terms of this theory, believing Wundt to be an introspectionist, an associationist, a dualist, and a believer in "mental chemistry." This conception of Wundt's thought now appears almost entirely false: It describes Titchener's own interpretation of Wundt, an interpretation that Wundt repudiated in print (Blumenthal, 1975, 1979, 1980).

Apparently the real Wundt thought that "systematic self-observation" was useful for investigating "simple sensations," but not for anything more complex. He used many behavioral measures of mental processes, but thought that higher mental functions, emotions, and social psychology were beyond the reach of the experimental method. Unlike Titchener, Wundt did not believe in the mere association of "mental elements," but emphasized rather the synthetic and creative aspects of mental life (Blumenthal, 1979). He was not an associationist at all, but rather believed in the effects of *context* on perception, thought, and action. Wundt was not a mind–body dualist; he believed that mind and body are two aspects of the same reality. He apparently believed after Schopenhauer in the primacy of "the will" as the fundamental mover in physical and mental matters. Blumenthal has suggested that Boring's upside-down account of Wundt represents the creation of a "myth of origin"—a way in which the experimental psychology of the 20th century could define itself in opposition to the psychology of its founder (Blumenthal, 1979, 1980). This resembles in some ways the manner in which modern psychophysics has reinterpreted Fechner as demonstrating the physical basis of experience. In both cases, 19th-century psychology was filtered through the views of the first half of the 20th.

Although psychological history clearly created a fantastic distortion of the real Wundt, it must be admitted that Wundt did at times use "self-observation," and some of his work does seem like an attempt to analyze experience, if not into basic elements, then perhaps into basic *dimensions*. For example, his short popular introduction to psychology (1912/1973) shows how one can analyze a series of clicks produced by a metronome:

. . . we have at the end of the row of beats the impression of an agreeable whole. If we wish to define this concept of "agreeable" more accurately, we may describe it as a subjective feeling of pleasure. . . . But feelings of pleasure are not the only ones that we observe in our rhythm experiments. . . . At the moment immediately following one beat, expectation strains itself to catch the next one, and this straining increases until this beat really occurs. At the same moment the strain is suddenly relieved by the realization of the expected, when the new beat comes.

We obtain therefore . . . feelings of pleasure and feelings of strain and relaxation in close connection with each other . . . This, however, is essentially changed if the rapidity of the beats is altered. If we chose intervals from 2½ to 3 seconds, we soon reach the limit where the strain of expectation becomes painful. Here, then, the former feeling of pleasure is transformed into a feeling of displeasure. . . .

Now let us proceed in the opposite direction by making the metronome beats follow each other after intervals of ½ to ¼ of a second, and we notice that the feelings of strain and relaxation disappear. In their place appears an excitement that increases with the rapidity of the impressions, and along with this we have generally a more or less lively feeling of displeasure. . . . We can also find the contrast to this feeling of excitation . . . by suddenly decreasing the rapidity of the beats to their medium rapidity again. This change is regularly accompanied by a very distinct feeling of quiescence.

Accordingly, our metronome experiments have brought to light three pairs of feelings — pleasure and pain, strain and relaxation, excitation and quiescence. (pp. 50–51)

Wundt argued that these three dimensions also characterize the experience of music, of color, and of emotion. Together with his students and collaborators he carried out a massive program of research starting in 1879, which dominated experimental psychology until early in the next century. Much of this work has been misinterpreted in the United States, especially through the influence of Titchener, and by the behaviorists' tendency to justify their perspective by pointing out perceived weaknesses in 19th-century experimental psychology.

It was apparently Titchener and Wundt's student Oswald Külpe (1862–1915) who developed the program of *trained introspection* by special observers, which received so much criticism from the behaviorists. For experimental science, the use of trained introspection as a primary tool for investigation presents several problems. One is that there are no checks on possible results. Different people may introspect differently: They may have been trained in different laboratories, or possess different talents and predilections. Further, the very act of self-observation probably interferes with the process that is being observed.

But it was likely the philosophical status of introspection that raised most questions in the minds of physicalistic critics. Are introspective reports "privileged"? Can they be contradicted by physical evidence? Are they reports of a reality different from the physical world? These philosophical issues had methodological consequences, as in the problem of individual differences. Some people are color-blind, others are not; some are tone-deaf, and others have perfect pitch; and there may be other, more subtle differences. Because the method of trained introspection, as articulated by Titchener and Külpe depended on the reports of highly articulate adults, it could not be used to study children, animals, or dysfunctional adults. John B. Watson made much of this limitation when he began his attack on the entire "consciousness psychology" of the 19th century. But of course his attack implied that *all* of 19th-century psychology was vulnerable to these criticisms, when in fact only Titchenerian introspection was.

The difficulty of replicating the experience of others came to the fore when one group of psychologists, led by Külpe in Germany, Binet in France, and Woodworth in the United States, made the observation that under some conditions thinking seemed to be possible without accompanying images — so called imageless thought.

Some [observers] reported visual images, some auditory, some kinesthetic, some verbal. Some reported vivid images, some mostly vague and scrappy ones. Some insisted that at the moment of a clear flash of thought they had no true images at all but only an awareness of some relationship. . . . Many psychologists would not accept testimony of this kind which they said must be due to imperfect introspection. (Woodworth & Schlosberg, 1954)

First, there seemed to be large differences between individual introspective observers. But worse, some observers reported no images at all during thinking. If thinking were possible without some conscious experience like an image, the entire consciousness psychology seemed to be in question. Like any metatheory, the consciousness psychology of the 19th century had to promise some degree of reliability, a reason to hope that its basic approach would enable psychologists to study the important issues. If thinking was to a significant extent unconscious, the mission of psychology could not be limited to studying conscious experience. The controversy about imageless thought was not just a matter of theory — the entire metatheoretical framework was at stake.

In a sense, we might say that psychology was in search of a consensual *canon of proof*, that is, a set of procedures whereby everyone could agree that some claim had been supported or disproved. Every scientific community has such canons of proof, however they may change during the development of a science. Numerous 19th-century psychologists, such as Helmholtz, Fechner, Wundt, and others, had very high experimental standards, but the evidence of yet others was more dubious. Behaviorists developed a standard of evidence that was so rigorous as to exclude all but the most well-demonstrated phenomena. From a scientific point of view, this may be a major contribution.

A related problem for 19th-century academic psychologists was the growing realization that unconscious processes had a powerful impact on the working of the mind. Long before Freud made the unconscious mind the centerpiece of his psychology, it was known that one could work on a problem — in mathematics, for example — keeping it in mind, forgetting it, and then suddenly, while thinking of something else, becoming conscious of a solution (*e.g.*, Ghiselin, 1952; Hadamard, 1945).

The fact that a solution to the problem suddenly becomes conscious suggests that it was worked out — somewhere — without direct conscious involvement. It follows that even those "higher mental functions" involved in solving complex mathematical problems are not entirely conscious, and that a psychology limited to conscious phenomena will not be able to investigate such events. In an age of computers, the idea that problem-solving can take place without awareness is not very startling. But to many people, well into the middle of this century, it was simply inconceivable that intelligent, symbolic processes could take place outside of consciousness.

When Hermann von Helmholtz in his *Physiological Optics* (1856–1866) suggested that the nervous system might be able to make "unconscious inferences" to fill in missing sensory information, a storm of controversy broke out (Boring, 1950; Warren & Warren, 1968). Helmholtz, who almost single-handedly discovered most of the basic facts in the physiology of hearing and vision, noted that perceptual experience does not reflect the physical stimulus as such — we always experience some *object* out in the world, rather than some stimulus impinging on eye and ear. Furthermore, there are many hundreds of demonstrations showing that perceptual experience is always *more complete* than the actual information coming into the receptors (*e.g.*, Gregory, 1966, 1970). The "blind spot" in the eye is one example. Even though there are no light receptors in the small spot on each retina called the "blind spot," we experience no gap in the visual field so long as the missing information can be filled in. But if we gaze at a single colored dot on a white piece of paper, moving the eye just so that the light from the colored dot projects exactly onto the blind spot, the colored dot will seem to disappear. The nervous system seems to infer missing information on the basis of the surrounding field. The existence of the colored dot cannot be inferred, because there is no information in the white surround that could suggest it. This and many other perceptual demonstrations led Helmholtz to conclude that the nervous system is unconsciously drawing conclusions that *go beyond* the information given.

It was deeply upsetting for many people to think that intelligent, symbolic thought processes could occur without conscious intervention. Helmholtz's suggestion aroused a storm of controversy, and he was forced to retract the paradoxical term "unconscious inference" (*Unbewüsster Schluss*) (Warren & Warren, 1968).

The idea of unconscious thought goes back at least to St. Augustine (Ellenberger, 1970; Whyte, 1962), but well into the 19th century many psychologists had insuperable objections to it. William James, whose *Principles of Psychology* (1890) is one of the high points of American psychology, had his own, unresolvable difficulties with the idea of unconscious processes. He reviewed 10 different "proofs" advanced by others of the existence of unconscious mental processes, and systematically rejected each one (James, 1890). Often he simply states that "brain processes" can account for the evidence adduced just as well as the hypothesis of unconscious thought. A modern computer scientist might say that there is no contradiction between the idea of intelligent activity and their physical basis in an organism or machine — that in fact, intelligence is only a higher-level description of brain processes. But this is a modern point of view. Like many of his contemporaries, James was caught in an either/or trap: *either* some process was conscious, *or* it was a physiological "brain process." And this dichotomy between conscious activity and the brain drove James toward a kind of mind–body dualism that he himself found intolerable. Once mind and brain are thought of as separate entities, the question arises as to how they interact, and this brings the discussion right back to the 17th century and Descartes. Thus William James, because he could not permit himself to conceive of unconscious mental processes, was confronted with a paradox that cannot be resolved. On this issue, James admitted with his customary charm, "our perplexity is extreme."

Many psychological thinkers speculated about unconscious processes even before Freud appeared on the scene (Whyte, 1960; Ellenberger, 1970), but few psychologists were comfortable with the idea. Even the unconscious processes that Freud postulated do not involve the kind of intelligent symbol manipulation that computers routinely perform today; the unconscious mind in Freud's theory is characterized by "primary process thought" — the kind of inchoate, irrational, symbolically charged images that we experience in dreams or drowsy states. Thus, as the 19th century was drawing to a close, more people than ever before were open to the possible existence of unconscious events. But even in the years just before Freud's *The Interpretation of Dreams* (1900/1953), the idea of unconscious processes was controversial, certainly as a proper topic of *psychological* investigation.

While the idea of unconscious psychological processes struck many people as paradoxical, the issue of consciousness itself presented a subtler problem. To the 19th-century psychologist, the existence of consciousness was a necessary assumption. That is to say, consciousness was always *presupposed* in psychological work, and never analyzed as such. The *contents* of consciousness were the subject of systematic self-observation, but consciousness itself could not be analyzed. Wundt acknowledges this in his writings: After defining psychology as the study of conscious contents, he notes, " . . . if we ask further, what is this consciousness which psychology investigates? The answer will be, 'It consists of the sum total of facts of which we are conscious'" (Wundt 1912/1973, p. 4). This kind of circularity makes it impossible, of course, to consider consciousness *as a problem to be investigated*. Even Freud, a thoroughgoing physical rationalist, wrote about consciousness as "a fact without parallel, which defies all explanation or description" (1920/1970, p. 21).

It is interesting to note that some behaviorists who rejected consciousness as a starting point for psychology were nevertheless able to see it as an important *topic* for psychologists to investigate. In this respect, behaviorism was able to make a major advance over earlier psychologists such as James, who by presupposing the existence of consciousness could not analyze it independently. Thus, Clark L. Hull wrote in 1937 that "to recognize the existence of [consciousness] is not the same as insisting upon its basic, i.e., logical, priority. Instead of furnishing a means for the solution of problems, consciousness appears to be itself a problem needing solution" (p. 855). Hull was unable to pursue this line of thought, perhaps because he did not have a theoretical language that would enable him to talk about it. But it is intriguing to speculate where his work might have led had he been able to follow through on this idea, treating consciousness as he would any other psychological concept. Indeed, in a way, this statement by Hull can be viewed as one of the high points of behavioristic thought.

In a sense, therefore, much of 19th-century psychology failed to deal with either unconscious *or* conscious processes. This failure, added to the difficulty of proving claims based on self-observation alone, indicates the limited nature of the progress made by 19th-century psychologists in the direction of a complete psychology.

Finally, some psychologists indulged in undisciplined speculation. Titchener at one point speculated that ants may once have been conscious, because they seemed to behave automatically. His reasoning was that consciousness is useful in exploring new actions, but we know from experience that once an action has been learned it becomes automatic and unconscious. Thus it seemed to him that the automatic actions of ants may once have been conscious. Others wondered whether amoebas were not conscious, given that some of their tropisms seemed goal-directed (Washburn, 1908). Such undisciplined speculation did much to bring 19th-century psychology into undeserved disrepute.

These were some of the limitations of the "consciousness psychology." By defining psychology exclusively as the analysis of mental contents, psychologists not only found it difficult to reconcile reports from different people, but further, their methods could not be used to study children, animals, and forms of psychopathology in which the patient could not observe his own experience. Nineteenth-century psychologists often de-nied the psychological reality of unconscious processes: Some, like James, consigned such processes to physiology — a position that makes difficult, of course, any attempt to look at the relationship between conscious and unconscious events. And 19th-century psychologists did not investigate consciousness as an independent entity, because their work required its *presupposition*. Many of the limitations of 19th-century methodology were already obvious to Wundt (though perhaps not to some of his followers), but if psychology was to be the science of conscious contents, then, by definition, there seemed to be no workable alternative.

There is also much to say in defense of 19th-century psychology. It recognized basic phenomena that occur, time and again, in psycholog-ical studies (*e.g.*, Blumenthal, 1977a, 1977b); it developed an exquisite sensitivity to some of the subtleties involved in research; and many of its findings have stood the test of time. In addition, the medical psychol-ogy of the 19th century made fundamental discoveries about perhaps the most dramatic and unexpected phenomena yet observed by psycholog-ical scientists — hypnosis, unconscious conflicts, hysteria, and split per-sonality (Ellenberger, 1970). Even Wundt's little experiment on sys-tematic self-observation with metronome clicks has been validated by later research. Where Wundt specified "pleasure and pain, strain and relaxation, excitation and quiescence" as universal properties of all sen-sations, Osgood, Suci, and Tannenbaum (1957) provided compelling evidence that nouns in a variety of languages can be consistently mapped into a three-dimensional space of connotative qualities, the dimensions being *evaluation, potency*, and *activity*. These dimensions are practically iden-tical to Wundt's: *Evaluation* is "pleasure and pain," *potency* is "strain and relaxation," and *activity* is "excitation and quiescence." Thus, systematic self-observation can lead to the same results we obtain from the sophis-ticated statistical techniques of behavioristic research.

Some historians in fact argue that cognitive psychology, which has largely superseded behaviorism, is merely a renaissance of 19th-century psychology. But there are some important differences. We are no longer as intensely focused on philosophical issues such as the mind-body prob-lem, as were James and Wundt. We no longer *define* psychology as the quest for understanding conscious experience, although that is increas-ingly a legitimate objective. We have much better theoretical and em-pirical tools than were available to psychologists in the 19th century. But no cognitive psychologist can read Wundt's little book (1912/1973) without recalling a host of modern studies that on the whole substan-tiate Wundt's findings. In practice, almost all experimentalists use a degree of self-observation in their work in the "context of discovery." That is to say, it is often useful for experimenters to go through the experiences their subjects will undergo in an experiment, or at least to try to imagine them. Many of the best-known experiments in psychology are persuasive precisely because they dramatize some point for the psychologist *as experiencer*. But today, self-observation is never accepted as *proof* of a subject's actual experiences without additional objective substantiation.

The "Consciousness Psychology" in America: Wundt, Titchener, and James

The first generation of American psychologists almost all traveled to Germany to be trained by Wundt, but there is much reason to think that physical proximity did not bridge the linguistic and cultural barriers (*e.g.*, Blumenthal, 1977a, 1977b). Conventional wisdom has it that American psychology revolted against Wundtian psychology, but it is now clear that the American understanding of Wundt was shaped by the work of Wundt's self-proclaimed disciple, Edward Titchener. So it is more accurate to say that with the coming of behaviorism, American psychology rebelled against *Titchenerian* introspectionism.

But even this view may leave something unsaid: namely the impact of William James, surely the greatest American psychologist of the 19th century. It was James who wrote the great textbook of American psychology, his *Principles of Psychology* (1890), which for several decades was required reading in psychology courses (sometimes in its abridged version, often called "Jimmie").

James (1890) epitomizes the best and the worst in 19th-century psychology. On the one hand, this two-volume work is simply filled with remarkable insights that are of great value to contemporary psychologists. On the other, James is deeply obsessed by the great Gordian knot of psychological thought, the mind–body problem. And he held to certain assumptions that made it effectively impossible for him to lay aside the philosophical issues and consider purely scientific issues in peace. First, James characteristically defines psychology as "the science of mental life," that is, of private experience. This definition automatically raises the question: what is the relationship between private experience and the *physical energies* we experience as sensation; the *physical actions* we perform in the world; and the *physical substrate* of consciousness, the brain? If private experience is the foundation of any psychology, as James wanted to believe, then the relationship between mind and body can take only two forms: *mentalistic monism*, the view that at bottom even physical things are manifestations of consciousness, or *mind*–body dualism, the view that there are two entirely separate worlds, the mental and the physical. Neither of these options was acceptable to James, nor would he back down from his insistence on the primacy of consciousness. A good part of Volume I of James's great work is devoted to an attempt to make sense of this paradox.

The difficulties James faced were made even greater by his unwillingness to recognize the existence of unconscious psychological processes. This makes it impossible for James to think of unconscious processes as mediating between external events and conscious experiences — it creates a chasm between the mental and the physical, forcing James to adopt a dualistic philosophy.

It may be impossible to know to what degree the first generation of American psychologists was influenced by James's great struggle with the mind–body paradox. Like James, the first "scientific generation" believed that psychology was the science of mental life. And like him, they believed that psychology must relate clearly to other natural sciences, most notably the physiology of the nervous system. Given these assumptions, they, too, became caught in the ancient paradox of the relationship between mental and physical phenomena. It is no wonder, perhaps, that the next generation welcomed John B. Watson, who severed this Gordian knot with a single blow by totally rejecting the conscious mind as a valid topic for scientific research. If James's impact on first-generation American psychologists was in fact as great as I believe, then William James may have been responsible for the remarkably rapid triumph of radical behaviorism early in the 20th century. Had he lived to see this triumph, he probably would have been appalled; yet his own struggle to provide a consistent framework for psychology, while retaining the primacy of consciousness, may have been responsible for John Watson's radical surgery on psychology's terms of inquiry (Baars, 1983b). Watson's behaviorism, for all its own paradoxical qualities, at least provided a consistent physicalistic framework within which scientific psychology could approach the world.

The Rise of Behaviorism:
The Revolutionary Impact of John Watson

With this background in mind we can now turn to the rise of behaviorism in the United States in the years just before the first World War. American universities before the war were much influenced by the German model, and American psychologists took their lead from what was then the most advanced form of scientific psychology in the world, the psychology of Wilhelm Wundt. Again, this was Wundt as understood via Edward Titchener's "introspectionism," with which Wundt was wrongly associated. When Titchener's influence waned under the onslaught of behavioristic criticism, so did the entire "consciousness psychology" in the United States.

But even before behaviorism appeared on the scene, Americans were ambivalent toward European psychology. As mentioned earlier, a number of Americans went to Germany to work with Wundt, but there seemed to be fundamental cultural contradictions between the Americans and Wundt (Blumenthal, 1977a, 1977b). William James also rejected the mentalistic philosophy of Kant and Hegel. He proposed in 1904 that the word "consciousness" be dropped — not because people do not have conscious experiences, but because the *word* "consciousness" suggests the existence of some single entity. (It should be noted that James also believed the word "brain" to be misleading, given that it is really only a collection of cells. Talking about that collection as though it were a single, unified entity was dangerous, he thought.) James was temperamentally opposed to the precise, systematic "brass instrument" approach of the German psychologists. But his classic textbook of psychology is full of gems of self-observation.

In the year before Watson's behavioristic manifesto appeared in print, G. Stanley Hall, who had studied with Wundt in Germany, voiced the American discomfort with Wundt:

We need a psychology that is usable, that is dietetic, efficient for thinking, living and working, and although Wundtian thoughts are now so successfully cultivated in academic gardens, they can never be acclimated here, as they are antipathetic to the American spirit and temper. (quoted in Blumenthal, 1977b, p. 13)

In the very next year, such a "dietetic" American psychology would be launched. (It is an intriguing fact that only a few years earlier, a kind of physiological behaviorism had independently appeared in Russia, with the work of Pavlov and Bekhterev.)

Numerous antecedents have been proposed for American behaviorism: the pragmatism of William James, the functionalism of John Dewey, the thinking of some of Watson's contemporaries such as Knight Dunlap, the physiologist W. J. Crozier, the biologist Jacques Loeb, and so on (Esper, 1964; Roback, 1964). In many ways behaviorism is simply a rigorous application of physicalistic philosophy to psychological matters, and physicalism was very much in the air. But overthrowing the whole Wundtian edifice and advocating a thoroughgoing house-cleaning to purge psychology of commonsense ideas — these things required more than just heretical thinking: They required a talented advocate as well. John B. Watson (1878–1958) was that advocate, tirelessly extolling the virtues of a behavioristic approach to experimental psychology, to child-rearing, to advertising, to Freud's psychoanalysis, to labor relations, and to the construction of utopias.

Watson's manifesto, "Psychology as the Behaviorist Views It," was published in 1913, and it caught on so quickly that Watson was elected president of the American Psychological Association two years later. Already by 1925 Watson could write that "Today, behaviorism is strong-ly entrenched," even though "it has not as yet replaced the older psychol-ogy" (p. 18) completely. The speed with which behaviorism caught on is astonishing. Boring (1950) remarks that in the years after 1910, "Some conservatives were Wundtians, some radicals were functionalists, more psychologists were agnostics. Then Watson touched a match to the mass, there was an explosion, and only behaviorism was left. Watson founded behaviorism because everything was ready for the founding. Otherwise he could not have done it" (p. 641).

Watson was a characteristic revolutionary personality: a brilliant, audacious, frequently troubled individual, constantly at odds with au-thority figures of all kinds (Cohen, 1979). He was born in rural South Carolina and brought up in a deeply religious Southern Baptist home. Until graduate school his education took place in religious institutions, and no doubt during these years he was impressed by the tenacity of the religious point of view in American higher education. In the small sec-tarian college that he attended, psychology was taught by ministers, who naturally taught about the soul and its participation in the divine scheme of things. When Watson was introduced to introspective psychology dur-ing his graduate studies at the University of Chicago, he saw only another version of this soul-psychology. Indeed, on the very first page of his book *Behaviorism* (1925) he stated his position clearly in terms of a revolt against religion:

. . . all schools of psychology except that of behaviorism claim that *"conscious-ness" is the subject-matter of psychology*. Behaviorism, on the contrary, holds that the subject matter of human psychology is the *behavior or activities of the human being*. Behaviorism claims that "consciousness" is neither a definable nor a usable concept; that it is merely another word for the "soul" of more ancient times. The old psychology is thus dominated by a kind of subtle religious philosophy. (p. 1)

Characteristically, he accuses people who promote religious ideas of being lazy and attempting to gain power by instilling fear:

No one knows just how the idea of a soul or the supernatural started. It probably had its origin in the general laziness of mankind. Certain individuals who in primitive society declined to work with their hands . . . became keen observers of human nature. They found that the loud noise from breaking limbs, thunder and other sound-producing phenomena, would throw the primitive individual . . . into a panicky state . . . and that in this state it was easy to train or, more scientifically, to *condition* him. . . . These lazy but good observers soon found devices by means of which they could at will throw individuals into this fearsome attitude and thus control primitive human behavior. For example, colored nurses down south have gained control over the young white children by telling them that there is someone ready to grab them in the dark. . . .

The "medicine men" of primitive times soon established an elaborate control through signs, symbols, rituals, formulae and the like. Medicine men have always flourished. A good medicine man has the best of everything and, best of all, he doesn't have to work.

I think an examination of the psychological history of people will show that their behavior has always been easily controlled by fear stimuli. If the fear element were dropped out of any religion, that religion could not long survive. This fear element (equivalent to the electric shock in establishing *conditioned reflexes*) . . . was variously introduced as the "devil," "evil," "sin," and the like. . . . Thus even the modern child from the beginning is confronted by the dicta of medicine men — be they the father, the soothsayer of the village, the God or Jehova. Having been brought up in this attitude towards authority, he never questions the concepts imposed upon him.

One example of such a concept is that there is a fearsome God and that every individual has a soul which is separate and distinct from the body. This soul is really a part of the supreme being. This concept has led to the philosophical platform called "dualism." All psychology except behaviorism is dualistic. . . .

With the development of the physical sciences which came with the renaissance, a certain release from this stifling soul cloud was obtained. A man could think of astronomy, of the celestial bodies and their motions, of gravitation and the like, without involving the soul. . . . Psychology and philosophy, however, in dealing as they thought with non-material objects, found it difficult to escape the language of the church, and hence the concepts of mind and soul come down to the latter part of the nineteenth century. It was the boast of Wundt's students, in 1879, when the first psychological laboratory was established, that psychology had at last become a science without a soul. For fifty years we have kept this pseudo-science, exactly as Wundt laid it down. All that Wundt and his students really accomplished was to substitute for the word "soul" the word "consciousness." (1925, pp. 3–5)

It is difficult to avoid the conclusion that Watson's own painful experiences in evangelical Baptist schools had something to do with his fervor in denouncing religion (Watson, 1936; Cohen, 1979). Science gave Watson a personally liberating ideology, as well as a promise of future salvation. Watson's writings echo the rhythm and excitement of the evangelical sermons he must have heard as a child, and his promises for the future — if only the world would adopt behaviorism — are nothing less than messianic.

No doubt Watson saw himself struggling against an overpowering, pervasive religious establishment, perniciously disguised in the introspective psychology. But this establishment was far weaker in psychology than it appeared; in the event, it melted away in a remarkably short time before the onslaught of behavioristic criticism. The long-term cultural trends were in Watson's favor, though perhaps he did not realize this at the time.

Behaviorism as an intellectual discipline forces psychologists to *distance* themselves from the everyday psychology that we all live. It is necessary to restate all of commonsense psychology in external terms. To use an expression coined by the behaviorist Max Meyer (Esper, 1966), behaviorism is the "psychology of the other one." It is significant in this regard that Watson had earned the first PhD in animal psychology given in the United States. The study of animals presented him with a viewpoint and method that he wanted to extend to all of psychology. As he later wrote (1930),

Behaviorism, as I tried to develop it in my lectures at Columbia in 1912 was an attempt to do one thing: to apply to the experimental study of man the same kind of procedure and the same language of description that many research men had found so useful for so many years in the study of animals lower than man. (p. 274)

The peculiarity of scientific psychology is, again, that scientists are conducting their research as observers, standing outside their subject matter, even as each scientist is ultimately an *insider* to the subject matter of psychology. Watson's solution to this dilemma was radical: let us pretend that we are ultimate outsiders, that we are studying animals and people only as bodies moving through space. In Watson's view, then, there is no room in psychology for anything that cannot be externally observed: no room for consciousness, purpose, thought, meaning, feelings, imagery, self, and the like.

In his straightforward application of physicalistic scientism, Watson was convinced that religion is the great enemy of science, and that if the scientific method — that is, physicalism — were applied with the utmost consistency, scientific solutions would soon be available to solve all psychological problems. To Watson, the concept of consciousness was the great villain — perhaps because if consciousness existed, the dominance of physicalism might be in doubt.

Edna Heidbreder (1933), one of the most thoughtful observers of the behavioral revolution, noted:

It is important to realize with vehemence and thoroughness with which the concept of consciousness is rejected [by Watson]. Mental processes, consciousness,
souls, and ghosts are all of a piece, and are altogether unfit for scientific use.
The existence of consciousness is a "plain assumption." It cannot be proved by
any scientific test, for consciousness cannot be seen, nor touched, nor exhibited
in a test-tube. Even if it exists it cannot be studied scientifically, because admittedly it is subject only to private inspection. Finally, a belief in the mental
is allied to modes of thinking that are wholly incompatible with the ways of
science. It is related to the religious, the mystical, and the metaphysical interpretations of the world. The notion of consciousness is the result of old wives'
tales and monks' lore, of the teachings of medicine-men and priests. Consciousness is only another name for the soul of theology, and the attempts of the older
psychology to make it seem anything else are utterly futile. . . . With the simplicity and finality of the Last Judgment, behaviorism divides the sheep from
the goats. On the right hand side are behaviorism and science and all its works;
on the left are souls and superstition and a mistaken tradition; and the line of
demarcation is clear and unmistakable. (pp. 235–236)

The Popular Appeal of Behaviorism

Some of the initial popularity of behaviorism in America can be attributed to the fact that it came on the scene just before the First World War,
at a time when isolationism (and later, anti-German hysteria) were sweeping the country. This home-grown product was believed to be vastly
superior to its ponderous Teutonic forerunner. Wundt did not help his
popularity in the United States when he wrote books to promote the
German side in the war, criticizing the English (and by implication,
Americans as well) as a nation of shopkeepers.

Further, we may guess that there was in early behaviorism a certain rebellion against the sheer amount of intellectual drudgery demanded
by 19th-century psychology, against the linguistic and philosophical
sophistication needed to understand its roots, and against the philosophical controversies in which some 19th-century psychologists seemed
always to be mired (Danziger, 1979). Indeed, behaviorists such as Watson also rebelled against major American thinkers such as James and
Dewey. James was dismissed as "unscientific" (Watson, 1925, p. 4), and
as for Dewey—the foremost thinker at the University of Chicago, Watson's graduate school—Watson wrote later that "I never knew what he
was talking about, and unfortunately for me, I still don't" (1936, p. 276).
Anti-intellectualism is a running theme in American history (Hofstadter,
1963) and in this sense behaviorism was a true native product. By denying any need for mental representations of the world, behaviorism simply
ruled out *knowledge*. During the 50-year period of behavioristic domi-

nance, psychology textbooks do not even mention the word. This is curious, because psychologists *are* after all intellectuals in pursuit of knowledge. Behavioristic psychologists were intellectuals who denied intellect.

Even this puzzle makes some cultural sense. American intellectuals have always tended to be on the defensive, always ready to answer the implicit question — "Well, what *good* is it?" Behaviorism had a ready answer for this. The mission of psychology was to improve people in the same way that physics or chemistry helped to improve the human environment. "Improving" people meant to make people happier, to be sure, but also more *productive*. Even in their own lives, radical behaviorists such as Watson and Skinner placed inordinate emphasis on visible productivity. Watson proudly recounted how even in his later years he built a barn with his own hands (Cohen, 1979), and Skinner connected his desk lamp to a cumulative recorder to keep track of the amount of time he spent working at his desk. Watson condemned his religious enemies for a disinclination to perform honest labor. Skinner's most traumatic year (his "Dark Year") came, when as a young man in Scranton, Pennsylvania, he tried to become a serious writer, while all his friends were doing *useful* work (Skinner, 1978, 1979). Thus, behaviorism gained acceptance in part because it promised practical efficiency.

Indeed, both Watson and Skinner defined the goal of psychology as the *prediction and control of behavior*, as if prediction and control were the only conceivable goals of science. Merely *understanding* human psychology meant little to them. For the radical behaviorist, no distinction can be made between science and technology. And so it happened that the psychology of James and Titchener lost ground with amazing rapidity because it promised nothing more than a deeper understanding of the human mind, whereas behaviorism was seen as a tool for changing people: In America at the turn of the century, there was no question which was the more favored choice.

All these factors must be acknowledged to explain the instant popularity of behaviorism — and yet they fail to explain why behaviorism was so much more than a fad, why it held on as the essence of a scientific approach to the study of humanity for more than 50 years. Let us look at the revolt led by Watson in more detail.

First, the behaviorism advocated by Watson could lay claim to an undoubted *objectivity* in its observations. "Even if there are states of consciousness for the introspectionist to examine . . . it is forever impossible for two observers to see the same thing. No one can see the thoughts and feelings of another person, and nothing that is open only to private inspection can possibly give rise to objective knowledge" (Heidbreder,

1933, p. 240). From our current vantage point, it may seem that behaviorists had to pay a high price for their objectivity, perhaps unnecessarily high. But this is in line with general scientific practice, which is always conservative. Most scientists would rather be certain about a few facts than *almost* certain about many. If even one premise of a scientific theory is uncertain, a whole theoretical edifice can come tumbling down.

Second, as Watson argued with some success, the behavioristic viewpoint seemed to have real *adequacy* in accounting for psychological phenomena. Everything in everyday psychology could be translated into behavior, presumably without loss of meaning. Although some of these claims may seem dubious to us now, they were always argued persuasively. For example:

Emotions are not matters of feeling or affective quality; they are (learned) bodily reactions . . . predominantly visceral. . . . Complex emotions are built up on the basis of the few unlearned reactions. Natively, fear may be aroused in an infant by loud noises, but the fear so aroused may be attached to an originally "inadequate" stimulus like a rabbit, if the child hears a loud noise every time he sees a rabbit. Through transfer and spread, the fear may become attached to other furry or hairy objects, to the room in which the rabbit was seen, to the person who held the rabbit. . . .

So too are the complicated system of habits and motor skills that Watson refers to as "manual habits." Manual habits include such specific skills as writing, typewriting, painting, and driving an automobile, and such generalized modes of behavior as make a man punctual, orderly, and persevering. Manual habits are built up on original "random" movements of the trunk, arms, legs, hands and fingers. . . .

"Laryngeal habits" is the behaviorist's phrase for thinking. Laryngeal habits (tiny movements of the vocal cords) are developed from random, unlearned vocalization, in exactly the same way as manual habits are developed from random movements of the limbs and trunk. Language is at first overt. By a process of conditioning, the child acquires words; and words, because they may be substituted for things and concrete situations, give him the power of manipulating his environment without making the actual overt movements. This is all that is meant by thinking.

Watson, by reducing images to implicit language responses, and affection to slight reactions set up by tumescence and detumescence of the genitals, maintained that both might be studied as bodily movements, and that there was therefore no portion of the subject-matter of psychology to which the methods of behaviorism were not adequate. (Heidbreder, 1933, pp. 248–251)

What about sensations? They, too, could be defined behaviorally. The sensation of a 1000-cycle tone, for example, could be defined as a distinct response to that tone, different from responses to lower and higher tones. So if one could induce an animal or human to act in a certain way whenever the 1000-cycle tone was presented, and to act differently when a different tone was given, the differential response was an objective version of the sensation.

Special mention should be given to the role of the "verbal report." The words spoken by a subject are recognized as a source of information,

> but at the hands of the behaviorist, the subject's comments on his own condition or performance receive exactly the same treatment as do any other overt reactions. Certainly they are not regarded as representing states of consciousness. If a person says "I feel sad," his statement is noted along with his drooping posture, as possibly symptomatic of the condition of his total reaction system. It is never accepted as a report on a "mental condition." (Heidbreder, 1933, p. 244)

Thus it was that behaviorists came to deny the *meaning* of language, treating a "verbal response" as nothing more than the sound of the words. Then, as now, behaviorists denied the need for "meaning" or "knowledge," or any kind of representation of the world. A complete statement of input–output relationships would serve instead as a completely objective and scientific substitute for such mentalistic notions.

One useful effect of this translation program was to force people to state their claims with precision.

> If I were to ask you to tell me what you mean by the terms you have been in the habit of using I could soon make you tongue-tied with contradictions. I believe I could even convince you that you do not know what you mean by them. You have been using them uncritically as a part of your social and literary tradition. (Watson, 1919, p. 10)

It was fairly easy to disprove the concrete and testable proposals made by Watson, or at least to show that there was no evidence *for* them. But many psychologists became convinced that even if love was not the "tumescence and detumescence of the genitals," then it was some other equally physical thing that would eventually be discovered by a diligent application of the experimental method. Thus, even when Watson's psychological claims were not believed, they still showed how a behaviorist *could* do psychology — and so the behavioristic metatheory remained untouched by the failure of Watson's particular hypotheses.

Recent radical behaviorism continues the tradition of translating commonsense ideas into presumably more objective concomitants. Skinner (1974) gives the following examples:

> "I miss you" could almost be thought of as a metaphor based on target practice, equivalent to "My behavior with respect to you as a person cannot reach to its mark" (p. 56) . . . a "lovelorn" person is unable to emit behavior directed toward the person he loves (p. 65) . . . when a person is "aware of his purpose"

he is feeling or observing introspectively a condition produced by reinforcement (p. 63) . . . If he has been punished by his peers, he is said to feel shame; if he has been punished by a religious agency, he is said to feel a sense of sin; and if he has been punished by a governmental agency, he is said to feel guilt (p. 69).

Though the explanations used in earlier and later behaviorism are somewhat different, the strategy of translating commonsense psychology into behavioral terms has not changed at all.

Several more important points should be noted about Watson's views.

Peripheralism

Being profoundly mistrustful of unobservable theoretical constructs, Watson yet continued to postulate their existence by seeking their observable analogues (as in the case of "laryngeal habits" and "genital reactions" to explain thinking and emotion). Such entities were thought to exist, not somewhere in the nervous system where Pavlov believed they were, but in the muscles and glands of the body. In fact, Watson was so suspicious of the central nervous system that he at one point proposed that the cerebral cortex was not a functional organ, because he associated it with consciousness (Cohen, 1979)! Of course, "peripheral" bodily movements were in principle no more observable than the operation of the nervous system, but peripheralistic claims gave the illusion of having their basis in behavioral observableness. This trend continued, especially in the work of Clark L. Hull, the most theoretical of the major behaviorists, and traces of peripheralism can be found in experimental psychology well into the beginnings of the cognitive period.

Emphasis on Learning

Watson's most famous words are in the following description of the infinite plasticity and manipulability of the human organism, written in the stirring language that typifies his writings (1930):

Give me a dozen healthy infants, well-formed and my own specified world to bring them up in and I'll guarantee to take any one at random and train him to become any type of specialist I might select—doctor, lawyer, artist, merchant-chief and, yes, even beggar-man and thief, regardless of his talents, penchants, tendencies, abilities, vocations, and race of his ancestors. (p. 82)

—a boast that is, to put it mildly, unproven to this day. This sort of claim was, however, profoundly attractive in the egalitarian New World.

Associationism

The behavioristic conception of learning has always been associationistic. As Edward L. Thorndike (1931) bluntly put it: "Learning is connecting. The mind is man's connection-system" (p. 122). Associationism has a history going back to Aristotle, and it has been a dominant theme in English and American thought. But earlier Associationists spoke of associations between *ideas*, whereas the behaviorists proposed that associations connect physical stimuli with physical responses. In order to demonstrate how such a view could explain all behavior, they turned to the physiological reflexes, as we noted earlier in this chapter. Unlike most behavior, reflexes appear to follow "billiard ball" causality, and the cause of the behavior — the stimulus — would appear always to be external and physical. The strategy of reducing all behavior to reflexes was suggested by I. M. Sechenov, the forerunner of Pavlov and Bekhterev. The problem with Sechenov's reflexology is, of course, that the great bulk of behavior is *not* reflexive but voluntary and apparently goal-directed. It was at this point that Pavlov's work suggested a rationale for believing that complex, voluntary behavior could be derived causally from a small number of simple, inborn reflexes.

The Conditioned Reflex

At the time he discovered the conditioned reflex, Ivan P. Pavlov was already world-famous for his classic work on the digestive system of dogs. Trained as a physiologist, he was enthusiastically in favor of the physicalist program for reducing psychology to physical quantities. In the course of his work on digestion he implanted tubes in the mouths of dogs to measure the salivation reflex to food. Eventually he noticed that the animals were beginning to salivate *in anticipation* of the food. Thus the salivation reflex seemed to be future-directed, which was of course the sticking point for physicalists who wanted to explain how reflexes could serve as a model for normal action. Pavlov noted that a mere reflex had somehow become anticipatory! How to explain such "psychic reflexes"? His solution was to show that any stimulus could act as a signal to the dog that food was coming, if it was presented reliably just before food. Thus when food was made *conditional upon* the sound of a bell, the dog would learn to anticipate the food and begin to salivate *before* it was actually presented. The reflex could be made conditional on any reliable signalling stimulus — Pavlov called such psychic reflexes "conditional reflexes." Due to the usual mistranslation, this term has come down to us as "*conditioned* reflexes."

Here at last was the solution to Sechenov's problem! Sechenov wished to claim that all nervous activity was reflexive, and here, finally, was a way to show the connection between simple physical causality and complex, apparently goal-directed action. It is very important to realize that an actual, detailed connection between reflexes and voluntary action has never to this day been demonstrated empirically. Indeed, since about 1930 there has been good physiological evidence against there being any such thing (Lashley, 1930). But the reduction of voluntary action to reflexes was *believed to be possible*, both by Pavlov's followers (*e.g.*, Razran, 1965) and by American behaviorists such as Watson. The importance of Pavlov's discovery was not so much scientific as programmatic — it fit perfectly into the physicalistic program for reducing human action to reflexes.

In both Russia and America, the meaning of the word "reflex" was sometimes stretched to include all behavior. Pavlov, sophisticated scientist though he was, was not above speaking of the "freedom reflex" as though he had just isolated it in his laboratory, and Watson speaks glibly of the "love reflex," which could be elicited experimentally by stimulating the genitalia of infants (Cohen, 1979; Watson & Raynor, 1928). In this usage the word "reflex" becomes equivalent to "causal sequence," "stimulus" to "cause"; and "response" came to mean the same as "effect." To say, as Sechenov did, that all behavior is reflexive, means no more than saying that the nervous system is subject to causality. "Stimulus–response" psychology, then, often came down to the faith that the nervous system behaves deterministically. Determinism is one of the metaphysical assumptions of almost all science, but because of the change in wording ("stimulus and response" instead of "cause and effect") it was frequently portrayed as an empirical *discovery*, as if psychologists in their laboratories had finally found the real causal relationships between perception and action.

In America, Watson leaped on the discovery of "conditioning" (a further corruption of the term "conditioned reflexes"), and all over the world Pavlov's discovery was greeted as a breakthrough. H. G. Wells wrote ecstatically of Pavlov as "a star which lights the world, shining above a vista hitherto unexplored" (quoted in Skinner, 1974, p. 300). Give Pavlov's findings, Watson could now argue that all human behavior resulted from pairing a few inborn reflexes with new stimuli. In fact, as Thorndike and Skinner pointed out later, Pavlov's experiments showed how *old* responses could be connected to *new* stimuli but not how to create entirely *new* responses. It therefore could not account for the development of new behavior. This deficit was soon remedied, however, by the arrival of a new kind of stimulus–response learning, called instrumental, or operant, conditioning (see pp. 62–66). But Pavlov had determined the principle of a learned stimulus–response connection. The physicalistic program had thus overcome its greatest obstacle. Starting with Watson, stimulus–response conditioning became the major focus for behavioristic research, and so it has remained until today (see any major textbook of the period, such as Hilgard & Marquis, 1940).

The Role of Heredity

Historically, behaviorists have tended to discount the importance of hereditary influences. Watson's claim about taking a dozen babies and conditioning them to be doctors, lawyers, beggarmen, or thieves illustrates this point very nicely. This tendency has begun to change in recent decades, but an almost exclusive environmentalism lasted well into the 1950s and '60s.

The Utopian Appeal of Behaviorism

As his words about the trainability of infants show, Watson was much concerned with using the new insights to change the world. Indeed, the final paragraph of his 1930 book, *Behaviorism*, was lyrical with promises for the future if only the world would turn to objective methods in psychology:

I am trying to dangle a stimulus in front of you, a verbal stimulus which, if acted upon, will gradually change this universe. For the universe will change if you bring up your children, not in the freedom of the libertine, but in behavioristic freedom — a freedom which we cannot even picture in words, so little do we know of it. Will not these children, in turn, with their better ways of living and thinking, replace us as society, and in turn bring up their children in a still more scientific way, until the world finally becomes a place fit for human habitation? (pp. 303–304)

And B. F. Skinner concludes his book *About Behaviorism* (1974) with a clear echo of this utopian sentiment: "In the behavioristic view, man can now control his destiny because he knows what must be done and how to do it" (p. 277).

Let us step back for a moment and examine in a broader context what Watson accomplished. A nonpsychologist may find it difficult to understand the tremendous power and influence exercised by behaviorists. Behaviorism was viewed as the one right way to do psychological science; every alternative was unscientific. Behaviorists taught two generations of American psychologists to lower their voices when speaking of "purpose" or "experience," "knowledge," "thinking," or "imagination." These words were effectively taboo, along with the rest of the common-sense vocabulary that applies to human beings. At the same time, behaviorists taught the need for precision and testability in theory and experiment. But beyond this educational effect on methodology, behavioristic philosophy possessed real teeth: The path of professional advancement was controlled by behaviorists (or functionalists, or operationists)—all of whom agreed on the same basic tenets. In America, almost all scientific journals in psychology were controlled by behaviorists, and tenure and promotion in most American universities were conditional upon at least an outward obedience to behavioristic method. Of course there were many varieties of behaviorism, many of them less radical than Watson's original formulation—but Watson's thoughts appear in different forms over and over again.

It is important to note again that behaviorism is not so much a scientific theory as a metatheoretical philosophy. Skinner (1974) has made this point quite clear: "Behaviorism," he has written, "is not the science of man, it is the philosophy of that science" (p. 3). That is to say, behaviorism is not something one attempts to test in the laboratory. It is critically dependent on a certain view of science, a view that seemed to receive general support from philosophers of science such as Bertrand Russell, the logical positivist group, the operationism of Percy Bridgman (1927), and the work of Ludwig Wittgenstein, Rudolf Carnap, and Karl Popper. Indeed, these philosophers often attempted to *prescribe* what science was, and what psychology should do if it was to be a science (*e.g.*, Savage, 1966). Generally, psychologists tried to follow the philosophers' prescriptions. Notice that because behaviorism is not a scientific theory but a presupposed framework, *it cannot be falsified by any experimental results*.

Logical positivism also has its roots in the spectacular advances of scientific thought in the 19th century, and the resulting withdrawal of religious and metaphysical thought. Like the behaviorists, logical positivists made much of the rejection of 19th-century "metaphysics" (*e.g.*, Ayer, 1946). In philosophy, the very word "metaphysics" came to have much the same pejorative flavor that "mentalistic" and "subjective" had in psychology. As late as 1966 the psychophysicist S. S. Stevens was strongly criticized by philosopher C. W. Savage for employing "mentalistic" terms such as "sensations," "judgments," and so on in his work on the perception of physical magnitudes (Savage, 1966; Stevens, 1966).

Psychologists such as Stevens and Boring technically did not consider themselves to be behaviorists but "operationists." That is to say, they followed the physicist Percy Bridgman's view that "in general, we mean by any concept nothing more than a set of operations; *the concept is synonymous with the corresponding set of operations*" (1927, p. 5; also see Esper, 1964). An operation is some physical action, such as laying a ruler along an object to be measured, or observing a needle deflect as a measure of voltage. This view permitted Bridgman, as a physicist, to claim that the theories of Newton actually concern the same concepts as the theories of Einstein, because they both used the same operations to define these concepts (but see Kuhn, 1962, for a different view). Philosophers since Plato have known the issue raised by the operationists as "the problem of particulars and universals": Operationists claimed that the real meaning of concepts resides in the *particular instances* of the concepts, and that abstractions (universals) have no more meaning than their particular instances. Arguments for and against this position are well known in the philosophical literature (*e.g.*, Plutchik, 1968). But in its effects, the operationist position was identical to behaviorism: As Skinner has written, "As far as I was concerned, there were only minor differences between behaviorism, operationism, and logical positivism" (1978, p. 161).

Today, all these philosophies of science appear to be increasingly dubious as descriptions of the way successful science is really done. A new generation of philosophers and historians have argued persuasively that successful science is far more messy, culture-bound and even propagandistic than the clean, rational conception of science promoted by the logical positivists and related philosophers of science. As the philosophy of science shifted its ground, it also took away many of the philosophical underpinnings of behaviorism. It now appears after all that there is no procedure for creating successful science that is guaranteed to work in all cases; that science depends as much on theory as it does on facts; and indeed, that whatever is perceived by a scientific community to constitute "the facts" will change with different theoretical preconceptions (*e.g.*, Putnam, 1975; Kuhn, 1962; Lakatoš & Musgrave, 1970; Feyerabend, 1975).

The history of behavioristic psychology illustrates all these points very nicely: It too, appears to be somewhat messy conceptually, culture-bound, and occasionally propagandistic. *In fact*, conditioned reflexes were never shown to add up to complex, voluntary behavior, but it was widely *believed* that they would, presumably because the resulting conception of psychology suited the general scientism of the times. Behaviorism, too, was often propagandistic and ideological. (Watson joined an advertising agency after leaving academia, and it is not surprising that he became highly successful in that field.) That behaviorism was culture-bound is shown by the fact that it remained largely confined to the United States until the Second World War. At the same time, a physiological analogue of behaviorism prevailed in the Soviet Union, and it, too, has remained largely confined to the Soviet sphere of influence. Meanwhile, European psychology produced psychoanalysis, Gestalt psychology, and the work of Piaget and Bartlett, largely in isolation from American and Russian work.

But one cannot have a successful science and openly admit that it is part ideology, part promise for the future, and part guesswork — one needs to claim legitimacy in terms of some conception of science and the search for truth. Behaviorism was increasingly deprived of this legitimacy as the philosophers of science changed their ideas. All this does not mean that behaviorism was *not* scientific, in some sense of that word. It does show that science, especially young science, is vulnerable to a host of influences that are not strictly empirical or even theoretical in nature.

There may be no other way to do science. Scientific work is often successful not because it is free from extraneous ideology, but because the scientific community has ways of correcting its own errors. Over a period of decades these mechanisms work to reduce the likelihood of false or ineffective approaches to the field. These self-correcting mechanisms include a constant appeal to verifiable evidence, explicit theory, mutual criticism, and not least, a constant turnover in active scientists, as young people entering the community attempt to make their mark. Against these self-correcting tendencies stand personal and institutional inertia of all kinds. Max Planck's remark that major scientific revolutions only advance when the older generation dies (quoted in Kuhn, 1962, p. 151) seems unduly pessimistic; it cannot be entirely true, because any scientific establishment includes people of different ages; obviously representatives of one particular age group do not all die at the same time. But clearly the constant turnover of scientists has something to do with the ability of scientific communities to correct themselves. It may be more accurate to say that subcommunities will split off from the main scientific community if there is strong resistance to their views, and such subcommunities sometimes come to dominate the entire field as the established view yields to age and retirement.

As I pointed out earlier, the danger inherent in the "official" establishment of behavioristic psychology was that the professional apparatus of science was put into place before the problems had matured. The natural sciences were never deliberately "established" in this sense — they simply grew as individuals became interested in certain issues, without any intention to create an entity called "science." But in psychology, an entire community of researchers depended for its income, careers, future prospects, and even self-respect, on the existence of something called scientific psychology; and the conception of psychology that resulted tended to show all of the inertia of an established science with few of its advantages.

Thus one important reason that Watson's view caught on in psychology is that behaviorism served to legitimize an entire profession — it created the "conceptual space" within which one kind of experimental psychology could be carried out. This may have been premature, but the normal scientific mechanisms for self-correction were also put into place, and ultimately did produce some corrections (see Chapter 4). It is difficult today to conceive of the psychological establishment before the advent of behaviorism as Watson must have perceived it: as overwhelmingly powerful, deeply superstitious, pervading popular thought as well as official psychology. If that establishment was as powerful as he imagined, perhaps a truly radical approach was the only possible one for creating a physicalistic psychology. Although many 19th-century psychologists emphasized good methodology, reliable observation, and intersubjective verification, the behaviorists gave unusual emphasis to methodology. They helped to promulgate a *consensual canon of proof* for psychological science. Much as one might disagree with their interpretations, it was always possible for anyone to check behavioristic findings. It is this emphasis on impeccable method — this "militant methodology," as Susanne Langer called it — that continues to give a degree of legitimacy to behavioristic work in the eyes of other scientists.

Behaviorism after Watson

Watson's direct influence in psychology was short-lived. He left academic work in 1920 — only 7 years after his behavioristic manifesto appeared — as a result of a divorce scandal. Surprisingly, no university in the United States offered him a job, possibly because any sexual scandal at this time was socially impermissible, or perhaps because psychologists were put off by Watson's constant appeal to the general public. In any case, unable to find work as an academic psychologist, Watson went into the advertising world, and soon rose to become vice president of the J. Walter Thompson agency. His book on child care (with his second wife, Rosalie Raynor) appeared some years later (1928), but even though it gained great popularity, it contains little new academically accepted information.

Watson continued to write for the popular press on a variety of controversial subjects, from sexual liberation to the reason why various people did not commit suicide after the market crash of 1929. His personal life became increasingly unhappy after Rosalie died, and he began to have frequent bouts of depression and drinking. But "respectable" academic psychologists had long ago rejected Watson as an active contributor, as he notes bitterly in his autobiography (Watson, 1936); and when he died in 1958, most obituaries mixed criticism with measured praise (Cohen, 1979). This is peculiar, because during all this time the behavioristic metatheory that Watson founded was going from strength to strength.

In 1933 Heidbreder described the rapid expansion of behavioristic influence:

. . . few psychologists call themselves behaviorists without qualification. Behavioristic psychology merges gradually into psychology in general, and strange to say, the result is not confusion. . . . The outcome is rather a communication between behavioristic and non-behavioristic psychologies that has resulted in enormous conquests on the part of the behaviorists by peaceful penetration . . . Indeed, one of the signs of vigor in this extraordinarily vigorous movement is the way in which it has managed to get its attitudes recognized by those who oppose its fundamental doctrines. Even its taboos are heeded, those especially perhaps. There is a tendency, even among psychologists who firmly believe in their right to take consciousness into consideration, to stress the objective records of their findings, and sometimes explain that, though in their own thinking they include consciousness, their statements hold equally for behavior with consciousness left out. Since the rise of behaviorism, introspectionism and the results of introspection are less likely to stand alone; they are supplemented and even supported by objective data. (p. 263)

There were critics, of course. Watson himself engaged in public debates with William McDougall, an English psychologist who tried to establish a purposive psychology. McDougall was outraged by behaviorism, but his outrage and contempt probably turned many people against him (Cohen, 1979). Further, McDougall's publically expressed interest in psychic phenomena made him appear less than an ideal advocate for a scientific alternative to behaviorism. As for Titchener, he appeared to view behaviorism with some amusement as philosophically unsophisticated. But he failed to publish his long-promised *magnum opus*, possibly because of the rising behavioristic tide. Other public critics included Roback (1964), and in later years, Arthur Koestler (1967) and humanists such as Abraham Maslow (1966). None of these critics had major standing within experimental psychology, and none proposed a promising alternative way to do experimental psychology. By and large, their criticisms fell on deaf ears.

Several varieties of behaviorism appeared after Watson left the scene in 1920 (Roback, 1964). Notwithstanding the differences between these and the Watsonian brand, particularly in their tendency to be less extreme in their rejection of consciousness and purpose, Watson's thought remained prototypical, and even his more extreme views are frequently echoed in different forms in the work that came after him. Of the many behaviorists of this period, the present chapter briefly discusses three: B. F. Skinner, who represented the radical wing after about 1930; Clark Hull, who was responsible for the greatest effort to establish an all-inclusive behavioristic learning theory; and Edward C. Tolman, who anticipated the cognitive response to behaviorism, and called himself a "cognitive behaviorist." Interestingly, each of these psychologists made a major attempt to solve the problem of purpose.

By 1930, the neuropsychologist Karl Lashley had already shown that the reduction of behavior to reflex arcs was without physiological foundation. "We have seen the notion of reflex paths," he wrote, " . . . is not only inadequate to account for the simplest facts of behavior but it is also opposed by direct neurological evidence" (1930, p. 2). Behaviorism was not to be stopped so easily however. The program of reducing complex, goal-directed actions to a few innate reflexes lost momentum after this point, but psychologists began instead to speak of "stimulus–response" behaviorism, whose aim was to reduce observed behavior to connections between stimuli and responses. In effect, the reflex-reduction program went on, but the stimulus–response sequences to which behavior was to be reduced became more abstract.

Neobehaviorism: Clark L. Hull and Kenneth W. Spence

The period after 1930 is often labeled "neobehaviorism," especially in reference to the work of Clark L. Hull (1884–1952) and his influential colleague Kenneth W. Spence (1907–1967). It was marked by intense enthusiasm for the behavioral approach to learning, which was thought to be the key topic for a scientific psychology. By "learning" was meant the kinds of associative change in behavior that could be studied conveniently in a variety of mazes and boxes, including the Skinner box.

Hull, in particular, attempted to develop a theory of behavior that would include motivations such as hunger or thirst, and which would be apply to a wide variety of animal species. Needless to say, this theory was designed to avoid any notion of mental representation — it would have to be stated completely in terms of observable, or potentially observable, physical stimuli and responses. Hull's theory was believed by many psychologists to be the proof of the behavioristic pudding—after several decades of intense experimental research, at last psychologists would have a general theory of learning. By the late 1940s there was great excitement as Hull's latest proposals became available to experimental psychologists. Each new idea was tested immediately in the laboratories, especially at Yale and the University of Iowa. Over this period, Spence alone supervised no fewer than 75 doctoral dissertations (Kendler & Spence, 1971), and in view of the fact that most of his students took academic positions and made contributions of their own, the sheer number of Hull–Spence students have shaped the field.

The typical psychology experiment in this period used the rat maze, consisting of a starting box, a maze of varying complexity, and a goal box containing food or water. An improvement in the animal's ability to find the goal box specified learning, and one of the basic questions was, of course, the problem of purpose—how the future event of eating in the goal box could come to cause earlier behavior. Hull's answer was that the rat began to move randomly through the maze, and would come to the goal box by chance. The act of eating in the goal box would be associated with immediately prior behavior, such as seeing the goal box from a distance. The sight of the goal box would, in future trials, serve as a stimulus for small, *anticipatory goal responses*, such as salivation and chewing. In turn, the anticipatory goal responses would associate to even earlier stimuli and responses, so that a chain of association would run backwards from the goal behavior to the stimuli and responses that typically occur in the starting box. When this associative chain was established, the rat in the starting box would be stimulated to run to the goal box by a simple series of associative links.

Furthermore, Hull argued, the behavior was not totally dependent on the availability of environmental stimuli. The rat could internalize the chain of stimuli and responses, because each response also had stimulus properties: In his notational system, each internal anticipatory goal response (r_g) also has some stimulus value (s_g), so that some of the rat's behavior is independent of external cues. This famous argument is reminiscent of the commonsense idea that people represent the world internally, so that they do not have to pay attention to the outside world all the time. But Hull insists that his r_g–s_g associations are *not* representations—they are merely physical stimuli and responses that become associatively conditioned to a behavioral chain that runs from the start to the goal box. In modern vocabulary, Hull's chain of stimuli and responses resembles a set of feedback loops.

In its final phases Hull's theory of learning also incorporated "drive" variables such as hunger and thirst, inhibitory factors such as fatigue or boredom, and the like. He postulated that a stimulus served to reinforce a response if it led to a decrease in a drive-state, such as hunger. It seems plausible that Hull's drive-reduction theory of reinforcement was heavily influenced by Freud's libido theory. Freud thought of "libido" as a non-specific psychic energy, in just the way Hull thought of "Drive." Hull is known to have discussed the libido theory in the seminars that led up to his book on drive theory (*e.g.*, Shakow & Rapaport, 1963). Indeed, Hull's very word "Drive" is the English cognate of the German *Trieb* used by Freud. (*Trieb* is usually mistranslated as "instinct.") If we translate *Trieb* as "Drive," and compare Hull's "reinforcement" with Freud's "pleasure," the connection becomes obvious. Both men claim that a decrease in some motivational tension leads to a rewarding experience that makes people and animals want more of the same. It is not clear whether Hull acknowledged Freud's influence on his own thinking, however.

Hull's behavior theory functioned in terms of an explicit "hypothetico-deductive" structure, a little like Euclidian geometry. Seventeen postulates could be combined into 133 specific theorems and numerous corollaries (Hull, 1952; Hull, Hovland, Ross, Perkins, & Fitch, 1940). Many of these theorems have great plausibility. They are stated in the form of algebraic equations, but these equations are mostly *discursive* (Miller, 1964). They often make as much sense when they are simply expressed in words.

To Hull, all behavior consists of stimulus–response (S–R) connections, which he called *habits*. A set of such S–R connections is a *habit-family hierarchy* — "hierarchy," because he thought the habits were ordered by the frequency with which they were reinforced.

Given his belief that all behavior is reducible to S–R connections, Hull postulated a set of *stimulus variables* and *response variables*. (In addition, Hull spoke of *intervening variables*, but these were entirely determined by the stimulus variables. They added nothing new to the theory, but only provided convenient labels.) Stimulus variables include S, the "stimulus intensity"; ω (omega), the amount of reward; N, the number of prior reinforcements; and C_D, the stimulus aspects of the Drive condition (for instance, hunger pangs). Response variables included $_st_r$, the response latency; A, the reaction amplitude; and n, the number of nonreinforced responses that would occur before extinction of the conditioned response. We will discuss Hull's theory primarily in terms of his intervening variables, because his basic claims can be stated most conveniently in these terms.

For any given stimulus and response Hull wants to determine the *reaction potential* (sEr), a measure of the potential that the stimulus has for eliciting a specific response. But sEr depends on *Habit strength* (sHr), *Drive* (D), *stimulus-intensity dynamism* (V), which is the change in the probability of a response as the stimulus intensity changes, and *incentive motivation* (K), determined by the amount of a reward that will accrue to a response. Taking all these factors into account, Hull expresses the formal definition:

$$sEr = sHr \times D \times V \times K$$

In commonsense terms, the expression states that the likelihood of an animal doing something depends on how habitual the act is; how hungry or thirsty the animal is; how intense the stimulus signalling the reward is; and how much reward may come as a consequence of the response. Hull maintains that if the product sEr is larger than some reaction threshold sLr, then the response will be made.

Using such equations, Hull tried to derive very specific and testable predictions. Along with Spence and a large number of students and colleagues, Hull's work became the focus of a widely shared program to create, for the first time in history, a truly adequate theory of behavior. Increasingly, during the 1930s and 1940s, Hull's attempt to build a comprehensive theory became the centerpiece of behavioristic research. Hull was sometimes seen as the Newton of 20th-century psychology, and the success of behaviorism as a whole seemed to be identified by many psychologists with the success of the Hull–Spence program. Laboratories throughout the country, but especially at Yale and Iowa, were pervaded with a heady sense of enthusiasm and impending accomplishment. Each new issue of *Psychological Review* was seized on with great enthusiasm as a new source of further experimental tests, and Hull's formulations were circulated in mimeographed form long before they appeared in print.

But as Hull's neobehavioristic theory of learning was tested more and more, it became apparent that it lacked adequacy and precision: Its testable predictions consistently failed, and each new failure led to new *ad hoc* stop gaps. At the time Hull's *magnum opus* appeared, shortly before his death (Hull, 1952), his students and collaborators knew that the entire project was deeply flawed (*e.g.*, Koch, 1954, 1959). The intense excitement surrounding Hullian theory turned to disillusionment and even despair. Experimental psychologists could not understand what could have gone wrong—they had religiously followed the scientific method (as taught by the philosophers of science); and yet, the enterprise was somehow not crowned with success.

The dramatic failure of Hullian theory resembles more than any thing else the "paradigm crisis" of Kuhnian theory in the years preceding the cognitive revolution. But although Hull and Spence were the most prominent figures in the major theoretical enterprise of behaviorism of the 1930s and '40s, they were not the only ones. In particular, we must discuss two others who were of great significance: Edward C. Tolman, who anticipated the cognitive revolution by several decades, and B. F. Skinner, the intellectual heir of John B. Watson.

"Cognitive Behaviorism": Edward C. Tolman

During the heyday of behaviorism the only major figure who advocated the possibility of mental representation was Edward C. Tolman (1886–1959). He anticipates, more than any other behaviorist, the cognitive point of view. For one thing, Tolman thought it necessary to postulate events other than stimuli and responses. Like Hull, he called these theoretical events *intervening variables*, to be inferred from observed behavior. But unlike Hull, as long as a persuasive case could be made for the existence of these entities, Tolman felt no immediate need to *reduce* his intervening variables to "nothing but" observable stimuli and responses.

For Tolman, perhaps the most important intervening variable was *purpose* (1932). Like any other behaviorist, Tolman was against vitalistic teleology, but he believed that purposes could be postulated without undermining the scientific world view. He also argued for the existence of "cognitive maps" to explain the spatial abilities of "rats and men" (1948). Such maps are, of course, one kind of mental representation. And finally, Tolman's behaviorism was *molar* — he did not believe that single muscle contractions were connected by conditioning to punctate physical stimuli. Rather, he pointed out, entire actions seem to be related to entire situations, and these actions are so flexible that they can only be specified by their purposes. Neither actions nor situations, he thought, could be reduced to very simple physical events without fundamentally distorting their character.

To the majority of "respectable behaviorists" these proposals seemed fuzzy or mentalistic. In experimental tests comparing Hull's ideas with Tolman's, the results were thought to favor Hull, especially because Tolman's ideas were believed to be *less parsimonious* — Tolman required one to believe in unobservable representations, purposes, and so on. The argument from parsimony was used with devastating effect against Tolman's theoretically rich approach. If one could explain behavior by observable, or potentially observable, stimulus–response connections, why bother to postulate entities that could not be observed? A great deal of ingenuity was devoted to finding ways to restate Tolman's evidence in stimulus–response terms, and in a surprising number of cases, stimulus–response formulations were able to explain the evidence cited in favor of Tolman's cognitive approach (see Hilgard & Marquis, 1940; Kimble, 1961). In the upshot, Tolman was often considered an interesting thought slightly eccentric figure, somewhat on the fringes of a truly scientific psychology.

B. F. Skinner: The Heir of John B. Watson

On the other extreme from Tolman, a true radical behaviorist in the mold of John B. Watson, was B. F. Skinner (b. 1904). Skinner is today the most famous living behaviorist, and it comes as a surprise to discover that before 1950 his impact was small. Skinner first truly comes to the fore in the 1950s with the failure of Hull's ambitious theory. In this period of disillusionment with theory in general, Skinner's antitheoretical approach seemed to many psychologists an attractive way out of the crisis.

Skinner did not begin to study psychology until graduate school. Before that time, his ambitions were literary, and as a young man Skinner wrote outstanding "psychological" short stories in the manner of Proust and Dos Passos. Indeed, as his autobiography makes clear (1976, 1979), he tried to become a writer, but failed. This failure occasioned a deep personal crisis, which was resolved only when he decided that his future lay in the direction of science. Vehemently rejecting literature, Skinner began to read Watson, Pavlov, and the physiologist Loeb. Reading Bertrand Russell converted him to behaviorism even before he had taken any courses in psychology; and as soon as he was admitted to graduate school at Harvard in 1924, he became the radical behaviorist of the psychology department, countering the regnant views of E. G. Boring and others. In the six decades since then, Skinner has held to radical behaviorism with remarkable consistency.

But even as a radical behaviorist, Skinner would be almost unknown today if it had not been for his laboratory work, which has had very wide influence. Appointed a Junior Fellow at Harvard, he developed all the basic concepts of what he called *operant conditioning* between 1930 and 1935. Operant conditioning was a method for carrying out the Watson program of behaviorism — to show that behavioral analysis could, in fact, account for all of human behavior, and to do so in a way that was far more effective and safe from criticism than Watson's approach had been. But first of all it was necessary to solve the problem of purpose.

Skinner denies the existence of purpose, but he has said that "operant conditioning is the field of purpose." Rather than speaking of mental representations or goals, he refers to "environmental contingencies of reinforcement." In ordinary language, we might say, when we see a dog sniffing at his bowl of food, that the dog has a goal of eating, but in Skinner's view there is simply a conditional relationship in the environment between moving toward the bowl, opening the mouth, and eating. Food is just a reinforcing stimulus, which increases the probability of any preceding response. A reinforcing stimulus is not a purpose, a reward, or a source of pleasure. Skinner eschews such mentalistic terms.

Reinforcement is defined circularly as any stimulus that will increase the likelihood of a response that precedes it. Having thus cut with a single blow the Gordian knot of mentalism, Skinner can proceed to apply his analysis to everything from the training of pigeons to the writing of poetry (Skinner, 1972). It is all grist for his mill—and, indeed, there is no apparently goal-directed behavior that cannot somehow be explained with this scheme.

Skinner's analysis of behavior has a number of advantages over the work of Pavlov, Watson, and others. First, it is a purely *functional* analysis. Skinner is not interested in reducing behavior to some sequence of causes and effects—the only object is to show lawful relationships between observables. In this respect, Skinner does not need to reduce everything to reflexes, or even to purely physically described stimuli and responses. A stimulus is defined by the way an organism responds to it, and a response is defined by how effective it is in gaining from the environment a reinforcing stimulus. By making the organism the measure of the stimulus, Skinner avoids having to specify the stimulus in physical detail. Second, unlike Pavlovian conditioning, operant conditioning can, in principle at least, explain any new activity that people or animals can perform. Such activities, Skinner claims, were operantly conditioned at some time "in the history of the organism." Of course, this explanation is largely a promissory note: In practice, no one actually searches back to see what it was, in the history of the organism, that produced some current behavior. But referring to "the history of the organism" permits Skinner to claim that one could do this *in principle* without appeal to such mentalistic constructions as "memory" or to neurophysiology. Third, contrary to Hull, Skinner claims that psychological theory is really unnecessary (Skinner, 1944, 1950). Because only lawful relationships between stimuli and responses are needed, it is not necessary to offer rationales for behavior. Understanding stimulus–response relationships will lead to prediction and control of human and animal behavior, and prediction and control is the goal of science.

Skinner's is a brilliant analysis, not only in the positive claims it makes, but in the problems it avoids. Skinner cannot be faulted for having the wrong theory, because insofar as he makes any theoretical claims, they are essentially circular. This circularity is not pernicious, because in particular experimental situations, variables such as stimulus, response, and reinforcement can be specifically defined. Nor can the analysis be attacked for having incorrectly specified the stimulus, the response, or the reinforcement, because all these are defined by reference to the concrete behavior of the organism and its observable relationships to the reinforcement contingencies (the things it must do to receive reinforcement). To say that Skinner's analysis circumvents a set of issues is not necessarily a criticism: A case can be made that many major advances in the history of science simply avoid problems that are not susceptible to a solution at the time. Thus Darwin avoided the problem of the source of genetic variation, and Newton avoided the problem of explaining "action at a distance." Skinner's analysis clears the ground, and makes it possible to carry out a coherent research program to specify the relationships between stimuli, responses, and reinforcers.

Even so, it is the effectiveness of operant conditioning that has made Skinner's analysis of real interest. Take any confined animal, and deprive it of food or water (or any other reinforcer) for a day or so. Then, whenever it moves any part of its body in a certain way (say, its tail), give it a small amount of food. Soon it will move its tail more frequently — the tail-moving response has been "conditioned by reinforcement." Now, only reinforce the animal when it moves the tail to touch its back. In a matter of minutes, most animals can learn that. Now, have it curl its tail, swing it up and down, or sideways. Any observable response can be shaped and increased in frequency by means of Skinner's procedure. Further, Skinner was able to automate this process by using a bar-press as a response and having each bar-press register on a moving drum. In this way it was easy to collect large amounts of data, and one could find out how often an animal would respond in order to get reinforcement, how temporal relationships between the variables affected responding, how animals would respond to shock compared with food, how they could learn a sequence of responses, or how they could learn to distribute their time among different responses and reinforcements.

Skinner developed this basic experimental approach in the years 1930–1935, and it has remained unchanged since then. Skinner and his followers have used these methods to investigate various features of his analysis, to assess the sensory capacities of animals, and to compare the capabilities of different animal species. Today, the technique of operant conditioning is used extensively in medical and physiological research, and for changing certain kinds of well-defined psychopathology. In fact, it has been useful in many cases where it is not important, or possible, to know about goals, rewards, or the experience of pleasure — all those thorny issues that Skinner so neatly circumvented.

Moreover, following in the footsteps of John B. Watson, Skinner advocated operant conditioning as *the* scientific approach to life. In his utopian novel *Walden Two* (Skinner, 1948), he advocated applying operant conditioning to the construction of entire new communities, in which reinforcement contingencies are not a matter of chance, but of rational design. Of course, in order to make reinforcement effective, some person or agency would have to have control over the supply of reinforcing goods, so that the members of the community could not have entirely free access. (Remember that in order for food to be a reinforcer, the animal must be deprived of food for some time.) This feature of operant utopia is not often remarked on, but it is the real sticking point, as the Romans well knew. *Quid custodiens ipsos custodes?* they asked: *Who will guard the guardians?* To this question it is not clear that Skinner has the answer.

It is an amusing exercise to reverse the radical behavioristic custom of translating commonsense psychology into behavioral terms, by making up a commonsense description of operant conditioning. Let's suppose that animals really do have goals, and that when they are hungry, they really seek food. That is to say, suppose animals have some kind of internal representation of food, some complicated set of related ideas about what is good to eat, perhaps even about what is nutritious. Such a representation, projected into the future, is a goal. Whenever such a goal is satisfied, the animal stores the procedure that led up to the goal in memory, and whenever it needs food again, it tries the same procedure that previously led to food. "So sticking my tail in the air seems to lead to food? Let's try it again!" Thus, moving its tail becomes a *subgoal* that must be met before the goal can be reached. Operant conditioning, then, would involve teaching animals to meet certain subgoals (*i.e.*, whatever the experimenter wants the animal to do). An experimenter would accomplish this by (1) finding out what the ordinary goals of the animal are (eating regularly is a good bet), and (2) preventing the animal from reaching its goal except by performing the subgoal.

This, in principle, is no different from a factory owner who will not pay his workers (pay being their main goal) unless they meet some intermediate subgoal that he finds to be of primary interest. Skinner's analysis has thus been called the psychological equivalent of wage-labor capitalism, and it does not appear to be new—quite a few economic and political leaders in human history have figured out these principles for themselves. (Nor is it obvious that humanity in general has profited from the times that these principles have been put into practice with total consistency.) Nevertheless, Skinner's analysis has been applied in more practical situations than any other method developed during the behavioristic period in psychology.

During the 1940s and early '50s, however, it was not Skinner, but Clark L. Hull who dominated behavioristic thought. We have already discussed Hull's attempt to build a grand theory that would cover all the major phenomena of behavioristic concern, and its evident failure. The crisis caused by the failure of Hullian theory was, in many ways, a watershed in the history of behavioristic psychology, with consequences for several decades of work in experimental psychology. Let us consider this crisis and its consequences in more detail.

The Crisis of Hullian Theory in the Early 1950s

In his study of scientific revolutions, Kuhn (1962) suggests that revolutions are often preceded by a period of crisis, and certainly the failure of Hullian theory suggests such a crisis. Hull's theory represents a point of convergence, in which the behavioristic movement focused on experimental tests of a comprehensive theory of learning. Learning was, of course, *the* critical topic for behavioristic psychologists, and learning was identified with the acquisition of stimulus–response relationships: conditioning, improvement in running a maze, or certain kinds of skill acquisition. Behaviorism had confidently promised that once a truly scientific approach had been taken to psychology, once the logical positivist prescription for doing science was followed consistently and "rigorously" (a favorite word of the times), progress would inevitably follow. At the same time, the behaviorists imposed narrow limits on the role of theory: the permissible theoretical mechanisms were usually limited to connections between discrete stimuli and responses. If we consider the construction of theory as a puzzle-solving task, the behaviorists had set up a puzzle, but taken away the freedom to move the pieces in any arbitrary way—one could only arrange them in pairs, or at most into chains of stimuli and responses. Psychologists already *knew* that behavior was "nothing but" stimulus–response connection; no other belief was scientific; and giving free rein to the theoretical imagination was *verboten*.

Some of our interview participants describe the heady atmosphere of excitement and certainty that pervaded the learning laboratories at Yale and Iowa at this time. When it became clear that Hullian theory was not going to work, that in fact the theory was so flexible that it could not be conclusively tested, the resulting disillusionment was proportional to the high hopes of only a few years before. What could have gone wrong? It was a difficult question to answer, because there was really no clear alternative to the approach pursued so diligently by Hull, Spence, and their students. In Kuhn's terms, there was a crisis in the "paradigm," but no alternative was in sight. From this time on, the behavioristic period began to take on a strongly negative and critical cast. There might be little agreement on what to do, but the sophisticated experimental methodology that was now spreading could still be used as a position from which to criticize various ideas and approaches. In the 1950s and early '60s, *Psychological Review*, the major theoretical journal, was filled with scathing attacks on various phenomena and hypotheses.

It was their respective answers to the question, "What had gone wrong?" that determined the paths taken in subsequent years by different experimental psychologists. When the cook spoils the broth, there are basically two possible responses: One says, "Too much," and the other, "Not enough." Too much salt, or too much cooking, or not enough vegetables, not enough spices.

In response to the failure of Hullian theory, B. F. Skinner (1957) responded: "Too much theory." Psychological theory is more than unnecessary to Skinner; indeed it is impermissible. If a theory refers to the organism, it is physiology, not psychology. If it refers to something other than the organism, it is not physicalistic and therefore unscientific. Coincident with the failure of Hullian theory, then, Skinner's star began to rise. His approach was effective in predicting and controlling behavior, at least in some situations, and it had few presuppositions to attack. Moreover, Skinner and his followers were remarkably good experimental methodologists, and his approach could be applied to important practical problems.

Starting in the 1950s, Skinner's approach (and Pavlov's as well) was applied increasingly to practical problems of behavior modification (*e.g.*, Ullmann & Krasner, 1969). Indeed, for the first time, the behavioral revolution now began to spread to the study of psychopathology. And just as Watson created the conceptual space for the experimental psychology profession, so did the new behavior modification psychologists create the conceptual space for clinical psychology. They had to struggle with the psychiatric profession for the right to treat patients, and the establishment of clinical psychology in the 1950s took on some of the character of a struggle for access to a market place. In this struggle, the side that could claim the greatest scientific legitimacy was likely to win. Behaviorism gave that legitimacy to the psychologists, while psychiatrists claimed legitimacy on the basis of psychoanalysis. Objective clinical outcome studies (mostly run by psychologists) cast doubt on the therapeutic effectiveness of psychoanalysis, and psychologists in this period made substantial inroads into the psychiatric domain. This is not to say that the struggle with psychiatry was carried on cynically, or only for financial and professional motives. Human motives are often mixed, and there was a crusading, idealistic spirit in this early clinical work that is reminiscent of Watson's crusade against religion and superstition. Clinical psychologists saw themselves as a vanguard, fighting for a truly scientific approach to human problems, and against untested mentalistic theory.

These, then, were the responses of behaviorists who held to the behavioristic faith, who said that Hull had, in fact, deviated from that faith. But others criticized the Hullian broth, not for being "too much," but "too little": "Too little physiology was known at the time." "Too little mathematical sophistication in Hullian theory." "Too little data for a general theory." Some experimental psychologists, such as Neal Miller, moved increasingly toward physiology, while others developed much more precise, limited, and mathematically sophisticated "minitheories" to explain data collected in a small number of very careful experiments (*e.g.*, Estes, 1975). The experimental psychology of the time is extremely conscious of methodology, statistical techniques, and all the possible flaws that can enter into an experimental design. There is enormous emphasis on method, and comparatively little on content.

And finally, some psychologists came to question behaviorism itself. Sigmund Koch, a former follower of Hull who had become an early critic (1954), edited a massive seven-volume book, reassuringly titled *Psychology: The Study of a Science* (1959). Psychology was still a science, but the insecurity that the behavioristic program was supposed to have alleviated was back again, a nagging presence. Koch was often scathing:

Ever since its stipulation into existence as an independent science, psychology has been far more concerned with being a science than with courageous and self-determining confrontation with its historically constituted subject matter. Its history has been largely a matter of emulating the methods, forms, symbols of the established sciences, especially physics. (1961, p. 630)

Koch thought that psychologists had rejected too many things, and that, in hot pursuit of scientism, psychology had lost psychology. And in a chapter on behaviorism caustically entitled "Psychology Out of Its Mind," Roback (1964) wrote that " . . . Psychology first lost its soul, then it lost consciousness, but no more than an individual who has lost consciousness for all time, can be said to remain a person, can psychology, without consciousness, exist as such" (pp. 264–265). But of course, consciousness was still taboo, and would remain so well into the 1970s.

Psychodynamics and Other Alternative Models for Psychology

But what rigorous scientific alternatives were available? Looking to Europe, American psychologists could see psychoanalysis, Gestalt psychology, and the work of Piaget and Bartlett. Metatheoretically, all the European movements were cognitive, in the sense that they postulated unobservable theoretical constructs to explain human behavior and experience. At best, their work seemed intuitively plausible, but often not even that. Methodologically, European work appeared unsophisticated, not nearly as "rigorous" as American research. American psychologists simply did not believe the data presented by most European psychologists, nor did they understand the theoretical framework in which these data made sense.

During the Second World War, a number of refugees from Hitler had come to the United States—indeed, starting at this time, American science in general moves into the first rank, stimulated by many such refugees—but they did not immediately affect the course of experimental psychology in this country. They were received kindly, and academic positions were found for many of them, but they seemed methodologically unsophisticated, appearing to jump to vast conclusions on the basis of little, and often conflicting, data.

The Freudians had great influence on medical psychotherapy, but little on academic psychology. This is in part because psychoanalysis is metatheoretically cognitive—it speaks of intentions, unconscious wishes, ego-defense mechanisms, and the like, which are unobservable constructs inferred from observations made in therapy. If psychodynamic ideas are cognitive, then it would be very difficult for psychologists operating within a behavioristic metatheory to test or even to understand them. And, indeed, psychodynamic theory has really never been put to a test using the rigorous experimental techniques developed during the behavioristic era. Some behaviorists (*e.g.*, Ullmann & Krasner, 1969) argued that psychoanalytic theory was untestable *in principle*, and this was no doubt true within the behavioristic metatheory. Presumably the cognitive metatheory might permit psychologists to define dynamic constructs with precision, and to test them rigorously. But as yet no general movement in this direction is noticeable (but see Erdelyi, 1985). Even today, one often hears criticisms of psychoanalysis as if it were a *refuted* theory; but since it has never been tested, it cannot be said to have been refuted.

Indeed, within the behavioristic movement there was a curiously equivocal approach to psychodynamics. Watson writes in his autobiographical chapter (1936) that

. . . In the Fall of the year in which I was graduated (from the University of Chicago) I had a breakdown — sleepless nights for weeks — a typical Angst . . . for three weeks I went to sleep only with the lights turned on. A sudden recovery and back to work. This, in a way, was one of my best experiences in my university course. It taught me to watch my step and in a way prepared me to accept a large part of Freud, when I first began to get really acquainted with him around 1910. (p. 274)

Of course, Freud had to be translated into behavioristic terms, which was done by speaking of the unconscious as the "unverbalized," and the Oedipus complex as the "incest complex." Indeed, Watson performed what is probably the only experimental test of the Oedipal notion on record, by performing mock-fighting and mock-lovemaking with his wife in front of their very young infant son, to see if the baby would exhibit jealousy (Cohen, 1979)!

Even Skinner's autobiography betrays a fascination with psychodynamics. As discussed, Skinner's first ambition was to be a writer, and he wrote in the manner of the psychological novel. In the first volume of his autobiography, Skinner performs a retrospective analysis on his own short stories, suggesting that a quarrel between a man and wife in the story could stand for his own struggle with his father. Later, Skinner discovered that when a tape recording of a sentence is repeated over and over, people would soon hear things in it that are not actually there. This "verbal summator," he noted, often resulted in apparently "significant" illusions by the people who listened to it (1979, pp. 174–176). This is, of course, the idea behind a projective test. And, finally, Skinner performs an analysis of his own writing of the utopian novel *Walden Two*. Much of the book consists of debates between the tough-minded scientist Frazier and the tender-minded Burris about the desirability of the operant utopia. Skinner remarks that only after finishing the book did he realize that both Burris and Frazier represented different parts of himself (see Chapter 3). Nothing could be more suggestive of inner conflict than writing a book in which two characters represent differing aspects of the author, especially when they spend much of the book arguing with each other! But as a behaviorist, Skinner cannot describe the situation in these terms; "inner conflict" is an inferred construct and, hence, unscientific. Nevertheless, Skinner comes very, very close to conveying exactly this idea in his autobiography. Like Watson, Skinner shows the same equivocal attraction to psychodynamic thinking, countered by his fidelity to the behavioristic point of view.

This ambivalence is also very clear in Hull, who, as discussed, apparently derived the idea of reinforcement as drive-reduction from Freudian theory. He announced the seminar that led to his learning theory as an examination of Freudian concepts of libido (Shakow & Rapaport, 1963), and it is difficult to doubt that the line of influence is quite direct. But it is largely unacknowledged.

Of all the prominent behaviorists of the 1930s and '40s, Tolman seems to be the most direct about his interest in psychodynamic concepts. The last few pages of his famous article "Cognitive Maps in Rats and Men" (1948) are devoted to a discussion of ways in which his viewpoint can incorporate dynamic ideas, including regression, fixation, displacement of aggression, and the contrast between the pleasure and reality principles.

In spite of all this interest, there was very little overt work on psychodynamic ideas during the behavioristic period. True, psychologists such as E. G. Boring and Neal E. Miller went through psychoanalysis, and came out with much greater respect for it. Miller collaborated with the psychoanalytic anthropologist John Dollard on an attempt to translate psychoanalytic theory into a behavioristic language, so that a concept such as "ambivalence" became "approach–avoidance gradient" (Dollard & Miller, 1950). Psychoanalytic thinking also influenced Jerome Bruner, who proposed in the 1950s a "New Look" in perception, in which motivation was thought to influence one's perception of reality (Erdelyi, 1974). But Bruner's attempt to create a kind of cognitive–psychoanalytic revolution fell out of favor when his experimental work was criticized for alleged methodological flaws. And when, in the 1950s, behavioristic clinical psychologists began to criticize psychoanalysis from a behavioristic perspective, and eventually began to contest the psychiatric profession for the legal right to treat patients, any rapprochement between psychodynamic and behavioral psychology became increasingly unlikely.

Gestalt psychologists such as Köhler, Koffka, and Lewin had more immediate impact when they came to this country than did the psycho-analysts. Indeed, the Gestaltists essentially established the experimental study of perception and social psychology, neglected topics during the heyday of behaviorism. It is interesting that the fields of perception and social psychology became effectively "cognitive" long before the core of experimental psychology did so. But in the 1950s, Gestalt psychology also seemed to be waning. The original German–Jewish immigrants who had brought it had few American students; their experiments were often only phenomenological demonstrations; and some of their more precise and testable hypotheses simply failed. Thus Wolfgang Köhler's theory that there were "brain fields" along the lines of the magnetic fields of physics was shown to be simply false (Lashley, 1930), although it has inspired some more recent thinking (Pribram, 1971).

Even before the refugee scientists came to the United States, the European psychologies had encountered a language problem. It is simply amazing how the critical terminology of European psychology was consistently mistranslated into English — almost without exception. It begins with Wundt, who was translated by Titchener as having said almost exactly the opposite of what he intended (Blumenthal, 1975, 1980). Titchener was an Englishman, and in his translation he apparently looked at Wundt through English associationistic filters.

But Pavlov fared no better: the Russian word that is usually translated as "conditioned reflex" should probably have been translated "conditional reflex," emphasizing the contingent "if–then" relationship between the neural stimulus and the response-evoking stimulus (Miller, 1962). In Pavlov's classic experiment the bell served simply as a *signal* that food would be coming. Some psychologists who thought of Pavlovian conditioning as establishing a two-way relationship between two stimuli, apparently tried to establish whether the presence of food would also signal the sound of the bell, which makes no sense at all if the word "conditional" is remembered. It is conceptually incoherent to think that what is being signaled can somehow signal the signal, as though the stopping of traffic could turn the traffic-light red.

As noted above, Freud's word for the sexual and other drives was *Trieb*, mistranslated as "instinct" at a time when American psychologists were vehemently rejecting the word "instinct" as unnecessary and hereditarian (*cf*. Bettelheim, 1983). But American psychologists had no difficulty with Hull's use of the English cognate word "Drive" — that seemed obviously sensible. Similarly, the German word for "ego" is simply *ich*, that is to say, "I." A German speaker cannot easily say, "*Ich glaube nicht an das 'Ich'*" ("I don't believe in the 'I'") — that sounds like a self-contradiction. But "ego" is a strange word, and one can easily imagine an American psychologist saying, as so many have, "I don't believe in the 'ego.'"

Even the word for "science" has a different meaning in German and French. The German *Wissenschaft* really means "scholarly discipline," and it applies to history and literary criticisms as well as to physics. The gulf that the English-speaking world perceives between "science" and other kinds of knowledge simply does not exist for speakers of other European languages.

The pattern of these consistent mistranslations almost seems deliberate, but a conspiracy theory is not necessary to explain them. It is simply very difficult, perhaps impossible, to avoid imposing one's own reality on the views of others. When those others are from other cultures, thinking within an intellectual framework alien to our own, the difficulty is compounded. The Italian proverb *Traditore — tradutore!* (to translate is to betray) makes this point eloquently. Furthermore, the social sciences in general seem to establish "myths of origin" (Samelson, 1974) "that evolve, consciously or unconsciously, in such ways as to serve the function of justifying their own present position in the course of history" (Blumenthal, 1977b, p. 17). In just this way, E. G. Boring, the foremost historian of experimental psychology, justified the psychology of his time by his questionable portrayal of Wundt.

So it was that behaviorism was largely insulated from any outside influences. When Hull's theory appeared to fail, no acceptable alternatives seemed to be in sight. Even as scientific psychologists were desperately seeking a new, positive program, the behavioristic metatheory armored them against any fundamental change by its own methodological sophistication. Behaviorists still *knew* just what science was supposed to be, even if psychologists were perhaps not doing it with obvious success. Maybe doing science was just much more difficult than Hull and Spence had imagined, or perhaps it would take many more decades to succeed. Perhaps more facts were needed.

There were some bright spots in this bleak picture. Perhaps the most significant signs of success were the empirical achievements of operant conditioning, pursued by B. F. Skinner and his followers, and the growth of behavior modification approaches in clinical psychology. (Behavior therapy is discussed in the following section.) Further, Charles Osgood, as discussed earlier, found a rich vein in his attempt to "measure the meaning" of words. Apparently, words could be judged consistently along a scale whose end-points were labeled by opposite adjectives. Thus the word *rock* would be consistently judged more "dark" than "light," more "down" than "up," and so on. A large number of such judgments were collected, and the data analyzed by the statistical technique of factor analysis, which determined the smallest number of dimensions of variation that could account for the greatest amount of the data. Osgood and his colleagues found that three basic dimensions could explain most of the data: Words were judged according to *potency, activity,* and *evaluation* (Osgood, Suci, & Tannenbaum, 1957). The same result has been obtained for many different languages and cultures, and it appears to be universally true. This is a significant achievement of behavioristic empiricism. It has all its characteristic virtues, such as reliability and generality of evidence, and also its characteristic flaws, especially in terms of its theoretical interpretations. Few language psychologists today believe that meaning has only three dimensions, or that it can be measured quantitatively in the way that Osgood and his colleagues suggested. But no one can dispute the evidence they presented. And we have already pointed out the ironic fact that Osgood's three dimensions of connotative meaning correspond directly with the three dimensions of experience found by Wilhelm Wundt, in an earlier age in the history of psychology, using a very different methodology.

But now one new element enters the picture: For the first time in the history of behaviorism, a major effort was mounted to apply some of the reliable laboratory findings in a practical setting, with considerable practical success. To this development of a true behavioral technology we now turn.

Behavior Therapy: A Vindication of Behaviorism?

The behavior modification movement, starting in the 1950s, stands as a major exception to the general decline of faith in behaviorism. Ironically, this "applied" success story began just as the feeling of disillusionment was beginning to spread about Hull's theory of behavior, the pinnacle of "pure" experimental psychology. But, of course, Watsonian behaviorism did not distinguish between pure and applied science—or rather, it viewed successful application as a primary proof of the scientific pudding. By this criterion, one could make a good case for the claim that behaviorism, far from failing, has actually succeeded in its primary stated goal. Much of the success of behavior modification has apparently been due to its attempt to apply in the clinic the kinds of reliable learning principles that had been worked out in the laboratory. Further, behaviorists emphasized in the clinic the same strongly empiricist approach that they taught in the laboratory. In most ways their applied work was far more successful than their earlier, purely scientific work had been (Krasner, 1962, 1973; Kazdin, 1978; Kalish, 1981).

In a retrospective paper, Krasner (1973) describes the motivation of this early work as deeply idealistic: "World War II veterans, children of the depression, and the war, [were] interested in social change" (p. 1). Elsewhere he also suggests that

A major characteristic of the postwar period shared by both the humanist and the behaviorist was the desire to create a better world. . . . This was a period of pervasive optimism . . . psychologists and psychiatrists in both the humanist and behaviorist streams stressing beliefs in individualism, freedom, and the dignity of the human being. (1978, p. 799)

He views Skinner's utopian novel *Walden Two* as part of this idealistic trend, although Skinner himself would, no doubt, take exception to words such as "freedom" and "dignity" to describe his own beliefs (Skinner, 1971). It is interesting to see how this idealistic strain echoes the idealism of Watsonian behaviorism, itself a postwar trend in a younger America.

Immediately after the Second World War, psychoanalytic thought was dominant in American psychotherapy. Indeed, most clinicians who helped to create behavior therapy were trained in psychoanalysis. As Krasner notes, for example, "If you asked what kind of psychotherapist I was, I would have to say that I was a psychoanalytically-oriented, eclectic psychologist" (1973, p. 2). In America, however, the clinical practice of psychotherapy was restricted to holders of medical degrees (a policy that Freud himself protested [1927]). Psychologists and others who wished to treat patients had to engage in a political struggle for the right to do so. Krasner writes:

One of the major meetings of the 1940s on the road to eventual licensing and certification for the psychologists was a protest meeting of strange bedfellows . . . psychologists, social workers, and the clergy . . . all of whom resented the interpretation that talking to people who have any sort of problem was restricted to the medicine man. . . . Psychiatry occupied the high ground which was the linkage between Freud, the physician, and the practice of psychotherapy. . . . If one were going to help people and help was the name of the game, what else was the clinical psychologist to do but muscle in on the psychotherapy business? Licensing and certification, to protect the public and the psychologist, was considered a basic necessity. (1973, pp. 2–3)

From a scientific behaviorist's point of view, classical psychoanalysis posed great difficulties. It was heavily theoretical, involving numerous unobservable constructs such as wishes, unconscious conflicts, ego-defense mechanisms, and the like. Its major works were written in a foreign language, with foreign philosophical presuppositions. The psychoanalytic community was structured around a central authority, Freud and his immediate circle, which was largely immune to serious criticism. This central group was surrounded by satellite communities, each loyal to a critic of Freud, such as Adler or Jung, and each accusing the others of misinterpreting the truth, or worse. There were no agreed-upon, consensus-building proof procedures, such as existed in physics or biology, and there was little interest in finding such procedures. There was no interest in experimentation. All of the theoretical constructs were based on interpretations of events in the psychoanalytic interview, which was inherently unique and complex, far too complex to approach in an atheoretical way.

Many of these characteristics of classical psychoanalysis were not just offensive to behavioristic empiricism, but in some basic sense, they seemed culturally "un-American." Here was a deeply intellectual theory, dependent on unchallengeable authority, whose primary purpose was not to change life for the better, but merely to understand obscure and powerful forces — and which took a fundamentally fatalistic view of life. Many of the same characteristics had led John Watson to reject the psychology of Wundt and Titchener: Not surprisingly, perhaps, they led the intellectual heirs of Watson to reject Freud.

We will select three names to epitomize three of the major streams of thought that converged to create early behavior modification: Skinner, Wolpe, and Eysenck. These core behavioristic influences soon merged with a "social learning" perspective advocated especially by Bandura (1969) and Lazarus (1971), and ultimately formed the modern field of behavior therapy, which has gone in many ways far beyond its early behavioristic roots. But let us look at those roots in some detail.

The Skinner influence led in several directions. First, a number of empirical studies encouraged some psychologists to think that practically all behavior could be viewed in terms of operant conditioning. Thus Greenspoon (1951) showed that one could increase the possibility that a human subject would use a certain word, or even a class of words, in a conversation, just by saying "um-hmm" each time the word occurred spontaneously. This finding seemed to be consistent with Skinner's account of language acquisition in his book *Verbal Behavior* (1957). In therapeutic contexts, it was shown that emotional statements, self-referring statements, early childhood memories, and the like, could be increased or decreased in frequency by reinforcement techniques used by the therapist, leading Krasner (1962) to suggest that a therapist is a "social reinforcement machine." If that were true, then the logical ap-

proach would be to turn the therapist into a deliberate, rather than accidental or misguided, social-reinforcement machine.

This line of thinking led to a second Skinnerian direction, the attempt to control patient behavior by means of operant methods. The first
study along these lines was reported by Skinner, Solomon, and Lindsley (1953), who successfully taught psychotic patients to pull a plunger
by means of operant conditioning. Other studies soon applied the same
techniques to the control of more practical behavior, such as self-care
in chronic psychotics, verbalization and eye-contact in autistic children,
and the like.

A third direction inspired by Skinnerian thought was a radical rejection of traditional psychotherapy, epitomized by criticism of "the
medical model" (Ullmann & Krasner, 1969). In general, the claim was
that psychoanalysis views a psychological problem as a disease state,
separate from the symptoms of the disease. Thus, anxiety may be a symptom of neurosis, but treating anxiety directly would be futile from a
psychoanalytic perspective, because it is not the real problem. To a
behaviorist, of course, the whole concept of "an underlying factor" is
unscientific, and this is, of course, the crux of the difference between the
cognitive and behavioristic metatheories. Ullmann and Krasner (1969)
believe that psychoanalysis is *in principle* untestable because of its reliance
on unobservable constructs, but this criticism seems to rest entirely on
a radical behavioristic or logical positivist view of science. This point does
not imply that psychoanalysis is *in fact* true, or even testable. It may or
may not be. It simply means that from the perspective of a cognitive
metatheory, one cannot rule out psychoanalytic constructs just because
they are not directly observable.

A second criticism of the "medical model" was that the very idea of
a *disease* is value-laden, not at all factual, and therefore not scientifically
testable. Certainly no scientific test can ever show that being anxious
or depressed is objectively good or bad. And it is certainly true that the
very act of labeling someone a "schizophrenic" can serve to stigmatize
the patient. However, historically, the ability to label underlying constructs has been an indispensable part of scientific theory construction,
and psychology is not likely to make progress without it. Social stigma
also accrues to people with physical diseases, but that does not make the
labeling process scientifically useless. We will see that the criticisms of
the "medical model" are largely criticisms of what we have called the
cognitive metatheory (see Chapter 5). From a cognitive point of view
these criticisms are not nearly as devastating as they must have appeared
to behaviorists in the 1960s and '70s.

The risk involved in the global criticisms of psychoanalysis is that the behavioral clinicians may have thrown out the baby with the bathwater, just as earlier behaviorists had done with Wundtian psychology. But there *was* a great deal of bathwater, and it was quite dirty. The disease categories derived from psychoanalytic thought were often ill-defined and unreliable. Psychotherapists *did* neglect symptomatic relief for their patients, predicting dire consequences if one treated merely the symptom. They also neglected the quest for more reliable proof-procedures, and many of their theoretical constructs were not tied unambiguously to observables. Psychoanalysts showed great resistance to the need for better scientific methodology, and although some of the behavioristic criticism now seems overstated, there was a dire need for some housecleaning.

Behavioral clinicians created improvements in all the "bathwater" categories enumerated above. They insisted on precise, observable definitions of psychological problems, made significant strides toward relieving problems that psychodynamic thought considered merely "symptomatic," created a methodology that made it possible to test clinical hypotheses rigorously, and in general insisted on clear evidence in a field in which reliable phenomena were previously hard to find. At the same time, as they developed in sophistication and were forced to confront the complexities of clinical reality, they went far beyond the rather simple models of pathology that originated in the laboratory.

The psychoanalytic movement itself seems to have changed only slowly in response to behavioristic criticisms, though it has lost considerable popularity. Psychiatry especially has moved more quickly in the direction of "biological psychiatry," as a result of the discovery of powerful psychoactive biochemicals.

Some of the psychodynamic resistance to experimentalism may be traceable to Freud's own attitude to experimental tests of psychoanalytic theory. In 1934 he wrote in a letter to S. Rosenzweig:

I have examined your experimental studies for the verification of the psychoanalytic assertions with interest. I cannot put much value on these confirmations because the wealth of reliable observations on which these assertions rest make them independent of experimental verification. Still, it can do no harm. (Shakow & Rapaport, 1963, p. 129)

Given the enormous personal influence of Freud in the psychoanalytic movement, his dismissive attitude, expressed in various ways, may have discouraged psychoanalytic interest in experimental research for decades to come.

A second major stream in early behavior modification can be traced to Pavlov and even Hull: It is the influence of the South African psychiatrist Joseph Wolpe. In contrast to Skinner's operant approach, Wolpe applied Pavlovian or "classical" conditioning techniques in the clinic, most notably with the technique of *systematic desensitization*, an effective treatment for phobias. From a Pavlovian perspective, a phobia is an overgeneralized fear response. The classic example is John Watson's child subject "little Albert," who was deliberately frightened by banging a metal bar loudly whenever he reached out to a rabbit. Afterwards, Little Albert showed fear of any small, furry object. If this interpretation can be extended to any exaggerated fear, then Pavlovian ideas point to a simple treatment: Furry objects must be experienced in the absence of fear. Wolpe was one of the first to apply this straightforward logic to real-life problems by having patients practice relaxation exercises while they were imagining a series of objects that increasingly resembled the phobic object, until finally they could think calmly about the fearful object. In this way snake phobics have learned to handle snakes, claustrophobics have been enabled to ride elevators, and people with a fear of heights, or of social contact, and the like, were helped to work through their fears. Since Wolpe's pioneering work, other techniques have been used with comparable success to treat phobias. It should be pointed out that in actual clinical practice, simple, isolated phobias are not common. Nevertheless, Pavlovian logic provided the first effective approach to a widespread problem that still creates great discomfort and suffering, and which can be severely disabling to some patients. The researchers and clinicians who developed these methods can feel justifiable satisfaction with their achievements.

The third paradigmatic name in early behavior modification is Hans Eysenck, the English psychologist who is still best known for his attack on conventional psychotherapy. Eysenck claimed that there is no believable evidence for psychotherapy's effectiveness (Eysenck, 1960), and for many years his conclusions stood without challenge: The hard evidence seemed to go against traditional, largely psychodynamic psychotherapy. His analysis has since been criticized as overly negative (*e.g.*, Smith & Glass, 1977), but in combination with the rise of Skinnerian and Pavlovian techniques and criticisms, Eysenck's arguments seemed devastating.

From a cognitive point of view, the behavioristic rejection of psychodynamics is not unlike earlier behavioristic rejections of commonsense psychology — of William James and Wundt, Gestalt psychology, Piaget, and all of the other metatheoretically cognitive developments in Europe. Since the cognitive shift in experimental psychology, all of these formerly disparaged movements have come into their own, and their contributions are now widely acknowledged in America. One might consider that psychodynamic thought has had more impact on Western thought in this century than all other movements *combined*. It would seem unlikely that psychodynamics has no contribution whatsoever to make to scientific psychology. More likely, theoretical constructs such as ego-defense mechanisms, unconscious wishes and conflicts, and the like, have not yet been assessed properly. Nevertheless, the behavioristic demand for clear and compelling public evidence for the effectiveness of psychotherapy is quite proper, and psychodynamic thinkers should devote much more effort to the whole issue of operationalizing psychodynamic constructs.

Since its early days, behavior therapy has become much more willing to embrace new ideas and techniques from almost any source. Today, most researchers are methodological behaviorists, but they see little need to force all effective treatment techniques into the mold of classical or operant conditioning. Their insistence on empirical testability has made behavior therapy a very flexible and fast-moving field. Clinical researchers have identified numerous phenomena that pose fundamental psychological questions, so that this "applied" field is feeding back issues to be resolved by basic psychology.

In 1976 Leonard Krasner wrote an article "On the Death of Behavior Modification: Some Comments from a Mourner." But it is very clear from his ironic commentary that even though the *label* may be dead, the fact of "behavior modification" is not. Nor should it be. It may be that the kind of atheoretical empiricism represented by much of the behavioral approach to therapy is of greater use in practical applications, where the goal of the treatment is clear and unambiguous. In fundamental psychological questions, where the criteria for success and failure are not so clear, the behavioral form of empiricism is perhaps less useful.

The Seeds of Change

Underneath all this activity within the behavioristic framework, the seeds of change were beginning to grow, though they were often difficult to discern. The very size of the profession militated against change — so many people had been trained in the "correct" way of doing science, so many had vested interests in careers based on these premises, so much was being published month after month. Psychology was no longer controlled by the small group of Ivy League intellects, well-educated and tolerant in outlook, who had started the whole enterprise around the turn of the century. The university system had expanded greatly, and each Western and Midwestern state now had university campuses with their own psychology departments, in which professional survival depended on publication. No longer could a small, elite group control the thinking of the whole field. Psychology had grown into a juggernaut, ponderously moving in its established direction even when its original motive force was gone.

In 1956, a rather small conference was held at Massachusetts Institute of Technology. It was not particularly well attended, and the conference proceedings were not widely disseminated. It must have seemed too specialized to many of the experimental psychologists who had even heard of it. The topics seemed irrelevant to empirical, scientific work. The participants included practically all of the people who were to play a major role in the cognitive revolution: George Miller, a Harvard psychophysicist who was increasingly interested in language and communication; Herbert Simon, an economist and political scientist by training, and his collaborator Allan Newell, who were now trying to program computers to solve problems of logic and to play chess; Noam Chomsky, an unknown mathematical linguist, holding a precarious position in the Electronics Laboratory at MIT; and David Green and John Swets, psychophysicists who were applying an engineering theory (signal detection theory) to human sensory functions. At the same time, Jerome Bruner, working with several colleagues, had just published *A Study of Thinking* (Bruner, Goodnow, & Austin, 1956), a book which makes no appeal to behavioristic conceptions of thinking. In these developments we can find all the major themes of the cognitive revolution that was just about to begin (see Chapter 4).

What Did Behavioristic Psychology Achieve?

In spite of the painful failure of Hull's theory, behaviorism was not by any means a complete failure, and some would agree that it was not a failure at all. Behavioristic psychologists were committed to a metatheory in which different laboratories could replicate each others' results. They were forced to be entirely precise and explicit in their laboratory work, and increasingly in their theoretical statements as well. The experimental method was applied conscientiously and with great honesty, self-discipline, and increasing sophistication. Indeed, perhaps the great contribution of behaviorism was the introduction into psychological method of the clear *possibility of failure*. When a Hullian prediction failed, it really failed, in contrast to predictions derived from less precise and more discursive theories, which could always be saved by some alternative interpretation. Experimental psychologists succeeded in introducing a canon of consensual proof, and this is perhaps the major accomplishment of the behavioristic period.

Someone who has never actually tried to test an idea experimentally may be inclined to scoff at the difficulties encountered by the beaviorists; but this would be unfair, and unrealistic as well. Submitting one's commonsense ideas to a precise, empirical test is often a shocking experience, one that is encountered by almost all fledgling psychologists. Very few commonsense hypotheses survive an explicit test, not necessarily because commonsense ideas are wrong, but because they are actually highly theoretical, and therefore dependent on unstated contextual conditions. Each commonsense claim about human psychology is supported by numerous unstated presuppositions, which are not made explicit in ordinary speech, because they are tacitly presumed by everyone. Phrasing these implicit presuppositions and qualifications explicitly enough to be tested is extremely difficult. And often, psychologists find that a commonsense idea is simply false when it is tested as a bare statement of fact.

Besides establishing a consensual canon of proof, behaviorism produced a number of other successes. Virtually all animal training uses conditioning techniques, methods that are especially useful in medical and physiological experiments. Skinnerian and Pavlovian techniques are widely used in the treatment of emotional disorders, and they have helped to relieve much human suffering. The same methods have made it possible to test the sensory capabilities of animals. Significant research on conditioning and motivation continues to be carried out by animal experimentalists, many of whom continue to consider themselves behaviorists.

There is no reason for such successful research programs to cease when the dominant metatheory changes, even though the results of such research might eventually be interpreted within the new framework. In a similar way, psychophysical research continued to thrive during the behavioristic period, even though it clearly dealt with the human experience behaviorism denied; the psychophysical research program was simply reinterpreted to fit the behavioristic mold (Stevens, 1966). There are numerous successful behavioristic research programs that will undoubtedly survive the current change in metatheory. History is not so neat and compartmentalized as our descriptions of it.

If one were to criticize behaviorism, it would not be for what it tried to accomplish, but rather for the things it found necessary to *deny*. Fundamentally, it denied the need for free theorizing, because all theory had to be limited to observable stimuli and responses. It denied all of the commonsense constructs without which none of us can get along in the world: conscious experience, thinking, knowledge, images, feelings, and so on. In fact, it rejected commonsense knowledge by fiat, rather than testing it and transcending it, as the other sciences had done. Fascinating topics such as hypnosis, altered states of consciousness, dissociation of personality, and the like, were almost completely neglected (Hilgard, 1977, 1980a, 1980b).

And certain ethical issues could not be recognized. If there is no such thing as conscious experience, then animals cannot have the conscious experience of pain — and thus it is all right to perform very painful experiments on animals (*e.g.*, Cohen, 1979; Singer, 1975). For example, in his studies on infant–mother attachment, Harlow was interested in finding out what it would take to permanently frighten an infant monkey away from a doll that served as an artificial mother. To test this, he had inserted into the doll's chest a variety of devices to repulse the baby monkey, including a sharp, spring-loaded prong, as well as several other similar devices. Clinical notes were taken of the infant monkey's reactions — it appeared that neither pain nor physical injury would permanently keep a monkey baby away from its artificial mother (Harlow & Suomi, 1970; Singer, 1975). And Watson himself did postdoctoral research on maze-running in rats, with the aim of determining *the* particular sensory mode that the rat used to learn his path through the maze. Watson systematically removed or incapacitated each sense modality — he blinded the rats, removed the olfactory bulb from their brains, deafened them, and cut their sensitive nose-hairs. Still the rats would find their way through the maze. Finally, Watson changed the layout of the maze itself, and this worked; the rats could no longer find the goal box. Thus, Watson concluded, it had to be the "kinesthetic" (muscle) sense that permitted the rats to find the goal box (Cohen, 1979). Work like this seems both scientifically and ethically questionable.

Behavioristic experimenters who inflicted suffering on animals were not deliberately cruel; no doubt they thought that the cause of science justified their experiments. Most of all, it was simply impossible within their point of view to conceive that animals could *consciously experience* suffering (Singer, 1975). Any ethical questions were simply incomprehensible. It is probably not reasonable therefore to criticize this kind of experiment for deliberate cruelty, but it *is* important to point out that one's psychological theory can dictate one's values, and in this way, it can cause us to ignore the very real suffering that may be inflicted in pursuit of apparently valid scientific objectives (Singer, 1975).

Experimentalists of the behavioristic period can also be criticized for severely limiting their perspective. In order to prove their scientific standing, they often seemed to adopt a "nothing but" attitude. Attention was "nothing but" stimulus selection; meaning was "nothing but" a small, potentially observable response; thinking "nothing but" subvocal speech. One can imagine an astronomer experiencing awe and wonder in viewing the night sky, or a biologist feeling entranced by the richness and complexity of a living organism intimately adapted to its environment. Such sentiments can hardly be admitted into behavioristic psychology, lest they bring back all the old, religious ghosts. Behaviorism does not encourage an experience of awe or beauty — or even irony — in contemplating the complexities of human behavior.

How does it all tally up? On the one hand, in the period of behaviorism, psychologists created a new scientific profession. They established proof-procedures able to command a true consensus in the scientific community, discovered a number of interesting facts, and in the case of behavior therapy, applied many of their findings to alleviate some real human problems. On the other hand, behaviorism, which was originally conceived as a way to *expand* the purview of psychological thinking, tended to create a great narrowing of perspective, as practically all of common-sense psychology was deliberately disregarded as unscientific for five decades. The personal dimension of human psychology was ignored; and along with it, some pressing ethical concerns were defined out of existence. Finally, the behavioral restrictions on theory probably prevented the development of psychological theory, and also served to emphasize the gap between psychodynamics (which is heavily theoretical) and "respectable" kinds of psychology. We are hardly in a position to judge, nor is it the purpose of this book to decide whether the pros of behaviorism outweigh the cons. It is important, however, to understand that our scientific knowledge of human psychology has been hard-won, and that the endeavor to know more is not without its drawbacks.

3

In Defense of Behaviorism

In this chapter we present interviews with five prominent behaviorists. The best-known behaviorist is, of course, B. F. Skinner, whose interview is presented first. Following Skinner is a well-known animal psychologist and public defender of radical behaviorism, Howard Rachlin. Next, representing the tradition of neobehaviorism — the tradition of Hull and Spence — are Irving R. Maltzman, who has done much to make the work of Russian researchers in the tradition of Pavlov better known in this country, and Howard H. Kendler, whose research often shades imperceptibly into cognitive psychology. Finally, to represent currently very influential work in clinical behavior modification, the chapter includes an interview with Alan O. Ross, a prominent clinical researcher with a behavioral bent, known especially for his contributions to the control of children's clinical problems.

B. F. Skinner: Founder of Operant Conditioning

B. F. Skinner's first serious ambitions were literary rather than scientific. Born in 1904 in Susquehanna, New York, he grew up in a small Yankee town infused with the turn-of-the-century American values of thrift, hard work, and Protestantism. Like many young men of his time, Skinner soon turned against religion in general as old-fashioned and superstitious, but he retained his respect for the Protestant work ethic. Also, like many of his contemporaries, Skinner was attracted to literature. His short stories received high praise from Robert Frost (Skinner, 1979), and Skinner might have had a future as a writer. In fact, after graduating college, he spent a year attempting to write seriously — and, according to his own account, failed. During this "Dark Year" (Skinner, 1976) he struggled with his ambition to write, and began to consider other possibilities:

I had apparently failed as a writer but was it not possible that literature had failed me as a method? . . . I was interested in human behavior, but I had been investigating it in the wrong way. Alf Evers [a friend] had said to me, "Science is the art of the twentieth century," and I believed him. Literature as an art form was dead; I would turn to science . . . for a long time I was quite ambivalent. At times I was quite violent: literature must be demolished. (1976, pp. 262–284)

A 1927 magazine article by H. G. Wells confirmed Skinner's decision to abandon literature and turn to the study of behavior. Wells had written of a hypothetical choice between saving the life of I. P. Pavlov and saving the life of George Bernard Shaw:

I have been amusing myself . . . with that amusing game of "one life belt." . . . If "A " is drowning on one side of a pier and "B" is equally drowning on the other, and you have one life belt and cannot otherwise help, to which of the two would you like to throw it? Which would I save, Pavloff [sic] or Shaw? I do not think it would interest the reader to give my private answer. But while I was considering it I was manifestly obliged to ask myself, "What is the good of Shaw?" And what is the good of Pavloff? Pavloff is a star which lights the world, shining above a vista hitherto unexplored. Why should I hesitate with my life belt for one moment? (quoted in Skinner, 1976, p. 300)

Like Wells, Skinner apparently chose Pavlov over Shaw. He read Pavlov, Bertrand Russell, John B. Watson, and the physiologist Jacques Loeb. Soon Skinner made the fateful decision to become a behaviorist (before he had taken any formal psychology courses), applied to Harvard for graduate study, and was admitted. From the very beginning he became the departmental behaviorist, a revolutionary position in a department then dominated by the grand old figure of E. G. Boring. Nevertheless, his talent and ambition were recognized, and his real intellectual odyssey began (Skinner, 1979). After receiving his doctorate in 1930, Skinner was admitted to the elite Society of Fellows at Harvard (which later was to produce his foremost public opponent, Noam Chomsky). His Junior Fellowship supported both Skinner and his research for a 5-year period (1931–1935), during which time he developed, in a sustained burst of creativity, all the major tools and concepts of what was to become known as operant conditioning (see Chapter 2). Since this period, comparatively little of fundamental interest has been added.

Skinner's newly discovered methods led to the demonstration of behavioral control so quickly and reliably that he could perform a multitude of experiments, thus establishing all the basic phenomena of operant conditioning. The definition of "the operant" as "the field of purpose" (without using the *word* "purpose," of course); the cumulative recorder; the bar press as a convenient, countable response; the use of response rate as a dependent variable; the discriminatory stimulus as one that "sets the stage for," but does not *cause* the response; the extension of reflex theory far beyond Pavlov's formulation; the discovery of schedules of reinforcement — all these belong to the early '30s.

Skinner's brand of behaviorism was not just methodological, but radical — that is, it involved an outright denial of the existence of private experience (see Chapter 1).

In spite of his commitment to an exceptionally rigorous brand of psychology, Skinner's love for literature reappeared at various points in his life. He wrote behavioristic analyses of the work of Joyce and Gertrude Stein, and attempted an analysis of Shakespeare based on word frequencies. His utopian novel *Walden Two* (Skinner, 1948), he comments, "was pretty obviously a venture in self-therapy in which I was struggling to reconcile two aspects of my own behavior, represented by [the two main protagonists] Burris and Frazier" (Skinner, 1967, p. 403). His recent autobiography (Skinner, 1976, 1979, 1983) abounds in literary flourishes, and even has a few psychodynamic analyses of Skinner's own early stories (1979). Perhaps Skinner's characterization of his early literary life as "a sort of behavioristic Proust" applies to his later life as well (Skinner, 1979, p. 16).

But of course Skinner is best known for his scientific work, and for his espousal of the philosophy of radical behaviorism. Even *Walden Two* (which ends in triumph for Frazier, his rigorously scientific *alter ego*) is not primarily a work of art, but a shot fired in the war for a behavioristic psychology. Already in the 1930s Skinner wrote his friend Fred Keller that the battle for behaviorism would probably take several decades, but Skinner was willing to fight that long with little doubt that his cause was right, or of eventual victory.

The following interview with Professor Skinner was done in June 1980. Skinner was then working on the third volume of his autobiography (published in 1983). Unlike the other interviews in this book, this one was not tape recorded, at Professor Skinner's request. The answers are based on written notes and should be considered to be paraphrases. On the other hand, most of the questions are structured around quotations from Skinner's works which obviously reflect his own words, and Professor Skinner has approved the final transcript.

Interview with B. F. Skinner

Q: I was very much impressed in reading the first two volumes of your autobiography by the literary quality of the writing. It was a pleasure to read. I noticed that the very first paragraph of Volume I (Skinner,

1976) starts with a description of the countryside around Susquehanna, New York, where you were born, and it is written to attribute all kinds of "mentalistic" motives to the Susquehanna River. You write that the Susquehanna "flows southwest and crosses into Pennsylvania a few miles below the town of Windsor. Almost at once it meets a foothill of the Alleghenies, which proves to be unbreachable, and returns to the hospitable plains of New York State. It flows west . . . and tackles Pennsylvania again at a more vulnerable point. This time it succeeds . . . " (p. 3). Words like "meet," "return," "hospitable," "tackle," and "succeed" are obviously anthropomorphic — they attribute to inanimate things our ideas about human beings. Your criticism for many years has been that we attribute these unobservable traits to human beings, to explain the observable behavior. Did you write this paragraph deliberately to be anthropomorphic?

A: Yes. There are some remarkable geographic features in that part of New York State, so that the Susquehanna actually flows away from the ocean at some points, and it seems as if it is trying to cross the Alleghenies without being able to.

Q: You have written that "Behaviorism is not the science of human behavior, but the philosophy of that science" (1974, p. 3). This definition shows the metatheoretical aspect of behaviorism, the way in which it tells you how to do psychology. In this sense, behaviorism is not something you discover in the laboratory, but a philosophy about the scientific approach to human beings. You also wrote that "As far as I was concerned, there were only minor differences between behaviorism, operationalism, and logical positivism" (1979, p. 115).

A: There are some differences, but the logical positivists at least insisted on the public nature of science, which is in agreement with behaviorism. Percy Bridgman (*e.g.*, 1927) was a good friend, and we talked for many years. Bridgman himself never properly used the notion that the operation *is* the construct. He never really got away from solipsism. You have to get back to behavior shaped by contingencies in the world, and to the rules that describe those contingencies. That does not just apply to psychology. In physics you are really talking about contingencies as well. *If* you do one thing, *then* something else will happen. Then physicists make up rules that describe these contingencies in order to communicate with other people.

Q: Your autobiography describes your years as a graduate student and Junior Fellow at Harvard, during which you had many debates with E. G. Boring about behaviorism. I had the sense that behaviorism seemed to be winning the day after some years, reading your description of it. How did this happen?

A: Behaviorism was never really dominant. When I came to Harvard as a student, the Psychology Department was at a low point. There were always nonbehaviorists at the Department of Social Relations, but Psychology had Boring and Lashley and Stevens. Boring became more of a behaviorist over time. Stevens became an operationalist later on, but he was always a psychophysicist at heart — he thought that there were two worlds, one mental and one physical.

Q: After the failure of Hull's ambitious attempt to build a theory of learning, you wrote a paper that became very well known, called, "Are Theories of Learning Necessary?" (1950). You argued essentially that they are not. In your view, theories in psychology should not refer to underlying constructs, but they can be used to summarize data. Would you still hold to that position?

A: Yes, I agree with that.

Q: But if we look at physics, for example, it seems clear that physicists refer to unobservable entities to explain the things that are observable. No one will ever see an electron, but electrons are useful to explain what you *can* see. Do you think that is right?

A: No good physicist talks about an electron as a thing, except for convenience. He uses equations instead, and equations are functional relationships between the things that can be observed.

Q: Over the past 20 years or so, behaviorism has lost a good deal of ground. Most academic psychologists who would have called themselves behaviorists several decades ago now consider themselves to be more cognitive. But whereas other varieties of behaviorism have declined, your own viewpoint seems still to be going strong. How do you explain that your work has survived so well?

A: Our work has been put to use. For example, operant conditioning led to the development of behavior modification techniques to help patients with various clinical problems. The power of the Experimental Analysis of Behavior emerged in the 1940s with Project Pigeon. We found that we had great certainty of experimental control using operant techniques such as shaping and scheduling.

Pavlovian conditioning was less useful. Watson tried to apply it, but with little success. In fact the famous case of little Albert is probably a case of operant rather than Pavlovian conditioning, because they waited till Albert reached out at the rabbit before they struck the bar which made the loud noise that frightened little Albert. Albert emitted some behavior, which was then punished. So the important thing is that operant conditioning has led to practical applications. In fact, I did the first work using operant conditioning on psychotics in the early 1950s.

Q: Very early in your career you set up an important definition of radical behaviorism. You wrote in 1931 that

it is . . . possible to be a behaviorist and recognize the existence of conscious events. . . . But I preferred the position of *radical behaviorism*, in which the existence of subjective entities is denied. (1976, p. 117)

Would you still agree with that definition?

A: Yes, I am still a radical behaviorist. Radical behaviorism can deal with private events, but it rejects the idea of subjective events existing in their own world. For instance, the body you feel is private, but not subjective. It is the external contingencies in the world that have changed me, but they have not been stored inside.

Q: Instead of saying that an organism has some internal states that *represent* the environment, would you say, instead, that an organism *adapts* to its environment?

A: No. Organisms do not adapt to the environment; it is the environment that adapts the organism. Species do not adapt to the environment — the environment changes the species.

Q: In *Walden Two* (1948) there is a running debate between the tough-minded scientist Frazier and the more tender-minded Burris about applying operant conditioning to the creation of a utopian community. In your autobiography you write that "I did not know until I finished the book that I was both Burris and Frazier" (1979, p. 296). Does the conflict between Frazier and Burris still exist?

A: After I wrote *Walden Two* I became Frazier, I suppose, and discarded Burris.

Q: One of the major criticisms of behaviorism has been that an emphasis on stimuli and responses ignores the rules that people seem to use, for example, in producing a new sentence. In a paper entitled, "Why I Am Not a Cognitive Psychologist" (1977), you have written:

Those who have acquired behavior through exposure to contingencies describe the contingencies, and others then circumvent exposure by behaving in the ways described. But cognitive psychologists contend that something of the same sort happens when people learn directly from the contingencies. They are said to discover rules which they themselves follow. But rules are not *in* the contingencies, nor must they be "known" by those who acquire behavior under exposure to them. We are in luck that this could be so, since rules are verbal products which arose very late in the evolution of the species. . . . Until the time of the Greeks, no one seems to have known that there were rules of grammar, although people spoke grammatically . . . there is no evidence that rules play any part in the behavior of the ordinary speaker. (pp. 1–11)

A: Rules are maxims, warnings, or governmental laws. These all describe contingencies. The rules are only as good as the contingencies, except in fields like logic where you have rules about rules, and there truth is tautological.

Q: As far as you are concerned, then, we are not justified in inferring underlying rules to account for observable behavior. In "Behaviorism at Fifty" (1963), you write that "Science often talks about things it cannot see or measure" (p. 952). Under what conditions do you think that would be justified? For example, from the behavior of the input and output of a computer, can we make inferences about the nature of the program? Much of the rationale of the cognitive approach would be that you can infer the program, and that psychology is in fact an attempt to infer "the program" that guides the behavior of human beings.

A: I've always thought that was nonsense. For example, you can make clay tiles, put impressions in the clay and store them — that is what is done rather more rapidly in a computer. But why put it inside the organism? It is the environment that made the impression in the first place.

Q: When you speak of rules as legal rules, maxims, and warnings, you seem to be talking about conscious rules. Many psychologists seem to think that there are unconscious rules, such as those that are supposed to be involved in generating a sentence. Would you consider this kind of thinking to be mentalistic?

A: If rules are simply representations of data in a *conceptual nervous system*, then my only criticism is that they aren't very useful. They do not represent contingencies of reinforcement. I'm saying you don't *store anything*. You change: That's very different from having anything stored.

Q: In the same article against cognitive psychology (1977) you wrote that "The variables of which human behavior is a function lie in the environment" (p. 7). Again, it would not be necessary to postulate anything inside the organism. But you might say the same thing in the case of an automobile — that the variables of which the automobile is composed start ultimately outside of the automobile. Yet it is useful to speak of a radiator breaking down inside of the car, without reference to how it got there.

A: But that is physiology. Physiologists are dealing with a blueprint of the engine. I deal with a blueprint of the contingencies. What cognitive psychologists move inside the organism is nothing but badly formulated contingencies of reinforcement. The contingencies don't go inside, so why put them inside?

Q: You have written of John Watson, the originator of behaviorism, that "Polemics led him into extreme positions from which he never escaped" (1959, p. 197). Howard Kendler has suggested that this criticism might apply to your work as well (1979). How would you respond to that criticism?

A: Fred Keller says that I make strong statements, and take them back only if I have to. But the claims I have made seem to me to have been borne out. There has been criticism — sometimes vicious criticism — of *Beyond Freedom and Dignity* (1971). But certainly the formulation of the operant and of reinforcement has held up remarkably well. Research and basic analysis go straight ahead.

Howard Rachlin: A Defense of Radical Behaviorism

Howard Rachlin (b. 1935) received his doctorate in psychology at Harvard in 1965. Although he describes his orientation as behavioristic in the mold of Skinner, some of his scientific research has been quite theoretical. For instance, he has applied ideas from theoretical economics to the question of how animals allocate time to different tasks, how they "decide" to forgo immediate for long-term rewards, and the like (Rachlin, 1974, 1980, 1981; Rachlin, Kagel, Battalio, & Green, 1981).

At the same time, Rachlin has been one of the foremost defenders of radical behaviorism in public debates, contesting both philosophical and scientific challenges to Skinnerian thought. The titles of his rebuttals suggest their contents: thus, "Skinner and the Philosophers" (Rachlin, 1979), "Reinforcing and Punishing Thoughts" (Rachlin, 1977a), and "Who Cares if the Chimpanzee Has a Theory of Mind?" (Rachlin, 1978). His *Introduction to Modern Behaviorism* (1970) describes ways in which behavioral techniques can be applied in everyday life. Professor Rachlin is married to the novelist Nahid Rachlin, and lives in New York City. He is a faculty member at the State University of New York at Stony Brook.

In the interview, Rachlin emphasizes the *usefulness* of the behavioral approach to psychology, and its distinct status from neurophysiology and philosophy. He is concerned that the ideas proposed by cognitive psychologists possess too much "surplus meaning" — that notions such as "memory," "attention," and "consciousness" carry with them an undesirable freight of unscientific implications that are better avoided.

Interview with Howard Rachlin

Q: How did you get started in psychology?

A: Actually, my bachelor's degree is in engineering. I worked as an engineer, and took evening classes in philosophy. I didn't like the work of an engineer, because it was very repetitive. I had sort of a positivistic philosophy, and I liked William James's pragmatism very much. That appealed to me, and gave me a sense of some order in the world. Eventually, after several years of taking courses at Columbia and the New School for Social Research, I just couldn't figure out what a philosopher *did*. What was the function that philosophy had? So I drifted away and got into psychology, got a master's degree in psychology, and then went to Harvard. I liked the idea that psychology combined the theoretical aspect of philosophy and the aspect of getting my hands dirty of engineering. But I didn't have any viewpoint in psychology — I didn't have any allegiances in psychology even after I got my master's degree.

I went to Harvard and people told me, "Well, don't get involved with Skinner. One thing we don't want you to do is become a Skinnerian." I said, "OK." I didn't know one from the other. In fact, at Harvard, even after I got my PhD I did not have a viewpoint. I did not consider myself a Skinnerian even after I got my PhD.

Q: Would you consider yourself a Skinnerian now?

A: I guess I would. I used to resist that, because Skinner himself varies. I used to vacillate between "No, I am not a Skinnerian," and "Yes, I am a Skinnerian, but Skinner is not a Skinnerian, so therefore I'm more of a Skinnerian than Skinner is."

Right now I consider myself a behaviorist. At Harvard I took some courses with cognitive psychologists such as Jerome Bruner and George Miller, and they were very excited about what they were doing. But I was more interested in my experimental work — not any theoretical aspect of Skinner, but in what I was doing experimentally. I was doing animal work, and was completely caught up in it — as an intellectual exercise, as a game. When I came to Stony Brook, I was challenged to defend behaviorism and Skinner, and when that happened more and more, I did more reading, and for me the behavioral world view gelled.

But philosophically, I have become more behavioristic. For one thing, I did not want to waste my philosophical background. So the opportunity came to write some more theoretical papers, and in that process, I began increasingly to see Skinner's point of view, not just as something that applied only in the lab, but as something that applies in everyday life. For example, I did some theoretical work on self-control.

Q: In talking about self-control, presumably you don't want to advance a notion of "self"?

A: Well, for example, suppose you're walking down the street and somebody taps you on the shoulder and says, "Here's an ice cream soda." What does it mean to refuse an ice cream soda? Now what sort of theory could handle that kind of behavior where you don't take something that in another context you would take? I was able to relate that to the work I had been doing with concurrent schedules of reinforcement, where the animal responds not to the immediate stimulus, but to some overall aspect of its environment.

Q: You obviously would not want to say that the person who is offered a tempting ice cream soda and "decides" not to take it is reflecting on the decision, or deliberating whether or not to take it.

A: I think that is a bad way of looking at decisions. I wouldn't want to use the word "decision" in a cognitive sense, but I think it has a role in describing behavior. A decision probably needs two characteristics: It needs an actual observable event with certain properties, and it needs what the philosopher Gilbert Ryle calls a "disposition" (Ryle, 1949).

Q: Suppose you have some engineers discussing how to build something: Would you agree that they consider different options — the pros and cons of different choices — and then make a "decision" at some point to do one thing rather than another?

A: I'd say that the description of the decisions of those engineers is a description of their behavior, not of anything that goes on inside their heads. They are exhibiting decision-making behavior.

Q: If they have blueprints of the machine they are building, that is an abstract representation of the machine. Their decisions really operate on the abstract representation of the machine. But you would not want to move that whole situation inside of somebody's head.

A: That is not the direction in which it goes. You go from the actual machine, to a photograph (which is a fairly concrete representation), to a blueprint, to maybe a few sentences about the machine. You get a more and more abstract representation. But I don't see that increasingly abstract line leading into the head. I just see it less and less in the immediate environment.

Q: In the case of a computer, we can say that it "has" an abstract representation of something outside itself. In artificial intelligence work, for instance, people have programmed representations of different semantic domains. Certainly many people seem to like this kind of metaphor today. But you feel this cannot be applied to people?

A: No. The history of psychology is filled with metaphors like that, and I don't see that this will work any better. Tomorrow somebody can invent a new kind of computer, a kind of computer where you plant a seed and a computer grows. And this new computer may have different properties from our present computer. All these models have a certain heuristic value, but I don't think you could take any of them seriously. I think that human beings are just not computers. You might say, well, this computer has a push-down store — let's see if human beings have a push-down store, too. And you might generate some interesting experiments. But then you turn around and say, well, if we can't do it with a computer, then we can't do it with a person, or if we do it with a person, it must have some analogy to the computer. That to me is a limiting rather than a helpful heuristic.

Q: If we don't look at a specific computer, but instead use the class of information-processing devices as we know them, might we be able to find some general properties that would tell us about the mind?

A: Well, we might be able to speculate about the nervous system, about the left temporal lobe. But that is not psychology, that's physiology. You might be able to use that to speculate about what the left temporal lobe is doing. But it is not very useful in explaining behavior at a molar level.

Take this analogy: You're Mario Andretti, the greatest racing driver in the world. To what extent does Mario Andretti know how the car is built? It may be useful to some extent, but there are many people who know much more than he does. But he knows how to drive the car. That is a different kind of knowledge. In psychology you can study behavior from a behavioral point of view and ask, What was the behavior? How do you manipulate it? How do you predict it? Here we are, treating each other as cars and predicting and controlling each others' behavior. To what extent does the knowledge of how the nervous system is built help you? Maybe a little.

Q: If you decide that science means getting insight about some phenomenon, rather than being about prediction and control, would you arrive at a different way of doing psychology?

A: You probably do. I think that you would. But I question the idea of just trying to get understanding without prediction or control. That leads to things like astrology.

Somebody who knows about the engines of racing cars may be able to tell Mario Andretti not to drive the car that day because there is something wrong with it. But that is a different level of knowledge than Mario's expertise, which is how hard you push the accelerator on a certain curved road, when to turn the wheel, and when not to turn the wheel. People at Mario's level I consider to be behaviorists. The engine people are doing physiological psychology. Cognitive psychology is also at Mario's level: Behavioral and cognitive psychology are directly competing. You can't resolve the conflict by saying that cognitive people and behaviorists are explaining things at different levels.

Q: Where do you think conflicts between behavioral and cognitive psychology might come to a head?

A: Well, to speculate mildly, perhaps in education. Maybe a cognitive psychologist and a behavioral psychologist will have two different ways to run a classroom. The only way to test science ultimately is by its application, I think. I don't think a science can exist for very long without application sooner or later. Science always needs to hold out the hope that application is just around the corner. If you and I couldn't walk into this room and turn the switch and get the electric light to go on, we would have that much less confidence in physics. The reason we think that physics is such a fantastic science is because it has a lot of practical consequences.

Q: What do you think has been the best application of behavioral theory in the real world, outside the laboratory?

A: I think in clinical psychology. Although it's pretty bad, it's been about the best. In things like phobias they've done a reasonable job, and also in managing psychotics in mental hospitals. It's not an inconsiderable accomplishment. On the other hand, the criticisms made of Skinner — that he exaggerates what we've accomplished in the laboratory and how easily it can be applied, I think are justified. I'd rather make the point that we don't really know anything — well, maybe better than zero. It's better to act on some information than none. But he probably feels that people won't pay attention if he makes that point.

Q: You were saying that behaviorism has had an impact on your personal life as well as on your scientific outlook. Would you give an example of that?

A: Let me give an example of where behaviorism has changed my everyday outlook. When I was a kid, one thing the kids in my neighborhood did was hitch rides on cars and trucks going by. There was one crazy kid named Eugene, who jumped up on top of a truck and was riding standing up on the truck. The truck went under the El and he was hit straight in the head, knocked off the truck, and was in the hospital unconscious for a long time.

One thing he did in the hospital is he kept on moaning about "Barbara, Barbara." Barbara was just a girl in the neighborhood who was rapidly developing. Everyone was sort of basically attracted to her, but being rough teenage boys, no one would admit it — it was a disgrace. It really worried me because, my God, here is this guy in the hospital bed — what if something happens to me, who knows what I'll blurt out? I mean, I'm going to blurt out such horrible things, it'll be out of my control, my "inner self" will come out, and people will know all the things that I *really* think.

Now that I'm a behaviorist, that doesn't worry me anymore. Because whatever I'll blurt out is not my real self, anymore than anything else. I've become reconciled that outer behavior is me, for good or bad. What I really want to do is there for everyone to see, so if I blurt it out, it won't be really me.

Q: You say that the line from concrete to abstract representation does not lead into the head. Are there lines that lead into the nervous system?

A: Yes, there are clear lines that lead into the nervous system, but that is not a cognitive issue, but a physiological issue. Certain things lead you to ask, What is the representation of something in the retina, or in the cortex?

Q: And physiology is a different domain of discourse.

A: I think it's necessary to separate physiology from psychology. People will argue that you can go from one level to another. If we knew everything we had to know about physiology, we might never have to talk about psychology, and possibly vice versa. We often cross the levels of explanation when we talk loosely about a physiological factor causing a behavioral change, or vice versa. But I don't think that is a useful way of talking scientifically, because it is confusing two levels. You give an explanation that is basically empty — it stops you from doing the appropriate experiments at the level of the problem. I think explanation by reference to another level is a way to get around saying "I don't know." People don't like saying that.

Q: But suppose you say that a virus is causing the symptoms of a cold: sneezing, coughing, feeling tired. That is explaining one level by another. Is that wrong?

A: I don't know if that is ever a useful scientific way of dealing with it. I have a feeling that even the medical researchers would rebel against that. They would want to say, "Well, you can call this a symptom, but in our lines of division, the virus causes half the sneeze and a quarter of the runny nose." And the division of the sneezes and the runny noses has nothing to do with the divisions I make in my science. I'm just dealing with viruses and how to reduce the population of viruses in certain localized areas. That's what I can tell you about. And your sneezes and runny noses you'll have to ask someone else about.

Q: What defines the domain of discourse? Why is one level different from another?

A: That's a good question. For my own use I rely on intuition. A level is some domain where causal relations hold. Within a level you can run experiments varying an independent variable and measuring the effects on a dependent variable.

Q: Now, you have done some theoretical work in which you use the concept of "value." That is clearly not something you can observe directly, but it does explain things that are observable. Value is not at the same level of analysis as a bar press.

A: That's a good point. No, it's not. It's probably a mistake — what

I would call an unavoidable mistake, or an unavoidable convenience — to talk about value. Value is not the real concept I want to get at. You could get rid of it. I would assume that if my theory were perfectly developed, you could get rid of value.

Q: So you could call it "Factor X," and then it comes down to the same level as a bar-press?

A: If it's wholly defined in terms of behavior it would. That's what I mean by value. All I mean is Factor X, the product of this times this times this. And these things are defined wholly as behavioral variables, such as a bar-press, or a rate of bar pressing.

Q: Would you ever draw inferences that go beyond what is observed?

A: Yes, I would draw inferences. I would say, even though I don't know anything about your past history, that you must have been reinforced for this behavior you do. That's not observable, even potentially. I couldn't even ask your relatives if you have been reinforced for doing whatever you are doing. I feel free to draw those inferences where my theory requires them, but not to draw inferences about entities in the head.

Q: Then the issue revolves around the ontological status of the inferences? Cognitive psychologists are willing to say that there is such a thing as "short-term memory," even though it cannot be observed directly, and you are not willing to say that such a thing really exists?

A: Well, I think that's part of it. You have an ontological commitment when you talk about memory, for instance. As soon as you say "memory," everyone gets a picture that there is something there.

But it's more the *consequences* of ontological status. It's the excess meaning that those unobservable entities often convey. It would be all right if you could do cognitive psychology without excess meaning. Tolman said that when he talked about "expectancy," he really meant such and such. If you could do cognitive psychology that way, it would be all right. But I couldn't do cognitive psychology that way, and I don't know who can. If you take out the excess meaning, then the convenience of using a word from our ordinary vocabulary would be lost.

Q: Part of the power of an abstraction is the surplus meaning, is it not? The fact that the abstraction leads you to ideas beyond the original data?

A: Yes, I agree with that. But in fact, when you say that a rat has an expectancy, and if you can predict what the rat will and will not do, that's all right. If you could actually do an experiment and find that, it's OK. But then you can't also mean that if the rat could talk it would tell me it hoped that there was cheese at the end of the runway. If you have surplus meaning, you are giving a promise that you can approach that abstraction in more than the way you are operationalizing it in the beginning. Now I would argue that this is generally a bad thing, because people will usually assume that a whole host of experiments would work if they were carried out — without ever doing the experiments. Once the experiments are done, then the usefulness of the central concept tends to disappear, because then you actually know what will and won't happen.

Q: How would you deal with something like consciousness? Do you think it exists or not?

A: That's an interesting question. I often ask students when I'm feeling in an argumentative mood to show me a rock — what criteria do we use to show that a rock does not have consciousness in the way a human being does? They never succeed in giving criteria, because humans can represent things, but rocks represent things too, obviously. Just like water will represent the cup you put it into, a rock represents the air around it, the temperature changes as a function of its environment, all sorts of so-called representations.

Q: But abstract representations?

A: Surely yes, abstract representations. The rock has an abstract representation of the temperatures around it. You could extract from it in an abstract form a map of the temperatures. A rock can't speak, but it can do whatever is cognitively necessary.

Or people will say that consciousness involves the greater complexity of people compared to rocks. I think we'd agree that physics has not reached the ultimate answer, physicists can't explain everything about a rock, so that the complexity of rocks is infinite as far as we are concerned. So you can't talk about consciousness as simply a greater degree of complexity. So all right, humans are complex in a different way from rocks — if that is all you mean by consciousness, the particular way that human behavior is complex, consciousness obviously exists. But most people mean by consciousness something *superior* that has evolved in humans, something independent of their behavior, and that's religion, not science.

Irving R. Maltzman: A Spirited Defense and Criticism

Irving R. Maltzman (b. 1924) received his doctorate in psychology at the University of Iowa in 1949 with a dissertation supervised by Kenneth W. Spence. His interests include verbal behavior, the effects of imaginary practice on performance, the Orienting Response (OR), and alco-

holism and addictive behavior (Maltzman, 1968). Because most work
on the Orienting Response has been performed in the USSR, Maltzman
has edited a selection of articles translated from Russian (Maltzman &
Cole, 1969). He also has an abiding interest in the philosophy of science,
from a distinctly logical positivist point of view. He admires the work
of philosophers such as Gustav Bergmann and Hans Reichenbach (1938)
and is quite critical of Thomas Kuhn (1962) and more recent philosophers
of science for taking a relativistic and "sociological" view of scientific work.
In 1966 Maltzman participated in the landmark Kentucky conference
on "Verbal Behavior and General Behavior Theory" (Dixon & Horton,
1968; Maltzman, 1968), in which many behavioristic researchers expressed a cognitive point of view for the first time, whereas Maltzman
upheld a strong neobehavioristic view.

      In graduate school at Iowa, Maltzman participated in perhaps the
most exciting period of behavioristic work. In regard to the controversy
between Tolman and Hull (in some ways a "protocognitive" controversy) Maltzman believed that "it was our mission at Iowa to demonstrate
that Hull was right and Tolman was wrong with respect to theory."
Maltzman thinks, however, that Tolman was a genuine behaviorist who
did not believe in unobservable goals, but rather believed in observable
goal-directed *behavior*. He also thinks that because of its youth, psychology
can be swayed by charismatic personalities such as Hull, Spence, and
Skinner. He uses his own research on imagery to illustrate the difference
between behavioral and cognitive methodology: As a behaviorist he iden-
tifies "imagery" with a score on an imagery questionnaire, rather than
treating it as something that is not directly observable.

      Professor Maltzman is sharply critical of cognitive psychologists for
what he perceives as imprecise use of theoretical terms, and for neglect-
ing issues such as drive, motivation, and conditioning. He has for many
years served on the faculty at UCLA, and is a former chairman of the
psychology department there.

Interview with Irving R. Maltzman

      Q: How did you become interested in psychology?
      A: When I was an undergraduate at New York University in the
'40s I took some classes with Leland W. Crafts, a student of Thorndike's.
He was an older gentleman at the time, and he had an enormous fund
of knowledge in the area of human learning. He had complete command
of the experimental literature, which at that time was still possible. He
literally knew every study that had been published in the general area
of learning.

I also read Guthrie's beautiful little book on learning (Guthrie, 1935), in which he discusses all the methods for changing what he called "bad habits" that have since been rediscovered by the behavior modifiers. Now it's called "flooding," "implosion," and "desensitizing," and so on, but Guthrie spoke about all of those things. And I read widely in the literature as an undergraduate, primarily Hull, because Hull was obviously the top-ranking figure at the time in the area of learning.

At the same time I took a minor in philosophy, and had a younger professor who was a student of Ernest Nagel at Columbia, and so I learned about logical positivism. I thought the best place to go to graduate school to learn a combination of experimental psychology and philosophy was Iowa. Kenneth Spence was there, as well as the philosopher of science Gustav Bergmann. I went to Iowa in 1946 and eventually got my PhD there. I got into psychology simply because I found it interesting, and I thought being a professor of psychology would be a marvelous way of life.

Q: Did you consider yourself a Hullian at the time?

A: Oh sure, how could you go to Iowa and get your PhD with Spence and not consider yourself a Hullian? Learning and learning theory was my major area of interest, and Hull was obviously the most influential and stimulating worker in the field at the time. I wanted to learn as much as I could about Hull when I got there, and Spence turned out to be a masterful teacher. We studied Hull intensively, but we also learned about every other learning theorist.

Q: Tolman at this time considered himself a "cognitive behaviorist." He was much more willing to talk about unobservable constructs such as "purpose" and "expectation" than people such as Spence or Hull. What was the Iowa view of Tolman at that time?

A: Tolman was misguided in his theory of learning, that is, S–S contiguity versus S–R drive reduction. He was wrong. You know, I think Spence had a great deal of respect for him as a pioneer methodological behaviorist. But he was just confused theoretically. He was wrong about drive reduction, about the nature of reinforcement, about the way in which organisms learn. There were presumably testable implications of the different theories of learning, and the testable implications of Hull's and Tolman's theory were contradictory, so one of them had to be right and one had to be wrong. But both were behaviorists. There was agreement on methodology. It was our mission at Iowa to demonstrate that Hull was right and Tolman was wrong with respect to theory. So we waited eagerly for each issue of the *American Journal of Psychology*, or the *Journal of Experimental Psychology*, to see what was going on, and then we'd run out and do an experiment.

Your question, however, suggests to me that you really do not understand what cognitive psychology and behaviorism are and how they may or may not differ. Tolman was a behaviorist in that all his theoretical terms are defined in terms of observable behavior and the conditions under which they occur. He is a cognitive psychologist because he uses intentional terms such as "purpose" and "expectancy." But, because he is a behaviorist, purpose for Tolman *is* a pattern of goal-directed behavior. "Purpose" does not refer ultimately to some unobservable mental or conscious process. Since Tolman is a methodological behaviorist and not a radical or metaphysical behaviorist, he does not deny the existence of consciousness, but leaves the analysis of such problems to philosophers. Hull agrees in all of the foregoing except that instead of using theoretical terms that are intentional in nature, he uses theoretical terms that are stated as *hypothetical* stimuli and responses, for example, "r_g-s_g." Whereas Tolman was a cognitive psychologist who defined his intentional, theoretical terms behaviorally, other cognitive psychologists do not. They believe that their intentional terms refer to some unobservable conscious process.

There is one more point I wish to make. Methodological behaviorists are not opposed in principle to the use of theoretical terms that refer to unobservables. Physics has such terms. But in contrast to psychology, these are part of a highly developed theory with explicit relationships to other concepts that do refer to observable events. Cognitive psychology has no such theory.

Q: It sounds as if your time as a graduate student at Iowa was very exciting.

A: Oh, it was an enormously exciting time, it was without question the most exciting intellectual period of my life. The place was a beehive of ideas and research and activity and stimulation. Everybody worked seven days a week — what else is there to do in Iowa City? So you go in on Sunday morning, and East Hall was just alive with people doing research. Spence would come in during the day, even on a Sunday, and most of the faculty were there in the evenings and on weekends. All the students were there, the clinical students as well as the experimental ones.

Q: Did you have a real sense of making progress and solving problems?

A: Yeah, right. The feeling was that there was real progress being made, and Iowa was at the forefront of that.

Q: Now at some point, a great disillusionment set in with Hull's theory, among some people at least. Did you experience that?

A: That started happening after I left Iowa during the '50s when Hull's book came out on his behavior system (Hull, 1952). It was just too grandiose. We'd get a mimeographed prepublication copy of his books with blanks in the equations of the laws of behavior. And the only problem was to fill in the empirical values for the blanks. It just broke down in its enormous detail, with all the exceptions to it. It became too comprehensive and at the same time he tried to become more and more specific. Finally, it just collapsed of its own weight. It became more and more apparent that his hypothetico-deductive system was just silly.

People just realized that it couldn't work in the grand manner. There was a multiplicity of factors that led to a change in the kind of theorizing that we engaged in. There were increasing criticisms of Hull's theory that it just wasn't working, and the latent learning issue kept dragging on. It became obvious that every time you got a negative result, you simply reinterpreted the theory and added some more assumptions. It was getting more and more cumbersome.

Besides, Hull died, and Spence moved and died, and they were very charismatic characters. Because psychology isn't a highly developed science, much of what you call theories in psychology are very dependent upon a particular individual's charismatic qualities, his ability to attract people and to excite them.

This is the reason for Skinner's success. He's a great PR man, and the reason there is such an interest in Skinnerian approaches to so many problems is not because there have been some great profound advances in knowledge, or some clearly established successes, but because the guy's a great publicist. He's got character, charisma, he's an enormous egoist — which you need in order to be a charismatic individual — and he developed a following. It's like a religion — this is what happens in psychology. So when the leaders of these movements die, the movements tend to fade. They don't have that vital source any longer. This is what happened to Hull.

Other factors were also involved: for example, the growth of physiological psychology. Olds (1956a, 1956b) showed there were "pleasure centers" in the brain, and that created problems for the Hullian drive-reduction theory of reinforcement. Hull, even though he had a biological orientation, ignored physiological psychology because there really was not much to know at the time.

Q: Was it Hull's idea that the constructs he postulated — little inner stimuli and responses — were potentially observable? That you could eventually find these things in the physiology?

A: Yes, this was Hull's orientation, that there were actual physiological changes going on. Spence was less physiologically oriented. He thought that the things Hull was talking about were just theoretical constructs, and calling it something physiological was really irrelevant. In this respect "expectancy" and "r_g-s_g" had precisely the same theoretical status.

Q: So the idea that the little stimuli and responses were really potentially observable — that they were little muscular and glandular events — wasn't taken very seriously by people at Iowa?

A: No, no. I think that Spence was right in that respect. But the point is that there was, in a sense, a denigration of physiological psychology and its potential. During the '30s and '40s there might have been some justification for that, because there really had not been any major advances in knowledge that were relevant to behavior and psychology, but as more was understood about the nervous system, that was no longer justified.

And finally, people just got interested in a lot more specific issues once they'd figured out that the grand theory was not going to work. They developed "minitheories" to cover limited problems. Then there was Skinner, who was claiming that he didn't have a theory at all and that psychologists shouldn't have theories. But this was more extreme.

Q: When you say that psychology is prone to charismatic leaders, and that when they leave the field, their ideas tend to fade, the one exception that comes to mind is Watson. He proposed behaviorism in 1913 and left psychology in 1920, but behaviorism remained dominant for another three or four decades.

A: Watson formed an entire system, an entire orientation toward psychology and what its goals *ought* to be, and not some particular theory of psychology the way Hull or Spence did. Watson permanently broadened the subject matter of psychology. The introspectionists such as Wundt and Titchener couldn't deal with animals or children, because they couldn't give introspections. There were other people before Watson who had said similar things, but Watson was a very effective spokesman, and because of his charismatic character he was able to inspire other people to adopt a similar point of view.

Q: Did Watson have to pay a price for his brand of behaviorism? Didn't he lose the ability to deal with personal experience, with imagery and purpose and so on?

A: Watson had specific hypotheses and theories that are different from his systematic approach to behaviorism. He had a frequency theory of learning and a peculiar theory of emotion, a theory of thinking and so on. You can be a behaviorist and accept none of those.

Q: So behaviorism is a metatheoretical viewpoint?

A: Well, of course, of course. Just as I indicated: Both Hull and Tolman were behaviorists. They had contradictory theories of learning. One of them was right and one of them was wrong, presumably, but they were both behaviorists. The same with Skinner and Guthrie and so on. Watson had difficulties with images; his theories for rearing children were silly; but that has nothing to do with behaviorism per se. You can be a behaviorist and have a totally different theory about all these things.

I'm personally interested in images and I'm a behaviorist. I use several objective tests of imagery. I don't see any difficulty in studying images. I could ask people just to describe some images, but I want to have a quantitative measure. So you can set up a questionnaire with questions about images, to get some numerical index of the strength of imagery, the controllability of imagery, and so forth. And what does this questionnaire test? It tests imagery.

Q: What does being a behaviorist mean when you study mental images?

A: The behaviorist says, "Well, I'm studying behavior. I have a score on this test, and that score is what I mean by the individual's image." How do I use that in an experiment? I'm interested in the effects of imagery on mental practice. What? A behaviorist studying mental practice? Yes, I'm studying how you can facilitate actual performance on a task by just thinking about a motor task, mentally practicing it. I've been interested in that kind of a problem ever since I was a sophomore.

And you say, "How do you define mental practice?" I define it in a behavioristic way. I present these questions to an individual and tell them what to do, and then I measure their performance. That's what I mean by mental practice. I'm measuring the effects of mental practice by looking at the individual's performance on a motor task.

Q: Doesn't the word "image" have meanings beyond just a score on an objective questionnaire?

A: You're implying that I'm not using the notion of imagery the same way someone else may. Fine, but I'm not excluding someone else's definition. Remember, all we can know of the other person's image is his behavior, including his verbal behavior. Why does referring to unobservables bug you, unless you have a precise theory that is falsifiable? If you had such a theory, I suspect it would "reduce" images to something else.

Q: Does "imagery" mean anything in terms of your personal experience?

A: This is an old question. Titchener in 1914 published a reply to

Watson's 1913 article — Titchener was obviously a very bright guy — in which he said in effect, "well, you know, Watson has the right to study anything he wants to, but it's not psychology as we know it. Maybe it's biology or technology." He used a very similar example to the one you used. He said, "Watson is talking about thinking in terms of muscle twitches. You know, changes in lips and larynx and so on. But how does he know about images and thinking in the first place? The fact that he knows about thinking can only come about because he is inspecting the elements of his consciousness."

My answer to that is what the philosopher Hans Reichenbach (1938) said many years ago. He said that you have to make a distinction between the *context of discovery* and the *context of verification*. You can do anything you want in the process of discovery. You can look cross-eyed at consciousness, smell bad apples, take cocaine, in order to get your ideas or hypotheses. Behaviorism is not concerned with the context of discovery, but with the context of verification — namely, that the concepts that we use will be of the same kind that the other natural sciences employ. "Psychology as the behaviorist views it," in Watson's (1913) words, is an objective experimental branch of natural science, and its theoretical goal is the prediction and control of behavior. Its hypotheses will be verified — put to public test or be falsified — according to the same procedures used in the natural sciences.

Q: Some people have talked about the cognitive approach as representing a paradigm shift. That seems to be somewhat controversial. What do you think about that?

A: One of the most obnoxious, misused terms in all of current thinking is "paradigm" and "paradigm shift." There's an article (Masterman, 1970) showing that Kuhn uses the term "paradigm" in his own writings in 21 different ways. What do you mean by a paradigm? Any psychologist comes up with some cockamamie little hypothesis or new experiment or some new kind of a metaphor and says, "There's a paradigm shift." I say that's bullshit. That wasn't even in general what Kuhn meant by "paradigm" or "paradigm shift." What has happened now is that there are new metaphors, metaphors of computers, metaphors of attributions. That's the problem in psychology; it's a new fad. Now, classic examples, such as Galilean physics and Einstein's theory of relativity — there's nothing like that in psychology, where all you've got is a bunch of metaphors and a couple of little experiments. There's a new way of talking about various kinds of phenomena, and in no fundamental sense is this a paradigm shift.

Q: There seem to be at least two very different meanings of "paradigm." One is just an experimental procedure, and another is a whole framework of thought.

A: Well, but the point is that the term "paradigm" was used by Kuhn himself in a great variety of ways. It is a highly ambiguous term. There's been a change in the kind of terminology used in psychology, and the kinds of problems people are interested in — and, in a loose sense, in the theoretical formulations. Now people use more intentional terms, more computer metaphors. But this is no guarantee that any real advance in knowledge or testable theory will occur. I haven't seen it.

Q: The word "imagery," for example, seemed distinctly out of favor from Watson's time until the middle '60s.

A: Yes, sure. But that doesn't represent a paradigm shift. There was a little research on it all along, and now it's become much more popular. This doesn't by any stretch of the imagination represent a paradigm shift in any sense that Kuhn used. Psychology has diversified and expanded the kinds of problems we're interested in, and this is healthy. And the ways of talking about these problems, the theoretical terms I used that weren't used before, I don't call this a paradigm. I think that using the term is arrogant, it's intellectually arrogant.

Q: Whether or not the word "paradigm" is appropriate for what has happened in psychology, it does seem that there has been one framework since 1913 that went through a relatively rapid change, perhaps in the middle '60s. Some people who now prefer to call themselves cognitive psychologists describe their experience that way.

A: Yes, so they've had a change of interest in the way they theorize about a problem. So, what about it? They are no longer S–R psychologists. But if they are not behaviorists, what are they? They use intentional terms, but so did Tolman.

Q: You were at the Kentucky conference in 1968 (Dixon & Horton, 1968; Maltzman, 1968), which is sometimes said to represent these people in transition. What was it like?

A: The conference was on verbal learning, and I was never really in verbal learning. I was there because of my interest in verbal behavior and semantic conditioning. There was clearly an influence from Chomsky at the time. It was a change in the orientation toward problems and issues that was due to Chomsky. [Thomas] Bever and some of Chomsky's other followers were there. And those guys were talking about this kind of shift, I don't remember if they used the term "paradigm shift." Guys who were right in the tradition of S–R verbal learning, like Jim Jenkins, changed. They adopted a different kind of theoretical orientation, began studying different kinds of problems. David Palermo was another one there.

So yes, there was a change. I guess there was a realization that the problems they had been studying had limited generality and interest, and here was a more fruitful way to study things. So sure there was a change of interests.

Q: Even though they no longer call themselves behaviorists, do you think that in fact they still are behaviorists? At least methodological behaviorists?

A: Did they ever call themselves behaviorists? Most people don't do that sort of thing. They are not S–R behaviorists, but you have to distinguish between S–R psychology and behaviorism. What characterizes S–R psychologists is the nature of the theoretical concepts they have. The theoretical concepts are conceived of as corresponding to stimuli and responses. But as I said, you can be a behaviorist and not use that kind of a theoretical formulation.

Q: How do you see the people who call themselves cognitive psychologists today?

A: Cognitive psychology doesn't use concepts that are couched in S–R terms, such as "r_g-s_g," "drive stimulus," and so forth. Tolman was a cognitive psychologist who talked about rats having hypotheses and expectancies. His theoretical terms are not hypothetical stimuli and responses. What are they? They are intentional terms. This goes back to a notion formulated by Brentano: Intentional terms are terms that refer to something beyond themselves (Brentano, 1874/1973). If I have an image, I have an image of *something*. In contrast, if I have an r_g, a fractional anticipatory response, that's not an r_g *of* something. This is the fundamental distinction.

In cognitive psychology there are theoretical terms that are intentional; they are "acts," as Brentano (1874/1973) called them. [Cognitive psychologists would call these "representations." — *B.J.B.*] An S–R psychologist doesn't use such terms. Now, you can be a cognitive psychologist using intentional terms and also be a behaviorist, the way Tolman was. Tolman was a behaviorist, because he would define his intentional terms by means of observable behavior.

Now you see, the problem is that most cognitive psychologists don't think about visible behavior. They just use intentional terms such as "thinking," "images," and so on, in a very vague way. They may not be concerned with, "How do I define these terms?" If they attempt to define them, they characteristically define them in terms of some observable operations, or some computer program, and so on. And then I say, well, they're behaviorists.

Q: If you were going to characterize the field today, would you say that there is more theoretical sloppiness than would have been permitted 20 years ago?

A: I think that psychology is in a really bad way today. I blame Kuhn and some of the philosophers of science who emphasize relativism. They are right that logical positivism was naïve in many respects, but now people think scientific proof is just sociological.

There are advantages and disadvantages. When we were students, there was an insistence: You declare what you are talking about operationally, and when you use a term, you take enormous care to stick with your definition. Now, the negative aspect of that was that there was also a lot of punishment for using different or new words, and a limitation on the kinds of problems you worked on.

Now today, you can study anything you want to, and talk about it in any way you want to, so that there's no communication. And I think there is an enormous amount of sloppy theorizing in many areas, which is seriously retarding progress. There is no critical analysis in many areas of what people mean by the theoretical concepts they are employing. Now, this varies enormously from one area to another. I'm talking in a general way now.

Years ago it was the big model, and now it's the model of the month. Every other experiment results in a new model or theory, and everybody now has their own theory. Years ago there was one country and a king, and now every little fiefdom or principality has their own prince, their own theory, and you have all these little knights and princes. They are all fighting about their little theory, and so on. I put all this at the feet of cognitive psychology.

One of the areas I'm interested in is alcoholism, not just laboratory alcoholism, but in the field. This is the major drug addiction problem in the United States and in the world. When you get cognitive psychologists coming at it, it's fascinating, because here is a profoundly important problem in drive, motivation, and learning. How does an addiction come about: Which people will literally kill themselves compulsively drinking? The same with smoking—literally kill themselves. Can't stop, even though they are destroying their bodies, getting cirrhosis of the liver, pancreatitis, and brain damage. Can't stop. It's a profoundly important problem in motivation, learning, and conditioning.

Here's one of the shortcomings of cognitive psychology—it's all intellectual. They don't recognize any problems like drive, motivation, or conditioning. They're worse than Hull in completely ignoring physiological correlates. But you have people with a cognitive orientation coming into the field of alcoholism and saying, "Well, the effects of alcohol are really nothing but attributions. What you expect or attribute to alcohol is what you get." Well, this is insanity. This alcohol kills you, and, you know, that's an attribution, people die from it? There are many problems where this simplistic kind of cognitive interpretation is made about real world problems.

So you see, cognitive psychology's opened up new problems in some areas, and so on. And other areas of psychology — it's set them back enormously. It has resulted in an enormous disregard for serious problems, where it approaches them in an unbelievably simplistic way.

Howard H. Kendler: Evolution Rather than Revolution

Howard H. Kendler (b. 1919) received his PhD in psychology from the University of Iowa under the direction of Kenneth W. Spence, but 6 years earlier than Maltzman, in 1943. He became well known quite early for his research into the issue of latent learning, culminating in his article entitled "What Is Learned? — a Theoretical Blind Alley" (Kendler, 1952). In this paper he argued, with considerable success, that the kinds of questions asked in the latent learning controversy were too imprecise to be answered by contemporary experimental techniques. Subsequently he and his wife, Tracy Kendler, became well known for their research on human discrimination learning (1975).

Kendler's interests extend broadly beyond his own research. For example, in 1971 he edited, together with Janet Spence, a book of neo-behavioristic papers in psychology (Kendler & Spence, 1971), and more recently he has written several historical papers (*e.g.*, Kendler & Kendler, 1975) and an overall perspective on the role of scientific psychology (Kendler, 1981). He believes that psychology has been called upon to do things that as a scientific discipline, it cannot do. Thus psychologists are sometimes asked to provide a scientific basis for value systems, or for an account of subjective experience — questions, he says, that are in principle out of reach of the scientific approach as we know it today.

Most interestingly perhaps, Kendler argues for an evolutionary rather than revolutionary view of cognitive psychology. The issue of internal representation, which he views as critical, has precedents in behavioristic ideas such as Hull's "fractional anticipatory goal response" (r_g–s_g). Altogether, Kendler views Hull as "a noble failure, who made many positive contributions to psychology."

In Kendler's view, all psychological research programs to date have "degenerated" (Lakatoš, 1970) — that is, they all have failed to achieve their promised objectives. Nevertheless, he believes that there has been some solid progress in areas such as "the powers of reinforcement, behavior modification, psychological testing, and developmental changes in human behavior." He advocates a "pragmatic behaviorism," in which one takes a tough-minded view of psychological data, but without denying such things as consciousness. Kendler believes that cognitive psychologists are basically employing a behavioristic methodology, but he believes that cognitive psychologists are less idealistic than behavioristic psychologists once were.

Interview with Howard H. Kendler

Q: How did you get started in psychology?

A: I went to college in 1936, in the deep Depression. My uncle happened to tell me about a friend who was a successful psychologist, and when I had to fill out the form at Brooklyn College for the major, I just filled in psychology. It was kind of silly — I didn't have any conception of it. I was actually interested in economics and biology, but I had such terrible courses in those subjects that when I finally took a psychology course and found it interesting, I decided to major in psychology. I took an experimental course with the Gestalt psychologist, Solomon Asch, and designed an original experiment on the *Einstellung* problem, the question of preparatory "set" in problem-solving tasks. I had a model that made a counterintuitive prediction — namely, that the longer the time between the training period and the test period, the more of a set effect one would find. It was the kind of theory I liked because it could be falsified — an unusual characteristic for many Gestalt hypotheses. Asch encouraged me to test my model, and even though my prediction was disconfirmed, the total experience was exciting and rewarding.

That experience, plus my romantic attachment to another psych major, Tracy Seedman, who later became my wife, encouraged the idea of going to graduate school. We decided to go to Iowa for graduate work, mainly because Kurt Lewin was there, but also because tuition and living expenses were so reasonable. We went to Iowa, and we both enrolled in a course with Lewin. Tracy took her MA with Lewin, but Lewin and I did not resonate to each other.

At the same time, we accidentally got into an advanced seminar with Kenneth W. Spence. Spence was very much a missionary for the neobehavioristic position of Hull. Unlike Lewin, he readily answered all my questions concerning differences between a Gestalt and a behaviorist orientation. Spence was extremely stimulating, and the intimate relationship he espoused between theory and research was most appealing.

When I visited Brooklyn College after a year at Iowa, I mentioned to Abraham Maslow, whose assistant I had been while at Brooklyn College, my preference for Spence's general orientation. Maslow's response, obviously aggressive (even humanistic psychologists can be aggressive!), was "Well, it fits your personality." There was some truth to that comment. Hull's analytic approach and his strong commitment to a tough-minded methodology appealed to what Maslow would probably diagnose as my "compulsive needs." It is interesting to note that Köhler (1959) acknowledged the superiority of American psychology in regard to questions of method and proof. I want to make it clear here that I don't mean to imply that Hullian theory *is* behaviorism, because as I wrote in my paper (Kendler, 1985), behaviorism should not be identified with any particular theory. It is a general methodological approach to psychology.

Q: In that paper you wrote that "There is more expected of psychology than behaviorism can offer" (p. 1). What do you mean by that?

A: Psychology is a multipurpose discipline in our society. In addition to answering questions about empirical matters, psychologists are also asked about the proper kind of life one should lead, the values one should adopt, the meaning of life, and so forth. A critical interpretation of behaviorism as a methodological orientation would lead to a conclusion that one cannot from an analysis of psychology come up with a scientific basis for value, in the sense of *logically* deriving ethical imperatives from empirical evidence (Kendler, 1981). Maslow and his followers argue that humans have a motive to become self-actualized, a state that involves the adoption of a scientifically "valid" set of values. Gestalt psychologists, too, were involved with a romantic, idealistic, metaphysical notion of ethics. According to his son Michael, Max Wertheimer (a founder of Gestalt psychology) believed in holism as a kind of religion—that the world had meaning and that humans were fundamentally good. For example, one reason that Gestalt psychologists were opposed to Freudian psychology was because of the "evil" drives Freud postulated. Some social psychologists who do action research suggest that psychology can somehow provide *valid*, as contrasted with *pragmatic*, answers to problems of social conflict as well as reveal the *true* "image of man." Finally, Skinner also bases his views on a prescriptive set of values, but I would argue that his position is more of an expression of his behavior as a social engineer than of behaviorism. He argues that the issue of values is a red herring. Fundamentally, Skinner argues for a kind of survival value— that society should survive. But a behavioristic interpretation would be that there is no logical relationship between facts and ethical imperatives. Consequently, psychology itself cannot offer society a scientific set of values, a valid blueprint for life. Psychologists scare me when they play the role of God, especially when they think they are qualified.

There is another aspect to the limitations of behaviorism. People expect psychology to offer a veridical account of human experience and consciousness. Sigmund Koch (1956) continuously raises this question, sometimes in relation to his own experiences of depression and to the broad field of esthetics — why psychology is incapable of coping with differences in human experiences because of inadequate methodological techniques. I can't see any way that natural science psychology can deal with his concerns, now or in the near future, although with certain technical developments of the science-fiction type it might. It is nevertheless a legitimate question. As a behaviorist, I have such concerns. I'd like to know how my phenomenological experiences compare with others'. But when I have such urges, I read novelists to whom I resonate, for example, Dostoyevsky and Bellow. They provide me with an intuitive grasp of the feelings of others and insight into the human condition.

Q: You are saying that behaviorism *is* scientific psychology.

A: You're not off base with that comment, but I have two reservations about the use of the term "scientific." First, the term "science" means different things. I tend to use it to refer to the methodological traditions of the natural sciences. But "science" can refer to the human sciences, for example, Vico, or mental sciences, for example, Dilthey. Natural science is quite different from the human and mental sciences, both of which have had great influence in the history of psychology, particularly on Wundt, Gestalt psychology, and humanistic psychology. Second, even if we restrict the word "science" to natural science I have to admit the absence of a clear demarcation between science and nonscience. But I agree that behaviorism represents an attempt to apply natural science methodology to psychology. Behavioristic methodology can reveal some of the causal aspects of experience, for example, depression, be they biochemical, or genetic, or the previous history of the individual. But the phenomenological experience itself — the feeling of depression — is presently beyond natural science methodology.

Q: You clearly think that behaviorism is still an important component of present-day psychology.

A: A student of mine, Roy Lachman, just co-authored a book on cognitive psychology and information processing (Lachman, Lachman, & Butterfield, 1979). It is an outstanding book. The book analyzes the historical background of cognitive psychology, and obviously Tolman's cognitive behaviorism played a significant role. Tolman was a committed behaviorist and sophisticated methodologist. Lachman argues that cognitive psychologists have adopted from behaviorism an objective (intersubjective) approach, the canons of natural science, and an operational analysis of experimental procedures. Many of the leading cognitive psychologists, for example, Posner, Shepard, and Garner, are using a fundamentally behavioristic methodology.

Q: You see a lot of continuities. Do you see important differences?

A: There are certain revolutionary and evolutionary components. For example, in my own mediational S–R approach (*e.g.*, Kendler & Kendler, 1975), a representational process assumed a major position. You can trace back the notion of representation in Hullian theory to the concept of the fractional anticipatory goal response, and back further to the early behaviorists' analysis of symbolic behavior of animals (*e.g.*, Hunter, 1913). One of the important principles enunciated in the cognitive revolution was the central role played by representational processes. The cognitive viewpoint is that this change was revolutionary, but within behavioristic learning theories, a similar development represents a continuity. Because cognitive psychologists perceived themselves as participants in a great, even holy, revolution, they interpreted their emphasis on representation as a truly intellectual insurrection. I view it as an evolutionary event. The revolutionary notion of many cognitive psychologists was a strategic gambit: Employ mental events as a source for fruitful hypotheses. The behaviorist revolution was directed against a mental psychology. They became suspicious of all introspective evidence. Cognitive psychologists reversed that trend. Interestingly, Tolman was very suspicious of introspective reports, but not of his own conscious experiences when formulating theoretical principles for rat behavior.

Q: Hull apparently claimed that the anticipatory goal response (r_g–s_g) is the kind of theoretical construct that is potentially observable. Do you agree with that?

A: No, I disagree if this implies that the validity of the construct ultimately depends on its being observable. Of course within the Hullian group you have to make certain distinctions. I think Hull himself was rather naïve methodologically. He was very ambitious, as all messiahs are. He had a powerful intellect, but some of his views are fundamentally different from those of his disciples Kenneth Spence and Neal Miller. Spence, a much more sophisticated methodologist than Hull was, emphasized the fictional aspect of theoretical constructs. They are fictions that serve as shorthand descriptions of empirical relationships. Neal Miller nicely balanced the needs of empiricism with those of theory. He was so damned pragmatic that he didn't worry too much about the formal demands of theory. He just theorized and let his creative intellect deal with the theoretical issues rather informally. Hull was more reality-oriented, more concerned with a reductionistic — physiological — interpretation of behavior. I would say that if you could really observe an r_g–s_g, fine, but if it didn't work out, and your theory could still generate deductions in agreement with the data, then you keep the notion, and be damned happy that it works.

Q: Who influenced you most in your own development?

A: Obviously Kenneth Spence played the most influential role, but Solomon Asch and Neal Miller exerted important influences. My views about methodology were influenced by the philosophers Gustav Bergmann, Ernest Nagel, and Imre Lakatoš, although I always perceived these issues from the perspective of an empiricist. My talented friend Sig Koch had an important impact on my thinking. He raised issues that are too easily ignored by research psychologists. Koch received his MA in the philosophy of science while studying with Herbert Feigl at Iowa. This predisposed him to look at Hull's efforts with great favor, if not enthusiasm. After getting his PhD in psychology at Duke he became very negative about Hull. This reaction culminated in a critical analysis of Hull (Koch, 1954) that had an important historical impact. His criticism was devastating with regard to the methodological and theoretical limitations of Hull. But most people did not appreciate that Koch was raising fundamental issues about *all* theories of behavior. This started me thinking about a broad spectrum of methodological issues that encouraged me to write *Psychology: A Science in Conflict* (Kendler, 1981). I responded to many questions raised by Koch, although I am sure in a manner that would not be acceptable to him. But getting back to his analysis of Hull, it should be noted that Koch concluded his essay by listing the significant contributions of Hull, for example, improved theoretical practices, useful hypotheses, useful experiments. Hull was a noble failure who made many positive contributions to psychology. I understand that Chomsky, for example, views Hull very differently from Skinner, because Hull was making a serious attempt at theorizing. Theorizing is an enterprise that concerns Chomsky, even though he himself, in my estimation, fails to offer a theory that even approaches the level of falsifiability that Hullian theory attained. Chomsky is primarily a rationalist, not an empiricist.

I was also very much influenced by the latent learning controversy in which I became involved when a graduate student. I did my master's thesis on it, and several studies afterwards. These studies were widely referred to. The problem with the latent learning controversy was that it really died at its own hands. The competing Hullian and Tolmanian views were inadequate to the task of offering a systematic interpretation of all the data. Anybody who writes or says that this controversy was resolved in favor of one of the two competing conceptions is deluding himself and misleading his or her audience. Perhaps the major contribution of the latent learning controversy was to demonstrate, as has since that time been repeatedly demonstrated, that purely "black box" theories were incapable of resolving controversies about fundamental behavioral processes.

Q: Could you define the issues for me?

A: There were several issues. The main one was whether what is learned is cognitive maps or stimulus — response associations. A secondary issue was whether reward was necessary for learning to occur. Many of the participants in the controversy failed to distinguish between these two separate issues. I later wrote a paper entitled, "What Is Learned? — a Theoretical Blind Alley" (1952), in which I argued that the question could not be answered because the competing theories could not generate determinate consequences that would be at odds with each other. It is not surprising, therefore, that the controversy was unresolvable.

The feeling among learning psychologists of that time, which I shared, was that the controversies were unresolvable because the theories weren't sufficiently precise. Attempts were made to make the theories more precise, but except for very specific mathematical models that lacked any generality, behavior theories have not been able to resolve their major disputes, for example, continuity versus noncontinuity theory, the number of memory stores, serial versus parallel processing. Consider the debate about whether human learning is basically associationistic or organizational. Postman (1971) argues that the difference is semantic, while for Mandler (1962) the difference is substantive. The historical evidence opposes Mandler's position.

The problem with these behavior theories is that repeated *ad hoc* modifications to the theory were required to cope with the impact of new evidence. To employ the words of Lakatoš (1970), the theory degenerates. Theories, or what Lakatoš prefers to call "research programs," can be progressive by predicting novel events. The neobehaviorism of Hull, Spence, and Neal Miller went through a progressive stage, with Hull predicting some novel learning — motivational interactions, Spence predicting some new discrimination learning phenomena, Neal Miller predicting some subtle conflict phenomena, and Tracy Kendler and myself integrating some developmental phenomena within an expanded neobehavioristic formulation. Although all of these findings, and others as well, represented progressive changes, the total neobehavioristic effort ultimately degenerated because of the incapacity of the general theory to incorporate the immense amount of data that was being generated. The general theory soon became buried under its numerous *ad hoc* assumptions. The early successes of "Hullian theory" turned into a later failure.

But I don't know of any behavioral theory that hasn't degenerated. Cognitive dissonance is a good example of a degenerating research program. Perhaps psychological theorists have been too ambitious. If I had to propose a frame of reference for how one should go about theorizing, I would favor a Darwinian strategy. Darwin may represent a better model for psychological theorizing than Newton or Galileo. At the time I was going to graduate school, Lewin was pretending to be a Galileo, and Hull thought he was a Newton. Imitating the cautious Darwinian strategy probably would have proven to be more productive.

Q: Skinner seems to model himself after Darwin to some extent. For example, the idea of responses being selected after occurring by chance, much as adaptive traits are selected by environmental pressures in Darwin's theory.

A: Only in terms of content, not in terms of strategy. A trial-and-error model — trial-and-error-with-accidental-success is a better designation — is characteristic of S–R formulations of animal behavior, and they bear a resemblance to evolutionary processes — selection by consequences. But this model should not be limited to Skinner alone. Darwin was an excellent theorist, formulating assumptions appropriate to the kind of data he had. Skinner is an unsatisfactory theorist even though he denies being one. He's very ambiguous. His strong statement about theory is that it is unnecessary. That is obviously wrong. In the weak form, Skinner says that at this stage of development, theories are not very useful to pursue. That's a reasonable statement. Hull certainly did not have the necessary data for his theoretical superstructure.

Neither do many modern cognitive theorists. All our behavior theories have blown up. Early successes, as I indicated, have turned into later failures. It finally occurred to me that it may not be precision that is needed, but perhaps there are just not enough constraints in behavioral research. These behavior theories progress to a point where they can't resolve their differences. Perhaps behavior theories have a limit to their explanatory ability. Perhaps the controversies that I have mentioned have to be put aside until they can be transformed into some kind of physiological model.

Q: So you see the resolution in physiology?

A: Possibly. Unfortunately not necessarily.

Q: Hull proposed that reinforcement was due to a drop in the total amount of "drive," the motivational energy. This sounds just like Freud's idea that pleasure is experienced when there is a drop in libido, which is also motivational energy. Is there a historical relationship?

A: Not a direct one. The general notion of some homeostatic-like mechanism operating, for example, hedonism, can be traced back to the Greek philosophers and probably before. Originally, Hull thought reinforcement resulted from a physiological need reduction. It certainly had some similarity to Freud's notion. The fact that both shared a general learning orientation made it inevitable that some psychologists would perceive a relationship between the two orientations. Dollard and Miller's *Personality and Psychotherapy* (1950) is a brilliant attempt to reconcile the two approaches. Neal Miller, who's one of the great neobehaviorists, went to Europe to be psychoanalyzed during his early career. He was always interested in Freudian theory, and he tried in this book to reinterpret Freud within a behavioristic frame of reference. It's an excellent interpretation, but it failed to have much impact for a variety of reasons: a reduction of interest in Freudian theory, the decline of Hullian theory, a disenchantment with general theories. To some extent Neal Miller himself was susceptible to these influences — as evidenced by the fact that he became a physiological psychologist.

Q: Has that been a trend among the neobehaviorists of the Hull–Spence period?

A: Becoming physiological? Yes, I think so. Neal Miller, Abe Amsel, Irving Maltzman [this volume], and Larry Stein have moved, to varying degrees, to a physiological orientation. This shift is not only characteristic of the Hull–Spence orientation, but is typical of the conditioning research area.

Q: If you had to list the major accomplishments of the period from 1913 to 1960 in experimental psychology, what would you list?

A: William Estes once wrote an article comparing the behavioristic revolution to the Copernican revolution, and I think this is valid in a certain limited sense. This reorientation to behavior as a dependent variable, rather than consciousness or the mind, has encouraged a lot of solid empirical research. It has not paid off in terms of the ideals that motivated experimental psychologists, who were searching for a general theory of behavior. The easy optimism that prevailed in the '40s that such a goal would be reached has been destroyed.

But at the same time we have a lot of information about the powers of reinforcement, behavior modification, psychological testing, developmental changes in human behavior. We're more sophisticated about the significance of species differences. All of these advances didn't come directly from Hull. In fact, in some cases he himself was an obstacle. He tended to ignore comparative and developmental differences by treating them purely as constants in mathematical formulas. But the entire behavioristic approach has yielded a lot of interesting and important information. It has led to specific theories, and to important applications. There's been progress, but unfortunately not of the magnitude that has occurred in genetics (which is also about 100 years old). But the progress is there.

Q: The big thing about the Copernican revolution, of course, is that people learned to look at the solar system from a less anthropocentric point of view. Instead of a geocentric universe, you got a heliocentric universe. Certainly behaviorism made people look at human beings from a less anthropocentric point of view — instead of asking about experience, we asked about publically observable behavior.

A: That's true. And your observation reflects a fundamental conflict within psychology. Which is more important? Behavior or consciousness? Do you want to predict behavior, or do you want a veridical picture of inner experience? Do you want a natural science of psychology or some form of a "human science"? An analysis of consciousness, as some cognitive theories have suggested, can yield interesting theoretical insights. But they can also be misleading, especially when dealing with motivational factors. I favor a *pragmatic behaviorist* approach. Our dependent variable is behavior. Don't let the mind–body problem ensnare you as it did John B. Watson. He got himself in an indefensible position when he adopted the absurd position that consciousness does not exist. Employ reports of conscious contents when useful, but never assume that such reports automatically reflect the "cause" of behavior.

Behaviorism has not been terribly successful in making people less anthropocentric when viewing others. There is much resistance to behavioristic methodology. The common gripe is that we are treating people like things, like objects, and that somehow you can't treat a person this way. You have somehow to realize that these are human beings with a consciousness like yours. I don't see where behaviorism has been very widely accepted, even within psychology, and certainly not outside of psychology. If you have taught introductory psychology, you know it's a very difficult thing to teach a behavioristic orientation because of the inability of students to escape from their own experience. They cannot resist the temptation to explain behavior on the basis of their own experience. Students seem to find it impossible to treat any kind of behavioral event, whether it be that of a rat or a human being, without attributing it to some mental events similar to their own. It's a very difficult thing for people to understand the behavioristic orientation. I don't mean to imply that people should not empathize with others. I suspect that the ability to follow the Golden Rule — Do unto others as you would have them do unto you — is dependent on empathy. This assumption can be treated in a behavioristic fashion. My argument is based on the assumption that one must behave differently as a natural-science psychologist and as an ordinary human being.

Q: That makes behaviorism a kind of intellectual self-discipline, a refusal to interpret, or overinterpret, the things that everyone can agree upon.

A: That's essentially correct. Unfortunately the methodological analysis is much more complex. You are right in suggesting that behaviorism represents a tough-minded approach to research.

Q: In your historical paper (1985) you wrote that the original claims associated with behaviorism were: objectivism, stimulus–response orientation, peripheralism, associationistic learning, and environmentalism. But in its seventh decade of life, what is left of these is only objectivism. Is behaviorism the same as objectivism at this point in psychology?

A: That's the thrust of my article. This was the core assumption of the behavioristic revolution, that the experimental operations are linked to observables, and behavior is the dependent variable. The litmus test of your theory has to be in terms of predicting some kind of behaviors, instead of trying to offer a veridical account of consciousness.

This may not seem very profound, but if you look at the time in which it occurred, in the context of a mentally oriented psychology of Wundt or Titchener or Külpe, or a functionalism that was confused about its goals, then behaviorism represents a radical change. It is important to recognize that this radical change was logically independent of the other behaviorist assumptions. As I said previously, Tolman is a critical case in the history of behaviorism. He was a very sophisticated behaviorist who accepted the need for objectivism, but not the other assumptions. To repeat myself again, many cognitive psychologists are employing essentially a behavioristic methodology.

Q: If we look historically at the failure of Hullian theory about 1950 as a kind of watershed, there were two kinds of responses to it. The immediate response, I think, was a deep suspicion of theory among experimental psychologists. Skinner certainly took the extreme position there in suggesting that theory simply was not needed at all. A more long-term response might be associated with Herbert Simon [Chapter 7], who might claim that Hull was not *sufficiently* theoretical. Hull failed, in this view, to use the really powerful theoretical tools that we see today in computational theories.

A: Yes, I fully agree with that. I once gave a talk at an APA meeting and said that Hull was the most influential theorist — this was after Hull's day — and some people started laughing. But then I said, his great influence was generated by his *failure*, not by his success. There were two reactions to his failure. One, as you've pointed out, was Skinner, saying that having a theory is wrong or unproductive. And the other was that Hull wasn't sufficiently qualified to theorize. He wasn't a good mathematician. This reaction came from people like Estes, who had tremendous admiration for Hull, but realized that his mathematical techniques were unsophisticated. One can argue that Hull's efforts led historically to mathematical modeling and an atheoretical approach. Simon's theoretical approach [Chapter 7] became prominent later on, emerging historically from the formal efforts of Estes. I cannot avoid commenting that the success of Simon's efforts in understanding human thinking has been overstated (Kendler, 1981).

Hull's work was actually a considerable improvement over that of his predecessors. Bitterman at one time was a critic of Hull, but now is more positive. He had a sabbatical during which he read successive issues of *Psychological Review*. When he came to Hull he felt it was like a breath of spring air. Ideas became much sharper, more scientific. I think that this improvement was, in part, a consequence of stimulus–response psychology. It helped anchor psychology to observables. It's unfortunate that S–R language became so controversial. To some extent it is the result of the tendency of psychologists to perceive difference among different paradigms solely in terms of revolutionary changes while ignoring evolutionary developments.

Q: One of the things difficult for people outside of the experimental psychology to understand is the experience of testing a very explicit hypothesis about some testable issue in the laboratory. To many people it's a shock to realize that things they consider to be "obvious" are in fact very difficult to demonstrate rigorously. You often find that nothing you expected actually comes out. That is an experience that people who don't do psychological experiments find hard to understand. This is the kind of experience that psychologists began to confront, perhaps around Watson's time, and it seems to be a formative influence for many psychologists.

A: Right. It's an amazingly exciting thing. This is the key to my interest. When I started doing research as an undergraduate, my whole life changed. It was a thrilling experience, which I find difficult to convey to contemporary students. I'm always depressed to discover how many students find this of no significance. When I gave up working with rats and got involved with human development, it became much more difficult to formulate assumptions and test their implications. The rigor of the predictions with rats seemed greater, and because of this, waiting for the results entailed more excitement. Human behavior is very complex, and I found myself doing more exploratory research in order to get enough information to formulate theoretical assumptions. The basic strategy we had in the early days was that if you can't explain rat behavior, you are not going to be successful in explaining human behavior.

Q: So you think that being excited about lab work, and making things testable — that these ideas are fundamental in the development of behavioristic psychology?

A: Yes. There was a tremendous emphasis on testability. I think that we were naïve — immediate testability is not the litmus test, because some ideas might be untestable at one time, but with technological advances might become testable. I think that behaviorists were too rigorous in their demands for testability, too intolerant of other ideas. At the same time, you must realize that there is a lot of stuff in psychology that is not even technically possible. It's just vague or transcendental. The basic demand for specificity and testability has an advantage over a tolerance for vagueness and untestability.

Being excited about experimentation played an important role in the personal development of many behavioristic psychologists, and I'm sure that it plays the same role among many cognitive psychologists. Although I do think that during the '40s and '50s we were much more idealistic than the younger psychologists of today. Psychology was a kind of calling, and perhaps we were unrealistically idealistic, but it was a great deal of fun. Today you see many bright people who view psychology as a kind of job. They do their jobs, publish their papers, but they are not terribly involved in the consequences, or in the future of psychology.

Alan O. Ross: Behavior Therapy in the Clinic

A reader who has gained the impression that behaviorism is a single, monolithic point of view may be surprised by some of Alan O. Ross's beliefs. Ross (b. 1921) has worked to build bridges between applied and basic psychology, focusing primarily on applications in child clinical psychology. In pursuit of this goal, he has used research produced by behavioristic as well as cognitive researchers, from operant conditioning to selective attention. Nevertheless, within clinical psychology he is strongly identified with "behavior therapy" — a label he finds rather misleading — and with the more "hard-nosed" groups within the clinical research community.

One may well question whether the terms "behavioristic" and "cognitive" have a different meaning in clinical psychology, and whether the distinctions between them hold at all. There are, of course, behavior therapists who are genuine behaviorists in the mold of Skinner and Rachlin, as described earlier in this chapter. But they tend to be rare. More commonly, behavior therapists are willing to make some inferences about underlying states such as emotions, perhaps because these inferences are so strongly compelled by our common sense in a clinical situation. Ross maintains in this interview that he is willing to make clinical use of children's "self-statements" — statements that children can be taught to make to themselves in order to control their behavior — though he is reluctant to infer that those statements exist if they cannot be observed. Further, he is quite worried that clinical research may swing back to the largely intuitive and implicit methods that many clinicians learned in a psychodynamic context. As he says, he has found "the land of milk and honey," and is reluctant to be thrown back into the desert. He is not averse in principle to testing psychodynamic constructs, though he does believe that this is not the role of clinical researchers but of investigators into the fundamental domains of personality, motivation, and emotion.

Alan O. Ross is the author of several influential texts in clinical child psychology (1959, 1974, 1976). As professor in the clinical group at the State University of New York at Stony Brook, he has also taught a number of behavioral clinicians and clinical researchers. In 1982, the Clinical Psychology Division of the American Psychological Association gave him its Distinguished Scientific Contribution to Clinical Psychology Award.

Interview with Alan O. Ross

Q: How did you get started in psychology?

A: I have liked children for as long as I can remember. In my freshman year in college I decided that I wanted to be a child psychologist. I had a poor advisor — which is not unusual — who gave me a list of graduate schools to apply to, supposedly good places to become a child psychologist. I applied to Yale and was accepted in 1949, and the first day I arrived I was asked what field I wanted to concentrate in. I said child psychology, and was immediately told, "We don't have a child psychology program here." Clinical psychology seemed to be the closest thing, so on that basis, I decided to study clinical.

At the Yale Child Study Center there were at that time a group of psychoanalytically oriented people, Freudians from the *Psychoanalytic Study of the Child* annual series, very conservative and orthodox. I did some work over there. Käte Wolf, one of the psychoanalysts there, assigned me to observe a set of twins at a nursery school across the street from the Center, but it was methodologically primitive. There was no observational coding system. I was just supposed to write down whatever I saw. Then they tried to develop a coding system *post hoc*, to put my random notes into some shape, but that never came to anything.

Q: Were you doing research based on psychoanalytic ideas at that point?

A: The general notion was to develop a personality test based on Freudian notions of child development. But I don't know what they were looking for. They had some vague notions about social interactions and what we would nowadays call "attachment," but I don't think they could possibly have gotten anything from the way they went about it. "Just go there and watch those twins." I remember they had a huge roll of paper somewhere on the first floor of the building, spread out on the floor, and they were putting all kinds of symbols on the paper to take these linear observations, and by running the symbols in parallel lines, they thought they could detect correlations between what the two kids were doing. But soon, the whole research group disappeared.

This was the year after the famous book by Dollard and Miller appeared, *Personality and Psychotherapy* (1950), which tried to interpret psychoanalysis behaviorally, and John Dollard taught psychotherapy in our program. The emphasis was very much on using learning theory words instead of Freudian words. In those days it was considered a breakthrough.

Q: Was it a breakthrough in your mind as well?

A: Well, inasmuch as it links psychoanalysis with psychology. Up to that point, things were more compartmentalized. In fact, in those days, psychologists weren't doing anything in the area of therapy. Most clinical psychologists were only doing testing. It was really out of World War II, and the emphasis within the Veterans Administration on the rehabilitation of psychiatric casualties, that the need for more personnel arose, and psychologists got involved with doing therapy. Before that point, you had to go to some psychiatrist to learn therapy. So in that sense,

Dollard and Miller's work represented a big change: Psychological words being used in a therapeutic context.

I had come out of World War II with a reserve commission, and when the Korean War started, the Army was beginning to call back its reserve officers. I thought I might be about to be called back, so I chose to enter an Army program in which I could continue with graduate school, do my clinical psychology internship in an Army facility, then finish the dissertation, followed by three years of service with the Army. I did my internship at Walter Reed Hospital in Washington, D.C. I happened to run into the head of Psychological Services for the Army one day in the swimming pool locker room at Walter Reed. So after I did my dissertation at Yale, I was assigned by the Army to Texas, one of the two places where the Army had child psychology clinics for the children of dependents. I became a clinical child psychologist for the Army — in fact, after two weeks, I became the chief psychologist for the clinic. The third year they transferred me to Frankfurt — which happened to be the place where I had been born — and I became the chief psychologist for the child clinic at the Army hospital there.

Q: What was your perspective on psychology at that time?

A: Well, I quickly discovered that the things I needed to know, nobody had ever taught me. For example, how do you interview the mother of a dying child? Or, how do you work with a dying child? That was one of the more traumatic experiences I went through. It was a fly-by-the-seat-of-your-pants situation. I guess I used a kind of neo-Freudian ego-psychology approach.

In 1955, my last year in Texas, I was driving North for a Christmas vacation, my family was asleep in the back of the car, and during the drive I got the idea of writing a book, to be called *Clinical Child Psychology* — a new term at that time. When I got out of the Army, I got a job in a child guidance clinic in New Haven, and finished the book, which was ultimately called *The Practice of Clinical Child Psychology* (1959). It was a neo-Freudian, psychoanalytic approach. Less of an emphasis on unconscious processes than classical psychoanalysis, and more attention to conscious ego functions. There was a good deal of focus on some of the defenses against anxiety that people use. I gave a lot of attention to early childhood experiences, but also a good deal of focus on mother–child interactions. It was the old mother-blaming approach — one would look at what the mother did that caused the child to behave that way. Looking back at it now, I find that I focused on *behavior* much more than was the custom in those days.

In 1956 I got an offer from the Pittsburgh Child Guidance Center, so we moved to Pittsburgh. By that time I had become rather disillusioned about my personal effectiveness in doing therapy with children. Back then, the typical therapy with children was to have the psychologist be the therapist for the child, and a social worker would work with the mother. Typically, I would be working with the child — but I kept feeling that I was a baby-sitter, a glorified, overeducated baby-sitter, and that any movement in the case was always due to the social worker having managed to get the mother to change her way of dealing with the child. That bothered me. When I came to Pittsburgh, I began to spend less and less time doing actual therapy, I think partly because of this feeling of ineffectualness.

I was on the board of the American Orthopsychiatric Association, and was asked to be a discussant in a symposium on learning difficulties in children. The organizer was an old, old psychoanalyst from New York. A number of people gave papers, and among them was one by some people from the Judge Baker Guidance Clinic in Boston — in those days, and even now, a cathedral of Freudian orthodoxy. As discussant, I was given some of the papers ahead of time, and the Boston people were arguing that a boy's problem in reversing the letters b, p, d, and q was related to the fact that an upright or a dangling extension in a letter was causing the little boy to be threatened by castration anxiety. This was written in such a doctrinaire fashion that I said, "My God, aside from the fact that it's implausible, it is terribly old-fashioned." Then I said to myself, "Now look, I'm a psychologist with a Yale PhD, and at Yale the big thing was learning theory. This symposium is about learning. What do I as a psychologist have to say about this issue?"

The answer was, "I don't know." But the question took me to the library, where I came across the very early writings of Hans Eysenck (1960), a Britisher who was also born in Germany; and the first work out of South Africa by both Joseph Wolpe and Arnold Lazarus. By golly, here were people who were using learning theory principles and applying them in the clinical situation — in quite a different way than Miller and Dollard had tried. That, to me, was a very exciting discovery.

It also happened that the very first study on counterconditioning was done at the University of Pittsburgh by Peter Lang and David Lazovik (1963) on snake phobia. Some of the grad students who were doing a practicum and internship in our clinic had been influenced by Lang and Lazovik, and so together we started to read everything there was to read about what became known as "behavior therapy." And we started to try some of it out.

Q: Why was that idea so powerful at that time to you, do you think?

A: It came at a time of disequilibrium — I was becoming disenchanted with the things I had been doing. In addition, I was having a very unhappy time with the head of this clinic, who was a psychiatrist. Back then, there was still the political problem, whether psychologists were really entitled to do therapy. There was always this thing that ultimately the only *real* doctor is an MD. In some cases the psychiatrists had to supervise the psychologists in doing therapy. No matter how senior the psychologists were, some young punk psychiatrist had to supervise him. I guess there was this undercurrent of "looking for a thing of our own." With behavior therapy, *we* had something to teach *them* — if we cared to, and we didn't decide that they weren't entitled because they didn't have the right kind of training.

Q: At that time, was there disillusionment with the theoretical assumptions of the psychoanalytic perspective?

A: My overreaction to the study on supposed castration anxiety in letter-reversal was sort of paradigmatic of my overall feeling that much of that is garbage. In the day-to-day work with people the metapsychology of Freud doesn't really enter in at all. I had begun to believe it less and less.

Ilse, my wife, was trained as a social worker at Smith College in a very orthodox Freudian program. In talking about our cases with each other, we shared the feeling that none of that was particularly useful or applicable. When somebody comes in with marital difficulties, Freudian theory can tell you really very little. So Ilse's experience paralleled my own. I suspect that the Freudian theory was very much a superstructure. In the day-to-day clinical activities, it had little relevance. This is not to say that theory is all that relevant today, but I do think that we have a little more basis for deciding where to go and what to do by referring to principles. Psychoanalytic theory was irrelevant.

Q: Is there any difference between clinical relevance and the abstract truth or falsehood of a theory? That is, is it possible for a theory to be true, at least in part, and still not help you in the clinic?

A: There are two levels of Freudian theory to be distinguished. Roy Schafer has written about this in his book, *A New Language for Psychoanalysis* (1976). He makes the point that the Freudian contribution is largely metapsychology — that all of the personality structure and developmental facts can stand by themselves, but that they have very little day-to-day relevance in the clinical setting. He urges the psychoanalysis to pay more attention to the actions of people than to the implication of their actions to the metapsychology of Freud, which is really at a different level of discourse.

Some people are looking for a *rapprochement* between behavioral and psychodynamic streams. If one wants to look for that, this may be the place where some convergence is possible. If we both look at behavior, well, we may agree on something. I guess it's a little bit like driving a car. You can drive a car quite competently without understanding the principles of the internal combustion engine. And you can teach a person to drive a car without teaching him or her about the principles of the engine. So, we were driving cars, but we kept running into the ditch. Now, we needed a new roadmap. I think I'd better stop this metaphor.

Q: To get back to your history: What happened when you began to apply behavioral principles in your clinical work in Pittsburgh?

A: Well, lo and behold, when we started applying some of these principles, all of a sudden, it worked! In retrospect, of course, the reason why the social workers were the crucial people in creating change, and I with my baby-sitting was doing very little, was because they were modifying behavior relevant to the mother–child interaction! And by having the child play with fingerpaints, and shoot dart-guns, and otherwise "get things out of his or her system" all I got were a bunch of broken windows in my office. I got close to heart failure when one kid tried to challenge me to see whether I would really let her jump out of the window! I was supposed to be so permissive, you see.

So I was beginning to be a behavior therapist. Meanwhile I had written another book called *The Exceptional Child and the Family* (1964), which is interesting, because I wrote it at a time when my theoretical leanings were already switching. But in that book I still deal with anxiety and the defenses against anxiety. Today, I would have enough to draw on so that I could probably do a book about what one does for people who have a very real problem — like a child born with a serious handicap — and how one helps them cope with this.

Toward the end of my Pittsburgh period the book called *Psychological Disorders of Children: Behavioral Approach to Theory, Research, and Therapy* (1974) had its beginnings. Up until that point I had been a full-time clinician, but I had always taught one course per semester at a university, and was always academically inclined. So in the mid '60s, when many universities started enlarging their faculties, and new universities were founded, there was a historically unique moment when senior clinical people were needed to staff these faculties. So some of us who had been in the clinical world for some 15 years could move laterally into tenured full professorships.

I was clearly interested in a clinical program with a behavioral orientation — hence, Stony Brook. This department's clinicians were basically all behavior therapists. And we represented a new orthodoxy: Nothing that was not derivable from laboratory psychology had any place in clinical psychology. And we prided ourselves on our purity, and very quickly developed a reputation for a monolithic behavioral program. I guess in some respects, the new convert is always the most doctrinaire. For obvious reasons, most of us had been trained in neo-Freudian therapy. Over the years since then, there has been a considerable blurring of the lines and I am unhappy about that.

One of the questions I had always asked myself and others is, To what extent is our background in the more psychodynamic tradition a prerequisite for being "good clinicians," regardless of orientation? The psychodynamic people would focus so much on the finer nuances of the interaction between the clinician and the client — can that sensitivity to nuances be taught in the context of teaching behavior therapy? Psychodynamic teachers would constantly ask, in supervising therapy, How did you *feel* when your client said that? Or, How do you think the client felt? At least in the beginning, when we were teaching our students to implement a certain reinforcement schedule, we'd be damned if we were going to ask about people's feelings! But when I look at some of these second-generation people who were taught only by us, they have turned out to be very good clinicians.

I still feel that we have not yet fully extracted everything there is to be mined from laboratory-derived psychological principles. To do what some of my colleagues are doing, that is, to turn to the Gestalt psychologists, or back to the psychodynamic tradition at this point, seems to me premature. In that respect I'm unhappy with the tendency to merge psychodynamic and behavioral perspectives again. There are whole areas of experimental psychology, such as the study of perception, which must have relevance to clinical work. We ought to mine that lode before trying other things.

It seems to me that clinical psychology is the application of scientific psychology. Psychology is the basic science for the mental health professions. In engineering, physics is the basic science; in the medical specialties, anatomy, physiology, biochemistry, and so forth, are the basic sciences. Our problem in the mental health professions has always been that we have been operating in the absence of a basic science. I don't think that any applied field can go very far without a basic science, or divorced from its basic science. It takes a lot of rather imaginative extrapolation to go and talk to the person in the perception lab, learn to read his or her literature, and make the connection to the clinic. I see clinical psychology as being in the critical position of having to build the bridges between the basic science of psychology and the mental health applications. This is the reason that I am sorry to see the development of clinical psychology as a strictly applied profession. If you divorce your training program from the psychological basics, then you lose the unique role of carrying basic research into the clinic and *vice versa*.

I continue to be sold on the "scientist–practitioner" model for clinical psychology. Being both scientist and practitioner seems to be very difficult for many people. There seems to be a temperamental problem. The temperamental qualities for being a practicing clinician may be quite different from the temperamental qualities that are required for doing hard-nosed laboratory research. Only relatively few people can do both, and I would like to select graduate students on the basis of their being able to do that, not on the basis of how many patients they will be able to cure in a lifetime. That's also important, but I think that there is a unique mission for clinical psychology.

Q: Why do you think that clinical psychologists have focused so much on bringing learning psychology into the clinic, compared with other kinds of basic psychology?

A: Well, the psychodynamic tradition greatly emphasizes the role of early learning in life, so there was a natural interest in learning. If Freud had been a phenomenologist, interested in how people perceive their world, then clinical psychologists might have been more interested in the perception area. But in fact, the question of how you acquire disorders can easily be viewed in terms of learning, and no psychoanalyst would deny the role of learning. How could you deny that?

There may also be similarities in the language. Joseph Wolpe, who is a psychiatrist from an analytic background, discovered the early Masserman (1943) studies on "neurotic" cats. Masserman had tried to create a clinical symptom in an animal analogue situation, and Wolpe started to develop his early thinking out of that. In my own development, the marriage between Neal Miller's learning approach and John Dollard's psychoanalytic approach may have played a role. Somewhere in the mid-'30s the National Science Foundation gave grants to a number of young, promising psychologists to go to Europe to be psychoanalyzed. Neal Miller was one of them. Robert Sears was another one (Sears, 1943). There was a book that came out of that program called *Psychoanalysis as Seen by Analyzed Psychologists* (Allport, 1953). The fact that Neal Miller went into this must have had something to do with his view of the relationship between his mentor, Clark Hull, and his analyst, Hans Sachs. So the answer to your question, Why do clinical psychologists look at learning theory? has to do with the experiences of a few, key individuals.

When Neal Miller came back from his analysis in Europe, he ran some experiments on the dynamic notion of displacement — rats who were shocked would begin to attack a doll or each other — and conflict — where rats who were shocked in a red box but not in a white box would develop some sort of conflict when the white box was made to more closely resemble the red box. At the same time, independently of Dollard and Miller, O. H. Mowrer came out with his own book bridging learning theory and psychoanalysis (Mowrer, 1950).

Q: What about drive reduction? Is there any relationship between Hull's drive reduction as the mechanism of reinforcement, and Freud's reduction in libido as the mechanism of pleasure?

A: I've often speculated whether the rejection of psychoanalysis by American learning theory of the '40s and '50s was due to a semantic problem. They had no use at all for Freudian stuff. Psychoanalysis could not be learned any place within a regular university psychology department. You had to go off somewhere else. I think that that rejection had to do, at least in part, with a semantic problem. The American psychology of Hull, *et al.* was very interested in drive. Freud had used the German word *Trieb* to describe the motivating force of the libido, and this word was unfortunately translated as "instinct." Now, American psychology had just come through a bad case of the instincts with the McDougall approach, where everything to be explained was explained by making up a new instinct (McDougall, 1923). So the notion of "instinct" was rejected very strongly, and the rejection of instinct about the late '20s and early '30s did make them look very kindly upon this foreigner Freud, who came just about then with his theory about "instinct"! If A. A. Brill, the translator, had used the word "drive" for *Trieb*, which is a much better translation, it might have been much more acceptable.

Q: Today a number of younger psychologists who were not trained as analysts are looking at the old Freudian literature, and they are beginning to see Freud as a cognitive psychologist — he talked about what it is that people do with information; he talked about underlying constructs that control observable things such as slips of the tongue and forgetting, and the like. Some of these psychologists are trying to build a bridge between mainstream academic work and at least some psychodynamic ideas (*e.g.*, Wachtel, 1977). Have you kept up with any of this?

A: No, I have not. I guess, as I said earlier, that when you are a convert to a new religion you reject any part of the old religion.

Q: You seem concerned that things will swing back to the old, very empirically sloppy ways of doing things. In the cognitive approach within experimental psychology, I do not think that people feel that they have become empirically sloppy. Rather, they might argue, they have the best of both worlds: In some sense they are as empirically tight and responsible as good behavioristic researchers, but they can also be theoretically imaginative.

A: But clinical psychology would then need to evolve its own theoretical structure, because it seems to me that if one construes psychology as the basic science for the applied field of clinical psychology, we ought to base ourselves on the developments within that basic science. The trouble is partly one of impatience. Pavlov and Skinner did their work before the early behavior therapists started their applications. In what is coming to be called "cognitive behavior therapy"—an interesting combination of words—the application is beginning to run ahead of the basic science.

Because of my skepticism about cognitive behavior therapy, I went to a two-day meeting on it; I wanted to see whether what I thought was happening was really true. And Edward Craighead, who is becoming one of the principal people in this field, gave a paper in which he frankly admitted that the cognitive behavior therapists are "looking for conceptual frameworks." Well, the conceptual framework for Joseph Wolpe was provided by Ivan Pavlov! Cognitive behavior therapy is an application in search of a conceptualization. And to my chagrin, the conceptualization Craighead proposed was the old attitude-change framework from social psychology, and he paraded out the old Carl Hovland studies on persuasive communication (Hovland, Janis, & Kelley, 1959). Now, having been at Yale when Hovland was working on that, I knew that even Hovland, toward the end of his life, thought that was a pretty bankrupt direction to go in. Their findings were very unreliable, and pretty meaningless. The behavioral changes they were trying to induce by their persuasive communications were largely changes in paper-and-pencil questionnaires. So this seemed like a pretty sorry conceptual framework for clinical psychologists.

It seems to me that there are cognitive psychologists nowadays doing important work, and it is there that people doing "cognitive behavior therapy" should be looking for their conceptual framework. And if there is no framework there yet, then maybe the whole thing is premature. That's what I mean by impatience.

When one gets away from one's basic science, one very quickly gets lost in all kinds of very fancy fantasies that have no foundation other than the clinical experience. And we've *been there*, you see. That is my concern. I have personally found that to be a rather frustrating existence. I have found "the land of milk and honey," and I hate to be dragged back out into the desert.

We have an outstanding training program here at Stony Brook, and particularly from the standpoint of a training program, you can very quickly, within one student generation—which is no more than eight years—turn the whole field around again into borrowing notions here and there and then later on looking for conceptual frameworks into which to order them. I would rather have us say in certain instances, "I don't know what to do about this clinical problem." For instance: A college student comes in with what he calls an "identity crisis." Well, I don't know what to do for an identity crisis, and I'd rather say to this student, "I don't know how to help you, go to the applied philosophy department, and see what they can do for you," than have me be forced to create *ad hoc* procedures for which I don't have a foundation in empirical fact.

Q: A lot of clinical psychologists seem to view behaviorism *as* experimental psychology, as exhausting the meaning of "experimental psychology." Would you be equally comfortable borrowing from cognitive psychology, which does not maintain the same assumptions as behaviorism?

A: I think the term "behavior therapy" was a very unfortunate invention, because it does imply that we can only use "behavioral" principles, that is, essentially principles from operant conditioning. I wish one could reinvent the term "applied psychology." I wish one could equate clinical psychology with the idea that this is psychology applied—*all* of psychology.

I have written a book on learning disabilities (1976), because I wanted to see if I could build a bridge from the psychological laboratory to another applied problem—namely, how to treat children with learning disabilities. And there is very little in operant and Pavlovian conditioning that has any bearing on a child's language disability. You can reinforce these children for reading the right word, but how do you get them to read the right word in the first place? For that I had to look at the experimental field of perception. After all, reading is a perceptual function to some extent.

And so I started to dig into the literature in that area, and found that the bridge had already been built for me by Eleanor Gibson (*e.g.*, 1969), who comes out of the perception laboratory and applies that to the problem of reading acquisition. It wasn't very hard for me then to take it one step further, and apply it to *difficulties* in the acquisition of reading.

Or take the issue of selective attention—if you want to perceive something, you have to attend selectively to a part of the stimulus field, and that becomes relevant to understanding reading disabilities also. It is possible to go back to basic psychology and bring it to bear on problems to go back to basic psychology and bring it to bear on problems in the clinic. But you have to have the patience and the stamina to learn a new language — I didn't know what the heck they were talking about when I first looked into the perception literature. But unless we who are interested in the clinical phenomena do it, nobody will. The perceptual psychologist is not likely to make that translation for us.

Of course it goes beyond just perception. In social psychology, attribution theory has many logical links into the clinic. In experimental child psychology there is a gold mine for me as a clinical child psychologist. So, yes, unfortunately we call it "behavior therapy." But I'd much prefer to redefine that as "the application of principles of psychology derived from empirical laboratory studies to the clinical situation." The other part of it, of course, is an ongoing, skeptical, principled hypothesis-testing approach to these applications. That, for me, is behavior therapy. I think we have just opened one seam in that mine of basic psychology, largely the learning theory stuff, and there is so much more.

Q: Then you would not consider yourself as firmly committed to the classical assumptions of behaviorism?

A: No, I'm not.

Q: Even though you are a "behavior therapist" by this strange quirk of terminology.

A: Right. That would be far too narrow, far too limiting for understanding the real clinical problems. Behavioral ideas have brought us a long way, but there continues to be many issues where you can't help in dealing with broader concerns. When I supervised a student a couple of days ago, the student wanted to shift from seeing a certain client every other week to seeing the client every week, for some superficial reason having to do with her schedule. And I had to ask, "How is this client going to perceive this?" "How is the client going to interpret your saying, 'I want to see you every week'?" Well, I don't have any operant words for this, but nonetheless it is an important question to ask. I suspect that the client might think to himself, "My God, she must think that I am a lot sicker than I think I am!" That is an important thing to be aware of. So I do need to go beyond the narrow metatheoretical issues of radical behaviorism.

Q: Are you an unusual behavior therapist in that respect?

A: Well, among my colleagues here at Stony Brook, I'm an oddball in the sense that I'm probably one of the more orthodox people. This is probably because I'm a child psychologist — the most operant people in our clinical group are the child psychologists. The child happens to be — pardon the expression — "an organism" that one can much more readily manipulate with contingent reinforcement than one can a great big adult. To get a mother to put a child on some kind of a contingent reinforcement schedule and to reward certain behavior is relatively easy. That's why I continue to be so sold on this approach. But if I have to answer the question, "Well, how do you get the mother to do what you want her to do?" then I have to depart a little bit from operant principles.

Q: How do the undergraduates view your psychology department?

A: They think we are a behavioral department. Of course, often I don't know what they mean by "behavioral." I suspect that what they mean is that this is not a humanistic department of psychology, and what they are learning in psychology is not what they thought they ought to be learning. Somehow the behavioral orientation of our clinical program, for which our department first became known, has created a "halo" for everybody else.

Precisely where do I stand? Well, my book *Psychological Disorders of Children* (1974), which was the first behavioral child clinical text, has just been revised for the second edition, and I have just seen the reviewers' comments on my last draft. One of the reviewers — it's fun to guess who it might be — I suspect I know who it is, but I won't tell you — seems to be in the forefront of cognitive behavior therapy. He takes me to task for not paying more attention to this development. I do pay attention to the Meichenbaum and Goodman (1971) stuff where children have learned to say something to themselves in order to gain some self-control, which, to me, is still pretty behavioral. But I refuse to speculate on whether they have thoughts inside their heads that parallel these empirical statements. Yet I can still apply this approach. But clearly, from the standpoint of that particular reviewer, I am expressing an "orthodox" point of view. And I'm not going to be very much influenced to change the manuscript in order to accommodate this person and his criticisms. I think I will let him write his own book.

Q: What does the phrase "cognitive behavior therapy" mean to you?

A: I guess originally it meant to me some derivative of this Meichenbaum and Goodman (1971) work on training children to talk to themselves to help them gain self-control. Of course, we've also managed to make room in our bed for the likes of Albert Ellis (*e.g.*, 1962) and his "rational–emotive" system, which fits in very nicely, but is a totally atheoretical product that sprang out of somebody's clinical experience. And I think if you take Ellis's work apart, in that approach you really have people restructuring their perceptions of things. We teach them to say to themselves, "This is *not* a catastrophe, it's just a pain in the neck!" One could probably find laboratory analogues where relabeling an object leads to its being perceived in a different way. But I would like to have seen the direction go from the laboratory to the application, instead of the application now going around to find a framework to which it might be related. So "cognitive behavior therapy" means getting people to think differently about themselves and their lives. But how one does that, and how one knows whether it has succeeded, those questions seem to me to be still anchored in observables. But that, I suspect, is not different from any laboratory cognitive psychologists, who also deal in observables, I believe.

Further, I am willing to speculate about mediating processes. I'm not a Howard Rachlin, although I find his approach a very stimulating and challenging way to try to do things. One of the most stimulating things I ever heard in connection with cognitive behavior therapy was this debate between Michael Mahoney and Howard Rachlin. I don't know who came out second best on that one.

Q: Most cognitive psychologists have not really addressed the emotions and the issue of emotional conflicts. That seems to be most relevant to the clinic. Why can't clinical psychologists go ahead and do their own "cognitive-style" research into these issues, and thus create their own "basic science" as a foundation for clinical work?

A: I guess the answer is, that they certainly could. The question to me is not, "Why couldn't they?" but "Why don't they?" It's a curious labeling problem. When Richard Lazarus, who was trained as a clinical psychologist, goes and performs research on stress and emotions, he is no longer considered a clinical psychologist. So, what defines a clinical psychologist? The answer may be in the labels people carry when they do certain things.

Q: If we consider research on personality, it seems that this kind of research is currently not closely associated with clinical psychology. But that is a very curious state of affairs — shouldn't clinical researchers work more closely with issues relating to personality?

A: Historically, different disciplines have their ups and downs. I think the study of personality is again on its way up, and there are clinical psychologists, such as Albert Bandura and Walter Mischel, who are in the forefront of this movement.

Q: In a sense, the label "personality" has become unpopular, but the issues have not gone away. Lots of questions regarding the emotions remain to be answered.

A: Clearly, you can think of the issues in terms of a triangle: the behavior, the cognitions, and the emotions. I think that to deal adequately with emotion, you would have to work very closely with a physiologist or biochemist to do various biochemical assays. I am not satisfied with testing emotions via a paper-and-pencil test or via very indirect measures of autonomic arousal, such as GSR and heart rate. I would like to do something like Schachter and Singer (1962), where you inject some biochemical factor in combination with psychological manipulations. Maybe the problem is the way our sciences are divided into disciplines — because the physiologists are across the street some place. I also wonder to what extent our recent recognition of ethical constraints makes it more difficult to do meaningful research on emotions. For one thing, I suspect you would have to do a lot of deception. For another, you often have to put things inside the body. So creative investigators may just shy away from those difficult topics.

Q: So you are saying that physiological measures of emotions are more important than physiological measures of other variables, such as beliefs or thoughts?

A: Actually, it is interesting that you make that point. I really believe, in general, that you can have a psychology without this reduction to physiology. And I wonder why, when you mention emotion, that I immediately start becoming a reductionist. I find it difficult to conceptualize emotions without thinking of things happening inside my body.

Q: As a therapist, if somebody comes in and says, "I'm extremely anxious," you treat that as an emotion, a cluster of things, not just the visible behaviors such as trembling or breathing quickly, and so on.

A: But you know, the way we deal with it in behavior therapy turns out to take a very direct detour through the body. I will relax the client's body in order to help his or her anxiety. That's where the behavior–cognition–emotion triangle comes in. If a person says I am anxious *about such-and-such* you can then start to work on their cognitions about such-and-such, and help them to redefine it and thereby remove it from whatever is making the client anxious. In children with school phobia, the treatment is to walk the children closer and closer to the school, and to reinforce their behavior of coming closer to the school. That's getting at it from the behavioral plane. In clinical work it is nice to keep the three points of the triangle in mind. We tend, I suppose, to take only one part of the triangle and focus on that.

Of course, some clinicians have in fact done research on anxiety, having to do with the fears and the phobias. I suppose this is where the arbitrary and artificial division between basic and applied research comes in. I believe that ultimately, knowledge will be advanced only by "basic research." Applications, of course, can be improved greatly by applied research. So when you say why don't clinical psychologists do their own research on emotions, that's the key: When clinicians do basic research on emotions, we no longer call them clinical psychologists! But as long as they do applied research on emotions, we call them clinical psychologists.

Q: Clinical psychologists seem to use the word "cognition" differently from cognitive psychologists. To clinicians, "cognition" seems to mean "thought," or "more-or-less conscious intellectual functions." Cognitive psychologists, however, mean by cognition either information processing, which includes essentially everything the nervous system does, including thinking, unconscious processing, emotion, perception, and the like; or they mean a kind of metatheoretical point of view on psychology that permits us to postulate unobservables as long as we can tie them down to observable measures. If that is true, then a cognitive clinician could deal with almost anything that people ordinarily talk about in a sloppy way — feelings, intuitions, and so forth — provided that they could tighten up the sloppy way of talking about it by using very specific operational and theoretical definitions. So we could take common sense and make it scientifically testable. Would that be acceptable from your point of view?

A: I suspect that I would accept that if it were 20 years from now. The reason is that clinical psychology needs to get that psychodynamic sloppiness out of its system. And when we have a generation of truly rigorous operationalizers, then I would be more comfortable to permit that. Otherwise, and what I see happening now, is that that approach now gives permission to go back into the psychodynamic thing. And the psychodynamic people are out there all the time, like Wachtel (1977), just hoping to connect with behavior therapists. There is a great deal of seduction in this, because it is far more intellectually interesting to operate in that conceptual framework than in a strict operationally defined way. I think the clinical situation, by and large, invites this kind of thinking, because you are constantly trying to figure out what this person is thinking. As a human being, you can hardly avoid that. In one way, I would like to see cognitive psychology itself establish its own rigor more visibly, and on the other hand, I would like us to get over our bad case of psychodynamic flu.

Q: What is the nature of the psychodynamic sloppiness you refer to?

A: It is the untestability of its constructs and the lack of falsifiability. From the view of traditional Western science, it is an unscientific frame of reference.

Q: So if it could be made testable, would that be acceptable to you?

A: You would have to reformulate it, but if it can be done, it would be all right. There is a deep source of ambiguity in their approach to observables. If you are not showing anger, well, you must be repressing it. If you are not doing whatever the therapist expects you to do, you must be showing resistance. So, whichever way the facts come out, they can explain it.

Q: One idea that obviously has been around long before Freud is that people sometimes deceive themselves, or that they might harbor two contradictory beliefs. Could that be incorporated into scientific psychology?

A: I suspect that is where Roy Schafer (1976) is going, with his idea of separating out the metapsychology and focusing more on the operationalizable notions. That is a welcome development, and I will observe it with interest.

Q: You seem to be saying that clinical psychology should be purged of some of the bad old sloppy thinking before it is ready to start dealing with whatever might be useful in the old approach. I can see your concern: In experimental psychology, behavioral thinking has been around since the 1920s, whereas in clinical work, the behavioristic trend is only about 20 years old. On the other hand, clinicians seem to have an easier time defining the criteria of success, whereas experimentalists are never quite sure when they have really succeeded in dealing with a certain problem.

A: Well, even in the clinic, the criteria of success are not so obvious. In fact, this is one of the attractions of behavior therapy. When you define the problem as some sort of behavior, if you remove the problematic behavior, you've succeeded. But if the problem resides in a person's "belief system," then I'm not at all sure when I can know that his belief system has changed. If the client says, "I no longer believe that my mother is a witch," how can I accept that? How can I be sure that he won't go home tomorrow and try to burn her at a stake?

The problem is that we don't have the measures to be sure what the belief is. This is where psychoanalysts can go on for five years doing psychoanalysis with a patient; because the goal is ill-defined you don't know when you have reached it.

Q: If there is any problem in the clinic that you think general academic psychology should work on, what do you think it would be?

A: To make thoughts visible — but I don't think it is for me to set up your agenda. You experimental psychologists investigate whatever you are interested in, and if there is a spinoff for me, I shall be very happy. Sometimes in science, if you set up targeted questions in the absence of the basic science foundations, you just steer people in the wrong direction. I suppose we could highlight problems that are not solved for people to look at if they are shopping around for interesting research problems. Maybe we need more articles in the *American Psychologist* to bring to the attention of the academic world some of the clinical issues for which we really could use more understanding.

4

The Cognitive Revolution:
The Rise of a Theoretical Psychology

Science is built of facts the way a house is built of bricks, but an accumulation of facts is no more science than a pile of bricks is a house.
— HENRI POINCARÉ (1913, p. 12)

Between 1955 and 1965 a quiet revolution in thought took place in scientific psychology. Even before 1955 there were many hints of this development, and much remained to be done after 1965, but for most opinion leaders in the field, this decade was crucial. The cognitive revolution was not a spectacular one — no one stormed the Winter Palace, not even metaphorically. Public fireworks were rare. Furthermore, unlike Watson's revolution, the cognitive shift was not self-conscious. No one announced its existence until long after the fact. Experimental psychologists did not set out to make a revolution. Many of them were surprised to find themselves breaking the prohibitions of the behavioristic metatheory, and did so reluctantly. The understanding of the cognitive revolution followed the event; it only emerged slowly, and even now there are some who will not agree that any "revolution" took place. Only now, in the 1980s, are the historical retrospectives being written (*e.g.*, Bruner, 1984; Kendler, 1979).

Most of the changes occurred silently. There was one major public controversy following Noam Chomsky's critical review of B. F. Skinner's work *Verbal Behavior* (Skinner, 1957; Chomsky, 1959); and some years later, public debates took place between these two men. But in 1957, Chomsky was still a little-known linguist, and Skinner, a respected but atypical behaviorist. Most of the milestone experiments in the cognitive revolution were published without fanfare, and changes were occurring even as their profundity was being denied. Many such changes seemed to proceed by a process of euphemism. Psychologists did not speak of "mental representation" at first, but of "memory"; not of "consciousness," but of "selective attention"; not of "the organization of meaning," but of "semantic features." In each case, the modest euphemistic term was defined operationally, by precise and reliable experiments, and the results were interpreted within narrow theoretical limits. But as the new ideas gained momentum, theoretical terms such as "mental representation," "meaning organization," and recently, even "consciousness" burst the boundaries of the experimental situations in which they were first defined. Soon, all these terms were extended far beyond any single experimental model or technique.

"Protocognitive" Psychologies

We have noted that the psychology of common sense requires a cognitive metatheory; in this respect the cognitive approach is hardly new. Most formal schools of psychology are metatheoretically cognitive, and their existence may have helped to bring about the cognitive revolution. This includes psychoanalysis and the various schools that derive from it; Gestalt psychology and its intellectual descendants in the study of perception; and the whole field of social psychology, started in America by the refugee Gestalt psychologist Kurt Lewin. The applied field of psychometrics began much earlier, and produced numerous tests of intelligence, aptitude, and personality characteristics while coexisting uneasily with academic behaviorism. To most behaviorists, such measures had no scientific standing, because the very constructs "intelligence" and "personality" were undefined. Among the cognitive viewpoints in Europe we must mention Jean Piaget's epochal studies of child development, the work of Selz and de Groot on problem solving and chess playing, and Bartlett's studies of memory. In the Soviet Union, Pavlov's followers, such as Y. Sokolov, began increasingly to talk in cognitive terms, and the earlier work of Y. Vygotsky and A. R. Luria has a distinctly cognitive flavor. In the 1940s Soviet cybernetics began to keep pace with Western developments, and psychologists such as N. Bernstein created a cognitive movement using cybernetic concepts. But there was astonishingly little communication between American and European psychologists, who were separated not only by language barriers, but by formidable differences in outlook. Even when European schools of psychology were transplanted to America, there was remarkably little visible communication.

In this connection we may also mention *humanistic psychology*, an American school of thought that has affected clinical practice, self-help techniques, and what may be called "recreational psychology." In all these aspects of popular psychology humanistic thought has been very influential. Humanism was originally conceived as a response to the pessimism of Freudian thought, and to the mechanistic quality of academic behaviorism (*e.g.*, Maslow, 1962; Rogers, 1970). Its orientation has been both optimistic and antimechanistic. On the other hand, though a native American product, its influence on American scientific psychology has been nearly zero. Humanism has flowered outside of academic psychology, but scientific psychologists in their official roles tend to see it as unscientific, and therefore outside of their sphere. What influence humanism has exerted has been very indirect (see, for example, the interview with Ulric Neisser in Chapter 6).

The Triumph of Behaviorism in the Clinic

Human history seems to abound with irony and paradox, and the history of psychology is no exception. One of the ironies is that between 1955 and 1965, just as cognitive psychology was emerging from the remnants of behaviorism in experimental psychology, exactly the *opposite* was happening in the applied area of clinical psychology! Psychopathology was largely neglected during the first three decades of behaviorism (though John B. Watson and others performed pioneering studies on phobias and habit-control). Instead, clinical work was dominated by psychodynamic theories, which presuppose a cognitive metatheory, postulating invisible entities such as wishes, fears, conflicts, and the like. As discussed in Chapter 2, during the 1950s behavioristic psychologists began to make a decisive move toward clinical psychology (Kazdin, 1978). These behavioristic clinicians were deeply critical of psychoanalysis. In arguing against psychodynamics, they made use of the classic behavioristic arguments against mentalism, concluding that psychodynamics was inherently unscientific. Like their forebears in experimental psychology, clinical behaviorists were determined to eliminate unobservable constructs (*e.g.*, Ullmann & Krasner, 1969).

The spread of behaviorism into the clinic had little effect on the "pure science" issues discussed in experimental psychology. Experimentalists continued to shift to a cognitive perspective, undeterred by the fact that their clinical colleagues next door were shifting the opposite way. For better or worse, experimental psychology is largely insulated from applied fields—the direction of influence tends to go from pure to applied psychology, rather than the reverse.

Today, the cognitive shift in experimental psychology seems to be reaching the clinical world, but in greatly modified form (*e.g.*, Mahoney & Arnkoff, 1978). We cannot go into these very interesting and important historical developments, other than to note their existence. Thus we return to the story of the revolution in mainstream experimental psychology.

The Role of the Theoretical Imagination

We have defined the cognitive metatheory as a belief that psychology studies behavior in order to infer unobservable explanatory constructs, such as "memory," "attention," and "meaning." A psychological theory is a network of such constructs, serving to summarize empirical observations, predict new results, and explain them in an economical way. Like behaviorism, cognitive psychology is primarily a metatheory for psychology, one that simply *encourages psychologists to do theory, relatively free from prior philosophical constraints.* No longer is it thought necessary for theoretical constructs to resemble visible stimuli and responses, or to adhere to rigid conceptions of theoretical parsimony. As simple as this change may seem, its impact on the practice of scientific psychology is pervasive. Cognitive psychologists do not assume that learning is necessarily a matter of associating observable stimuli and responses, that conditioning is a fundamental form of learning, or that inherited factors are of minor importance in human action and experience. Nor do they assume that consciousness is merely a byproduct of the ordinary, physical functioning of the nervous system. One of our interview participants calls this "the liberation"—permission to use one's theoretical imagination free from prior constraints.

It is not unscientific to speak of the "theoretical imagination." In one way or another, scientists have always employed imagination to account for their observations: In Dalton's time, the atom was almost entirely an imaginative construction; Darwin imagined the continuity of descent between the species; and Newton had to imagine gravitational forces emanating from the sun to keep the planets in orbit. A witty remark attributed to the prominent physicist Richard Feynman makes this point about the centripetal forces of Newton's theory: "Before Newton," Feynman has reportedly said, "people thought that angels were pushing the planets in orbit around the sun. But now we know that the angels are pushing the planets *into* the sun!" In their way, the centripetal force vectors of Newtonian physics are as imaginary as angels; but they are scientifically useful and perhaps indispensable (Jammer, 1957).

Indeed, behaviorism itself was fundamentally an act of theoretical imagination, one that had psychologists for 50 years pretending in their professional lives that goals, memories, and images did not exist, even while they freely used commonsense psychology in their private lives. Behaviorism was a *metatheoretical* act of imagination, but one that prohibited the use of the theoretical imagination in the actual practice of scientific psychology. By the same token cognitive psychology is an act of imagination that permits wider latitude in imagining explanations for behavior. Whereas behaviorism taught psychologists to respect public empirical evidence, the cognitive metatheory may make it possible to do good theory. This involves a learning process, of course. The tools needed to do theory do not spring up instantly, any more than the tools for experimentation did after Watson's revolution. A new metatheory can clear the way, but the new opening must be exploited by hard, thoughtful work.

Consider what would happen if scientists were not allowed to use their imagination freely — if they could not imagine that some undiscovered fact were true, or that some inconvenient observation were false. Galileo's work is an interesting case in point, given that he has often been considered a model of the hardheaded empiricist, who presented plain facts that his theological opponents literally refused to see. Some modern historians of science view Galileo's contribution somewhat differently. Apparently, Galileo's facts were not quite as solid as subsequent generations have thought, and his opponents themselves could cite numerous facts in their favor (Feyerabend, 1975, and others). Many of Galileo's arguments for the Copernican solar system were actually quite false, but his overall conclusions were correct. In this light it becomes clear that Galileo's claims really involved a daring act of imagination. Conclusive empirical evidence in his favor only became available more than a century after his death.

Now imagine what might have happened if tough-minded experimentalists had dominated the physics of Galileo's time in the same way that behaviorists dominated psychology in this century. Consider Galileo's famous (though probably apocryphal) experiment of simultaneously dropping a musket ball and a cannon ball from the Leaning Tower of Pisa, and noting that both objects hit the ground at the same moment. This presumably showed that the mass of an object does not affect its rate of acceleration in gravity. But a good experimentalist would quickly refute Galileo's demonstration by dropping from the Tower a feather, a hot-air balloon, and a musket ball. Now, which would fall fastest? Obviously, the feather would encounter more resistance from the air than the musket ball, while the balloon would actually float upward! Is this an unfair experiment, because it neglects the effects of air resistance and buoyancy? Not really; even to conceive of air, and of its possible absence, required in Galileo's time a profound act of imagination, a leap that scientists would not be able to justify until several centuries later. The whole point of Galileo's experiment depends on our imaginative ability to pretend that air does not exist, and that the effect of gravity can be considered separately from the effects of air.

Without this imaginative leap, an entire experimental profession might have developed, collecting a multitude of facts about falling objects. Good experimentalists would not stop with testing feathers and hot-air balloons. As conscientious believers in empirical fact, they would perforce investigate other factors: the wind-speed and ambient temperature, the weather and the time of day. Soon they would have collected enormous numbers of facts, but without gaining any *insight* into the problem of gravity. Facts alone do not make a science; indeed, thoughtless fact-gathering can interfere with the work of science. It has now become commonplace in the philosophy of science to say that "the facts" cannot even be perceived *as* facts without some theoretical framework, explicit or not (*e.g.*, Kuhn, 1962, 1970; Lakatoš & Musgrave, 1970).

The Computational Metaphor and the Role of Experiments

But why were psychologists granted more theoretical freedom in the 1960s and '70s, when a few decades before, a psychologist such as Tolman was considered unscientific for talking about "purpose" and "cognitive maps"? Answers to this question must ultimately come from our interviews, but we may suggest two general reasons for the liberalization of theory: First, developments associated with the theory of computation led some psychologists and neurophysiologists to view the nervous system as a kind of information processor, a theoretical metaphor that made it legitimate to think in terms of goals and representations. Second, the experimental methodology developed by behavioristic psychologists provided proof-procedures whereby nascent cognitive thinkers could make compelling arguments for ideas such as "attention," "imagery," "mental representation," "unconscious inference," "goals," and the like. Computational theory provided a guarantee that the theoretical imagination did not exceed the bounds of physical possibility, and experimental demonstrations made a compelling case that computational ideas could apply to human beings.

The cognitive revolution took place in many places at the same time, and involved a number of areas, including memory, language, imagery, and attention. In each case, careful and reliable experiments forced psychologists to adopt a more theoretical stance than was permitted before. This chapter sketches these transformations in several areas, including mental representation, attention and consciousness, the problem of serial order, and the problem of inferring underlying structure and process. Space permits no more than a sketch of these events, however. More details may be found in any modern textbook of perception, human learning, or cognitive psychology, such as Norman (1976), Bransford (1979), Anderson (1980), and especially Neisser (1967). Other important perspectives on this historic metamorphosis are presented by Posner and Shulman (1979), Newell and Simon (1972), and Bruner (1984).

Behaviorists in general did not contest these developments publically, perhaps because they emerged clothed in the guise of simple, unadorned facts, using the accepted proof-procedures that the behaviorists themselves had pioneered. This chapter discusses only a few instances of public controversy. Finally, the chapter briefly traces the careers of five psychologists who figured prominently in the revolution: Charles E. Osgood, a neobehaviorist who tried to extend Hullian theory to encompass the concept of linguistic "meaning"; James J. Jenkins, who at first tried to pursue a behavioristic approach to verbal learning, failed, and then became a pioneer in exploring cognitive alternatives; George A. Miller, the most visible leader of the cognitive revolution, who exerted great influence by always staying one step ahead of the rest of the field; Jerome S. Bruner, less concerned with communicating with other experimental psychologists, and whose work was consistently far ahead of the rest; and Herbert A. Simon, whose work of the 1950s is only now entering the mainstream of cognitive psychology. In terms of their adherence to the behavioristic perspective, these men represent a spectrum ranging from the most conservative (Osgood) to the least (Simon), with the others ranged in between. Of course, "conservative" does not mean either "good" or "bad" in science; it is the interaction between adventurous souls and their hard-nosed colleagues that provides scientific work with the necessary mixture of daring and certainty, and a successful science will encourage the whole spectrum of scientists to thrive.

The Computational Rationale for the Cognitive Revolution

The persuasive mechanism of the cognitive shift was empirical rather than theoretical. Psychologists used experimental evidence to persuade themselves and each other of the need for change. It may seem peculiar, therefore, to start the story of this historic transformation with issues usually associated with the foundations of computer science. Nevertheless, it is important to be clear about these ideas. First, developments in computational theory led to the invention of the computer, which became the dominant "machine metaphor" of the cognitive shift. No one seriously maintains that humans resemble digital computers, but the nervous system needs to solve many of the same problems that must be solved by computers in performing similar tasks. Second, it is important to understand computational theory because it applies not merely to contemporary computational hardware; rather, it specifies mathematical principles that apply to an infinite class of symbolic devices. If nervous systems are specially adapted to represent and symbolically transform the world of the organism, then the abstract principles of symbol-manipulation must also apply to it. As a full-fledged realization this idea is rather recent in cognitive psychology; during most of the cognitive revolution it certainly was not accepted. Nevertheless, it is the most cogent scientific rationale for the revolution available today, and we may speculate that some unstated intuition like this may have played a part in the historical developments. Of course, the public proof-procedures used by psychologists were always empirical; but underlying these experiments were some strong commonsense intuitions about human beings. When these intuitions are rigorously analyzed, one arrives at something very much like a computational conception of human psychology (*e.g.*, Fodor, 1968). We will discuss the computational rationale of the cognitive shift before describing the actual story of the shift.

Information, Automata, and the Foundations of Mathematics

I am using the term "computational theory" very broadly to refer to the cluster of mathematical ideas that led up to the modern computer, its programs, and its higher-level languages. Some of these ideas go clear back to Aristotle's logic and to the set theory developed by George Boole in the 19th century. Russell and Whitehead's symbolic logic (1910) played a role, as did the 19th-century movement toward specifying the foundations of mathematics. About the beginning of this century, it became clear that any mathematical system can be expressed in symbolic logic, and that logic itself was largely reducible to Boolean set theory. When mathematicians and engineers discovered that electrical circuits could be modeled with Boolean set theory, it was only a matter of time before they realized that electrical circuits could also then *represent and compute*

Boolean equations. But if electrical circuits could compute Boolean equations, they could also calculate symbolic logic expressions, and thence any mathematical formulae whatsoever. Furthermore, developments in mathematics made it clear that mathematics was not limited to numerical expressions — any symbolic pattern could be an object of mathematical analysis. In summary, these developments in the foundations of mathematics implied that electrical circuits could "act out" any precise set of instructions, whether they involved logic, arithmetic, or even natural language.

The Concept of Representation

"Representation" seems to be a commonsense idea. Ordinary words such as "knowledge," "thought," "feeling," "plan," and "description" express the idea that we can somehow model aspects of the world in our minds and in our speech. Like other commonsense ideas, the concept of "representation" is a good deal more subtle than we may suppose. It raises considerable philosophical difficulties. In philosophy there is a large technical literature on these difficulties, which I can only mention here. (For instance, some philosophers maintain that the mind–body problem emerges whenever one entity represents another.)

Certainly in behaviorism and logical positivism there was great resistance to the idea that people can represent things about the world "in their heads." The concept of an internal representation was often ridiculed with a *reductio ad absurdum* argument, the so-called "homunculus theory." This argument, which dates back to Aristotle, starts by supposing that people represent an object (say, a chair) internally. How does the nervous system deal with such a representation? Surely, the argument goes, there must be something that inspects the representation of the chair, or acts upon it. This "something" is just like a little inner man, a homunculus. But how does the homunculus know what to do with this information? Surely it needs to represent the representation somehow. But *that* representation in turn needs some little homunculus to act upon it, *etc., ad infinitum.* Thus the idea of mental representation seemed inevitably to lead to an infinite regress.

Today no one can maintain this argument anymore. Computers have become so commonplace, and the business of representing some part of the world in a computer code has in many instances become so trivial that the homunculus theory has itself become absurd. The existence of the computer provides a concrete proof that the commonsense notion of representation is indeed viable, even with all its attendant philosophical difficulties.

Mathematical Machines

Starting in the 1930s the English mathematician Alan Turing studied a remarkably simple, imaginary machine, consisting merely of a tape, and a head that could make marks on the tape, read them, and erase them (Turing, 1950). Suppose that such a simple machine had an unlimited amount of time and tape to work with — are there any limits to the mathematical functions it could compute? Turing proved that even this simple machine can compute any mathematical function whatsoever. This means that any device which is formally equivalent to Turing's machine will also be able to model any imaginable relationship that can be stated explicitly. An electronic digital computer is really just a large, fast Turing Machine, able in principle to compute *any conceivable symbolic relationship*. But of course, unlike Turing's imaginary machine, a physical computer has only finite time and memory.

In the 1940s, spurred on by the World War and its demands for automatically controlled radar-tracking devices, mathematicians and engineers developed various kinds of computers, as well as formal theories for describing information and cybernetic feedback. *Information* was at first defined mainly for the purpose of measuring the carrying capacity of telephone lines and the like (Shannon & Weaver, 1949), but this precise definition is directly relevant to fundamental questions in physics and biology. The mathematical definition of information is simple but profound. Basically, it states that information exists when a signal reaches a receiver, enabling the receiver to make a *choice* within a set of alternatives. One might recall in this respect the game of Twenty Questions, in which an answer to a question provides real information only when it permits a player to reduce the number of possible alternatives. A player may get many answers that provide no real information at all. In physics, the very basic notion of entropy — the tendency of energy to dissipate — is defined simply as the inverse of information, and in biology, the genetic role of DNA can be expressed in terms of information transmission. Thus, information is a foundation concept in the fundamental sciences.

The smallest conceivable unit of information is one that enables the receiver to discriminate between two alternatives, and this amount of information is called a "bit." Any larger amount of information can be expressed in bits, because any number can be restated to a numerical base of two. Thus a message may be represented as either + or − , where + could mean, for example, "go to war," and − , "make peace." If there are four choices, say, "go to war," "make peace," "exchange ambassadors," and "protest to the U.N.," the alternatives can still be denoted with only two bits of information (− − , + + , − + , + −); and so on. All the axioms of Boolean algebra can be represented by a small number of bits, and only a few more are needed to symbolize the fundamental axioms of symbolic logic. Once this is done, any other mathematical symbol-system can be easily represented in terms of bits of information, and any physical system able to represent strings of pluses and minuses can then be used as a medium, able to "act out" the operations of any mathematics whatsoever. Thus, a computer can act out arithmetic operations, but also logical deductions, analyses of syntax, representations of objects in space, or control of the movements of a robot, as long as these events can be represented in terms of some explicit set of symbols and operations. Current computers use electrical switching circuits to do such things, with "switch open" versus, "switch closed" to represent plus or minus. But the same information may be equally well represented by magnetized pieces of metal, the position of the beads of an abacus, the position of gears in a mechanical calculator, or any other convenient physical system, including neurons. From the very beginnings of information theory, it was clearly understood that information could be defined *free of any particular physical medium of representation*.

In this way, computers are at once physical and nonphysical. They are physical machines. But the use and significance of computers is not in the switching circuits as such, but in the fact that these circuits can flexibly encode information. A certain piece of information may start as a mark on paper, be transferred mechanically to a hole in a paper tape, to a magnetized bubble, to an electrical pulse running down a wire, or to a radio signal echoing off the earth's ionosphere; it may be stored indefinitely as a magnetized region on a metal disk, and finally end up as a beam of electrons activating the phosphor on the screen of a computer terminal. All these media are different from one another, but the user is not interested in the physical medium, only in the outcome: whether the message is "make peace" or "go to war." In this sense, information is not precisely physical; *as information*, it exists only with reference to the set of alternatives held by the receiver (Bakan, 1980; Szilard, 1929/ 1964). And it did not take long before engineers and mathematicians began to think that human beings might also be viewed as bearers and transmitters of information.

Human Beings as
Information Processors

Human beings in general show a similar disregard for the medium of information, and a decided preference for information itself. Most of the time, when we hear someone speak a sentence, we will forget the exact words within a matter of seconds (try to recall the first sentence of this paragraph). But we will usually be able to *paraphrase* the forgotten sentence. A paraphrase is of course another sentence that preserves the meaning but not the form of the original. The "same" sentence can be spoken in a man's bass voice or a child's falsetto; it can be sung, printed, handwritten, or tapped out in Morse Code; between long-time friends, meaning can be conveyed by a look, a gesture, or even by an unexpected silence. In all these cases it is *not* the physical event that is important, but only the information it conveys.

Further, people tend to confuse two physically different events that bear the same information. Physically different sounds that signal the same phoneme of a language may be perceptually indistinguishable. And in memory, we tend to confuse physically different sentences if they carry similar meaning (*e.g.*, Bransford & Franks, 1971). But adults rarely confuse physically similar sentences if they *differ* in meaning.

The nervous system itself is responsive to information rather than to physical energy as such. Even a single neuron, if it is stimulated by a certain electrical pulse train, will adapt to that *particular* stimulating frequency, but not to any other. That is, it will soon stop responding to the incoming stimulus, not because it is "fatigued," but only because the repeated input conveys no new information. We can show that the adapted neuron will still respond to a *new* stimulus by stimulating it with a different electrical frequency, which will make it respond again. Thus it seems to "recognize" the old stimulus and distinguish it from any new stimulus. In informational terms, a repetitive stimulus becomes redundant to the neuron — it carries no more information.

At a far more complex level of neural integration, every sensory tract in the nervous system adapts to redundant stimulation, so that incoming energy patterns that carry no new information are ignored. And at the highest level of integration, people lose awareness of predictable sensations, of well-learned automatic actions, and even of the meaning of repeated words. All these neural systems begin to activate again when new information becomes available. In general, mere physical input does not usually provide the nervous system with information, and without information the nervous system does not respond. A stimulus must convey some news, some signal that is not redundant (Bateson, 1979; Soko-lov, 1963).

In the 1950s, it seemed natural for psychologists and neurophys-iologists to investigate how information theory could be used to under-stand human beings (*e.g.*, Miller, 1964; Garner, 1962). Less than a decade previously, cybernetic theorists had provided a formal proof that normal physical systems could behave in a goal-directed fashion, finally resolving the controversy over "teleology" that had been debated since Aristotle (Rosenblueth, Wiener, & Bigelow, 1943). The "problem" of pur-pose, which had shaped the theories of Hull, Tolman, and Skinner, was shown to be no problem at all. Meanwhile, Turing's imaginary machine had led other mathematicians to work out a theory of such mathematical machines, and this "theory of automata" soon led Noam Chomsky to a formal proof of the inadequacy of existing behavioristic theories of lan-guage (Chomsky, 1957, 1959).

Already by the late 1940s, the conceptual apparatus existed to pro-vide a formal justification for cognitive psychology. An engineer who wanted to discover what a cybernetic machine was doing, or what pro-gram was being run on a computer, would not look only at the inputs and outputs of the machine (the stimuli and responses), but would at-tempt to describe its *functional* innards — does it have the goal of main-taining a certain constant temperature? Does it compensate for changes in a target that it is tracking? Does it compute a theorem in formal logic? These questions are best described not by reference to the physical states of the machine, but to the way in which it functions — a higher-level of description. In fact, the engineer's description of an information machine begins to sound just like our commonsense way of describing a human being: It is stated in terms of goals, knowledge of the world, decisions, predicted gains and losses, and sometimes even intelligent strategies.

Levels of Reality in the Computer

There are a number of legitimate and useful ways of analyzing the func-tioning of any computer (Newell, 1981): At the physical level one can study the machine as such (the *device* level), and somewhat more abstract-ly, one can view its elements as electrical circuits (the *circuit* level); as memories with transfers between them (the *register–transfer* level); in terms of the program (the *symbolic* level, the most familiar one); and even fur-ther, in terms of the system architecture (the *configuration* level). According to Newell (1981),

Each level is defined in two ways. First, it can be defined autonomously, without reference to any other level. To an amazing degree, programmers need not know logic circuits, logic designers need not know electrical circuits, managers can operate at the configuration level with no knowledge of programming, and so forth. Second, each level can be reduced to the level below. . . .

Thus each level can be treated as functionally autonomous *and also* as reducible to the next lower level.

If this is generally true of biological information processors as well, then one can see how a similar relationship might hold between psychology and neurophysiology — psychologists would seem to operate at the level of programs and system architecture, while neurophysiologists work with neurons, neural pathways, centers, and the like. Although this is a bit simplistic, it suggests one way to view the relationships between psychological concerns and the underlying physical system. In principle, psychological functions might also be treated autonomously, with emphasis on the unique properties of psychological regularities, without in any way denying the possibility of reducing the psychological level to neurophysiology. That reduction may be possible, but it is not necessarily useful (Fodor, 1968). To oversimplify a bit, psychologists may be primarily concerned with the "programming" of the human nervous system, rather than with the lower-level hardware.

"Machine metaphors" are not new to psychologists. Even in the 17th century, French thinkers were fascinated by the lifelike robots that were built for the amusement of the aristocracy, and Descartes himself suggested that the human body was just such an automaton, interacting with the divine soul by way of the pineal gland. To Descartes, the soul was the seat of reason, and reason was *not* a mechanical affair. But several centuries later, behaviorists such as Watson and Thorndike thought of learning in terms of a telephone switchboard, as a mechanical connecting of stimuli and responses. Sigmund Freud, probably the most creative theoretical psychologist to date, employed numerous mechanical metaphors to describe the "vicissitudes of the libido" in its various transformations, though Freud acknowledged these as merely metaphors, to be exchanged for more precise neurological descriptions when they became available (Erdelyi, 1985). Machine metaphors are common elsewhere in science as well. For example, the Newtonian solar system looks much like the elaborate clockwork mechanisms that were popular in Newton's time, and indeed, mechanical models inspired by Newton's theory were soon made. For psychologists, always looking for reassurance that their theories refer to some physically possible reality, the lure of machine metaphors is well-nigh irresistible.

Psychological Resistance to the Computational Metaphor

Nevertheless, the new computational ideas were not welcomed with open arms. In the early 1950s, George A. Miller inspired a number of psychologists to investigate information theory as a way of looking at human beings (Miller, 1956), but the results were never completely satisfactory. Behavioristic metatheory still required that the elements of the information system (the sender, receiver, and information-channel) be observable. Thus the stimulus could be treated as a sender, the response as the receiver, and the human subject as the channel. With some exceptions, this application of information theory was unproductive. In retrospect, it seems that information theory posed a challenge that psychologists were unable to meet at the time: If a human being processes incoming stimuli as information, the question suggested by information theory is, "What is the context of alternatives that the information helps to reduce?" This is equivalent to asking what representations people maintain of the world around them, and this question could not be tackled squarely until some years later. The mathematical theory of information presupposed that the context of alternatives was already known; but this is precisely what psychologists needed to discover.

Between 1946 and 1953, the Macy Foundation sponsored a number of meetings among mathematicians, psychologists and other social scientists, and neurobiologists, to explore the emerging parallels between machines and living organisms (Heims, 1975). The regular participants included anthropologists such as Gregory Bateson and Margaret Mead; mathematicians such as Norbert Wiener (the major founder of cybernetics), John von Neumann, Warren McCulloch, Walter Pitts, Julian Bigelow, and Arturo Rosenblueth; Gestalt psychologists such as Kurt Lewin, Wolfgang Köhler, and Heinrich Klüver; sociologists and social psychologists such as Paul Lazarsfeld and Alex Bavelas; neurophysiologists Hans Lukas Teuber and Ralph Gerard; and psychoanalysts such as Lawrence Kubie, and briefly, Erik Erickson. Few, if any, behaviorists attended the Macy conferences. The results were apparently mixed. A number of the leading thinkers in each field attended the conferences repeatedly, and we may suppose that they found the meetings worth their while, but the impact of the new computational theories did not seem to affect the scientific work of most participants (but see McCulloch & Pitts, 1943; Bateson, 1979).

But in 1956, only three years after the last Macy Conference, another conference was held in which all of the core ideas of the cognitive revolution were already contained. The participants included George A.

Miller, soon to become for several decades the most identifiable leader in the cognitive movement; Noam Chomsky, who was about to initiate a cognitive shift in linguistics that would profoundly influence many psychologists; David Green and John Swets, who were applying an engineering theory to human psychophysics, destined to have major impact; and perhaps most fatefully, Allan Newell and Herbert A. Simon, who were then helping to develop the first higher-level computer languages: They would soon be using these new languages to model human performance. Within the next few years, Newell and Simon showed that computers could be programmed to play chess, prove sophisticated logic theorems, and even simulate some important properties of human short-term memory (Newell & Simon, 1972). Over the next several decades, the number of simulations of human intelligence increased dramatically, and the resulting field of Artificial Intelligence is today having increasing impact in experimental psychology. But this is getting ahead of the story. The seeds were there in 1956, but any widespread impact on psychology was very much in the future.

The rapid advances in computational theory had a pervasive *but indirect* impact on the course of scientific psychology. Even today, most psychologists know little about the mathematical arguments originating from information theory, cybernetics, or the theory of automata. Contemporary psychologists seem to take for granted such ideas as "information," "cybernetics," and "computation," without making them explicit. But when these ideas were first proposed, psychologists were committed exclusively to an empirical proof procedure, and felt deeply suspicious of any theoretical argument. Very few psychologists became directly involved with computational theory, and those who did were often not considered to be doing psychology. The suspicion of "arm-chair theory" kept most experimentalists from becoming directly acquainted with the new ideas, especially because these ideas were not easy to test empirically. Some of this suspicion of theory remains in force today, even among cognitive psychologists. To some extent this is normal. Mature sciences often show a similar tension between experimental and theoretical scientists. But in psychology, the claim to be scientific seemed to rest *entirely* on the existence of experimental proof-procedures. Experimentation was treated with far more respect than theory, so that there was a profound imbalance between the influence of facts and the influence of ideas.

Some Indirect Influences of Computational Theory

A number of cognitive psychologists reject the analogy of computational processes for human functioning (*e.g.*, Neisser, 1976; Gibson, 1966). But even those who reject a computational metaphor still profit from the concrete "existence proof" provided by the computer. The brute fact of computers helps to create the possibility of doing theory, because we can talk about the functioning of the computer abstractly, without being limited to physical stimuli and responses. Thus the mere existence of the computer has a liberating influence on the theoretical imagination, even for psychologists who do not believe in a computational metaphor.

Ideas that may seem obvious today were much less so a decade or two ago. Computational ideas have spread only gradually, and a formal connection between computational theory and psychological theory was not made until the founding of "cognitive science" in the late 70s. At the beginning of the cognitive revolution, experimentation was still the *sine qua non* of scientific psychology. The computer showed perhaps that representations and information processing were possible, but this possibility rarely convinced psychologists that human beings did *in fact* have representations and goals, or that they did something very much like the processing of information. The real burden of proof for the cognitive revolution was carried by a remarkable series of experiments, which very gradually brought an intensely skeptical community around to a more theoretical point of view.

The Cognitive Revolution: Persuasion by "the Respectable Experiment"

The major mechanism for change in experimental psychology is the persuasive experiment. This is not necessarily true for more highly developed sciences, in which purely theoretical arguments can be more persuasive than empirical observations. Einstein's famous paper on relativity triggered a revolution in the Newtonian physics of the previous two centuries, but it was only 11 pages long, and contained no empirical evidence whatsoever (Einstein, 1905). It merely posed a "thought experiment," asking, "How would the world look to an observer in a vehicle traveling near the speed of light?" A theoretical argument such as this can be persuasive only in a scientific community that views theory with the greatest respect. The behavioristic psychology of the 1950s, however, was deeply suspicious of theory and greatly enamored of experiments. As a result, the theoretical implications of the critical experiments in the cognitive revolution were realized silently, because they could not be stated openly within the accepted framework.

Therefore we must be cautious in discussing the critical experiments.

It is important to place them in their historical and theoretical context — that is the purpose of this book — and yet, we must keep in mind the fact that most psychologists at this time were ahistorical and antitheoretical. Wundt and James had anticipated many of the issues raised by the new cognitive experiments, but in the '50s they were considered unscientific, and their books simply were not read. Many ideas that seem so obvious today were unacceptable, even inconceivable, to serious experimental psychologists at the time. Each new "cognitive" experiment was seen as just another isolated contribution, not creating the coherent whole we see today.

I have noted that the word "cognitive" is ambiguous: For our purposes it refers primarily to a metatheory that encourages one to infer unobservable theoretical constructs from empirical observations. It is rather confusing that the shift toward the cognitive metatheory originated in a field of psychology that is also called "cognitive" — the field that is most concerned with functions such as language, thought, and attention. In a way, this is an historical accident: In principle, at least, the cognitive metatheory could have started in any other part of empirical psychology (and in fact, one could argue that it started first in social psychology). But the cognitive *metatheory*, like the behavioristic one, applies to all of psychology, and indeed today it is rapidly spreading to the rest of scientific psychology.

Yet the cognitive metatheory and the study of human cognition cannot be entirely separated. The study of human cognition provided the empirical domain in which the success or failure of the cognitive metatheory was to be demonstrated, just as the study of conditioning was to be the proof of the behavioristic pudding. A metatheory cannot stand on its own; it must promise not only a plausible approach to the science, but also point to a set of succesful applications of its approach. In just this way, "cognitive psychology" (in the narrow sense) provided a test-case for the cognitive metatheory.

There is a third, rather old-fashioned sense of "cognitive," meaning "conscious, or potentially conscious intellectual activity" such as thinking, problem solving, or memory. This is emphatically *not* the meaning used by modern cognitive psychologists; to them, cognitive functions are roughly synonymous with human informational processes, which can be either conscious or unconscious. Indeed, it has only recently become clear (again) that the overwhelming bulk of effective information processing in the nervous system is unconscious. Nevertheless, this old-fashioned meaning of "cognitive" as "conscious processes" continues to create confusion (*e.g.*, Zajonc, 1980; Baars, 1981).

The Theoreticians' Dilemma: Adequacy versus Testability

The persuasive force of the cognitive revolution was carried almost entirely by "the respectable experiment": By dint of sheer accumulation of novel experiments, the realization slowly dawned that psychological theory would have to become far more abstract and powerful than before. This is true even though explicit theoretical statements in these experiments were always strictly limited. The metatheory still held that science proceeds by small and continuous accumulations of facts, rather than by large, rapid insights. In fact, the theoretical tools needed to accommodate the new facts were developing in tandem with the experimental work—not in psychology as such, but in the new field of Artificial Intelligence. Until recently these new theoretical tools were not considered to be part of scientific psychology. Some Artificial Intelligence researchers thought of their work as a kind of theoretical psychology, but they gained only grudging acceptance among psychologists, often several decades after their work was published (Newell & Simon, 1972, historical addendum). Until very recently, those psychologists who worked in Artificial Intelligence were simply not considered to be doing scientific psychology. For one thing, the computer programs that were able to simulate intelligent functions such as language comprehension or visual recognition were far too complex, interactive, and fast to test empirically.

Unfortunately, the theories that emerged from the experimental laboratories had the opposite problem: They were extremely simple and economical, able to explain certain experimental results, but usually not much more. As Chomsky showed so devastatingly, behavioristic theories of language could not even explain some elementary properties of language (Chomsky, 1957; Bever, Fodor, & Garrett, 1968). Until very recently, *all* experimentally-based theories in psychology failed the test of adequacy—they simply lacked the power to explain even the basic properties of the domain they were supposed to explain. Thus, theories of language could not handle the relationships between paraphrases (such as active and passive sentences with similar meanings). And theories of perception could not explain perceptual constancies—those aspects of perception that allow us to consider an object to be "the same thing" no matter what its orientation and distance. This lack of explanatory adequacy did not make these models useless, because they could always handle the direct results of experiments. But it made them largely irrelevant to the job of explaining perception, memory, or language in the real world.

Over several decades of work, Artificial Intelligence researchers developed computational systems that came much closer to adequacy. Thus, Artificial Intelligence systems were able to do the sorts of things that human beings do with language: answer questions, resolve ambiguities, generate paraphrases, and the like. But these more adequate theories were so enormously complex that they could not be tested with the proof-procedures used by experimental psychologists. A fundamental dilemma arose between theoretical adequacy and empirical testability: One could do experimental research in language, and feel secure as a scientist, at the sacrifice of theoretical adequacy; or alternatively, one could build very large and complex interactive computational systems that could simulate many aspects of human linguistic functioning, without being able to test these ideas experimentally. This fundamental dilemma in cognitive research has not yet been resolved. Although the gap between theory and experiment has narrowed somewhat over the past few years, even a very recent textbook of cognitive psychology reflects the doubts of experimentalists concerning the value of complex computational theories. As Lachman, Lachman, and Butterfield (1979) write:

Their colleagues have mixed feelings about the global modelers. On the one hand, most information-processing psychologists concede that they are asking the right questions. On the other hand, there is some objection to the movement away from traditional experimentation on the part of some modelers. The global modelers are similar to linguists in their willingness to use rational argument, and they are similar to artificial intelligence specialists in their willingness to be pragmatic for the purpose of implementing parts of their models on computers. To at least some information-processing psychologists, these are character flaws. (p. 437)

A long time lag between theory and empirical testing is not unknown in other scientific fields. We noted before that Galileo's theory was not really tested for 150 years after his death, and in this century in geology the theory of continental drift was not taken seriously for 50 years after it was first suggested. Many similar examples could be cited in other fields. But a great time lag between theory and experimental confirmation is always uncomfortable.

The Cognitive Revolution Proceeded Atheoretically

Thus the revolutionary experiments had to appeal to experimentalists on largely nontheoretical grounds. This may seem strange. To most people in the natural sciences, the idea that experiments can be evaluated without reference to theory may seem peculiar or even incoherent. But experimental psychologists had learned through hard experience that models built to account for one set of experimental findings usually failed to generalize to new results, and that any attempt to generalize to the world outside of the laboratory was likewise doomed to failure. The more ambitious the theory, it was believed, the less likely it was to succeed; and Artificial Intelligence theories seemed ambitious indeed. Suspicion of theory seemed justified by experience.

As a result, experimentalists developed their own criteria for evaluating data: Were the results precise and quantifiable? Were they replicable? Did they show simple functional relationships between the variables? Did they open up new areas of empirical inquiry? The most influential experiments of the cognitive revolution had these empiricist virtues. Quite a few of them appealed to experimentalists because they demonstrated linear relationships between the variables measured. There is no particular reason why psychological functions should be linear, but these kinds of results seemed to guarantee a kind of simplicity that inspired confidence. Straight-line graphs were very persuasive pieces of evidence (*e.g.*, Sternberg, 1966; Cooper & Shepard, 1973; Bransford & Franks, 1971).

Almost every mature science shows a tension between experimentalists and theoreticans. Experimental scientists often complain that the theoreticians simply ignore inconvenient evidence, whereas theoreticians tend to believe that experimentalists cannot see the larger picture. This tension can be healthy and creative, providing that there is also good communication.

A remarkable article in the journal *Science* illustrates this tension vividly in the case of biochemistry:

At the 1958 Conference on Biophysics, at Boulder, there was a dramatic confrontation between the two points of view. Leo Szilard (Nobel Prize-winning physicist and biochemist) said: "The problem of how enzymes are induced, of how proteins are synthesized, of how antibodies are formed, are closer to solution than is generally believed. If you do stupid experiments, and finish one a year, it can take 50 years. But if you stop doing experiments for a little while and *think* how proteins can possibly be synthesized, there are only about 5 ways, not 50! And it will take only a few experiments to distinguish these."

One of the young men added: "It is essentially the old question: How *small* and *elegant* an experiment can you perform?"

These comments upset a number of those present. An electron microscopist said, "Gentlemen, this is off the track. This is philosophy of science."

Szilard retorted: "I was not quarreling with third-rate scientists. I was quarreling with first-rate scientists."

A physical chemist hurriedly asked: "Are we going to take the official photograph before lunch or after lunch?"

But this did not deflect the dispute. A distinguished cell biologist rose and said: "No two cells give the same properties. Biology is the science of heterogeneous systems." And he added privately, "You know there are *scientists* and there are people in science who are just working with these oversimplified model systems — DNA chains and *in vitro* systems — who are not doing science at all. We need their auxiliary work: They build apparatus, they make minor studies, but they are not scientists."

To which Cy Leventhal replied: "Well, there are two kinds of biologists, those who are looking to see if there is one thing that can be understood, and those who keep saying it is very complicated and that nothing can be understood . . . You must study the *simplest* system you think has the properties you are interested in."

As they were leaving the meeting, one man could be heard muttering, "What does Szilard expect me to do — kill myself?" (Platt, 1964, p. 350)

And so it goes. The fact is, of course, that theory and experiment are both indispensable, and that it is often useful if they are to some extent pursued independently of each other.

But in psychology, only one-half of this dialectic existed. There simply was no credible theory. In the absence of accepted theory, it was never clear which experiments had important implications. When such implications did become clear after a decade or two, many previous experimental findings suddenly seemed obvious, trivial, or irrelevant. Atheoretical empiricism is a costly way to do science.

We will discuss just a few of the many hundreds of experiments that created the cognitive revolution: experiments bearing on mental representation; on linguistic meaning, attention, and consciousness; on the problem of inferring structure and process; and on the problem of serial order in behavior. For additional detail the reader is referred to any standard text in cognitive psychology, human memory, or psychology of language (*e.g.*, Neisser, 1967; Norman, 1976; Anderson, 1980; Bransford, 1979; Newell & Simon, 1972; Clark & Clark, 1977; Blumenthal, 1977b).

The Issue of Mental Representation

Many cognitive psychologists study memory, and memories are clearly representations of the world. In some reasonable sense my memory of yesterday's breakfast is a representation of that event. With a little effort I could generate an image of yesterday's toast and orange juice, which an outside observer could verify by comparing my verbal description of the image to a photograph record of yesterday's breakfast. My mental image and description can serve as plans for tomorrow's breakfast as well, indicating that representations can also describe future states. Plausible commonsense? Yes, but not acceptable psychology, even to memory psychologists until well into the cognitive revolution. Psychologists were not comfortable with the idea of internal representation, even though they willingly spoke of all kinds of memories. Radical behaviorists considered the idea of "memory" to involve a scientifically unwarranted inference (see Chapter 3, Skinner and Rachlin). Behaviorists preferred to speak of "learning" rather than memory, because a memory is not observable, whereas learning was thought to be definable behaviorally.

On the other hand, computers have memories, and of particular significance, they have buffer memories. Buffers are small, local memories that are used whenever two events that arrive at different times must be related to each other. Buffer memories are always needed if the speed of processing inside the computer is different from the speed of external information. Take the word "they" for example, in the first sentence of this paragraph, "they have buffer memories"; in order to comprehend the sentence, the reader must understand that "they" refers to "computers" in the previous clause. Because the word "computers" was read a half second *before* the word "they," it is natural to suppose that the first word was held in some temporary store, so that when the pronoun "they" arrived, it was matched with its referent. A buffer memory is that kind of temporary holding bin. A significant part of the cognitive revolution began when evidence began to accumulate for the existence of such temporary holding memories in the human nervous system.

Wilhelm Wundt had already performed experiments using brief exposures of a grid of letters, and he reported that trained observers could report only three to six briefly glimpsed letters (1912). Imagine that the following grid is exposed for a few tenths of a second:

t   f   v   x

o   a   z   l

q   c   e   g

People invariably claimed that they could see more letters in a glance than they could report! It seemed as if the very act of recalling the letters or of pronouncing them, or perhaps the sheer effort of holding them long enough to say them, interferes with the memory for what was actually seen. In one of the landmark experiments of the cognitive shift, Sperling (1960) developed an ingenious way to circumvent this difficulty—to measure how many letters people can actually see, no matter how many they report at any one time. He presented an array of 12 letters in a 3 x 4 arrangement for about one-tenth of a second. Immediately afterwards he sounded a tone, signalling the observer which row of letters to report.

The results showed that people can report the letters from any arbitrarily designated row in this experiment, but not much more than that. We can be sure that the observers consistently perceived for a moment *more* than they could report, because they could name all the letters in any arbitrary row quite accurately. Because the reporting signal was given after the display was turned off, there was no way for the observers to know beforehand which row would be designated. Given that any arbitrary row could be reported, we must infer that *all* of the information in the display was briefly available to the subjects, in spite of their inability to report all the letters in any one exposure.

The Sperling experiment is extremely precise and reliable, and it compels the inference that we have just made: People can remember momentarily more than they can report. To explain this, we are forced to imagine a kind of memory store in which more can be held than the observer can talk about. But if that is so, then the experimental operation of reporting the letters from memory *cannot be a direct measure* of the memory that is being inferred. Operationist philosophy would hold that the measure is the same as the construct, and many psychologists apparently believe this (*e.g.*, Stevens, 1966). But Sperling's results suggested to some psychologists that we may sometimes be obliged to infer a construct that goes beyond the measuring operation — in this case, a visual buffer memory, whose contents cannot be fully reported at any one time.

Another construct, called "short-term memory," has much the same methodological status. Wundt and James had noted that people could report no more than about six separate stimuli in any sensory modality, but psychologists had largely ignored this phenomenon for more than 50 years. Starting in the mid-1950s, people such as George Miller and Herbert A. Simon began to draw attention to the massive evidence for this fact. In a charming paper entitled "The Magical Number Seven, Plus or Minus Two: Some Limits on Our Capacity for Processing Information," Miller (1956) wrote,

My problem is that I have been persecuted by an integer. For seven years this number has followed me around, has intruded in my most private data, and has assaulted me from the pages of our most public journals. This number assumes a variety of disguises, being sometimes a little larger and sometimes a little smaller than usual, but never changing so much as to be unrecognizable.

People can report only seven (plus or minus two) unrelated words or arbitrary numbers in immediate memory; this is why telephone numbers are limited to seven digits. In judging anything from "size" to "degree of happiness," we can reliably use only about seven judgment categories on a scale. We can accurately estimate in a single glance the number of no more than seven objects. Thus, "short-term memory" seems to be drastically limited.

But there is a peculiar amendment to this observation: As Wundt had already noted, it does not matter what *size* each item in the short-term memory is. We can remember some seven letters, syllables, or multisyllabic words, and somewhat less than seven short, idiomatic sentences. This short-term memory, therefore, has the same capacity for seven separate, unrelated items, no matter how lengthy the items themselves are. If we think of short-term memory as a container, say a shoe box, we can immediately see the problem: What kind of a shoe box will take seven shoes of *any* size — either seven baby shoes or seven giant boots?

Miller gave a partial explanation in terms of "chunking"; the capacity of the short-term memory buffer appeared to be limited to roughly seven chunks of any size. By recoding ("chunking") letters into words and words into sentences, more efficient use could be made of this capacity. But a real explanation of this phenomenon had to await a deeper understanding, not of short-term memory, but of long-term memory.

The buffer memories discussed so far are only temporary holding bins. Obviously, people can remember some things for years, and under optimal conditions perhaps any experience can be retrieved long afterwards (*e.g.*, Bransford, 1979; Williams & Hollan, 1981). Evidence was soon discovered that items held in short-term memory tend to move into long-term memory, especially if people actively try to integrate the newer items into existing knowledge. The great difference between short-term and long-term memory seemed to be the fact that long-term memory was highly organized. The evidence for this is as follows:

It had long been known that if people are asked to say any words that come to mind, their responses will seem obviously connected to each other. The word "book" may be followed by "volume," "space," "container," "Coke bottle," "bottle-fed babies," "breast-fed babies," "baby carriage," "carriage-house," and so on. Each response seems related to the next. This free-association technique has been used extensively in psychoanalysis since the beginning of the 20th century, to encourage trains of association that people would normally avoid. Indeed, the early experimental work on free association was done by Carl Jung.

But evidence from free association did not fit the experimental design criteria of experimental psychology, because the connectedness between the words could only be known *post hoc*; *post hoc* designs did not fit the assumptions of the statistical tests needed to support experimental claims. Only if all conditions were specified in advance could one draw statistically valid conclusions, or so it was thought. (It is noteworthy that this re-

quirement entirely rules out new observations, that is, results not anticipated in the design.)

How could a respectable experimental psychologist test the possibility that people would spontaneously organize words in memory? Psychologists such as Bousfield (1953) taught their subjects lists of words
belonging to different categories (such as animals, furniture, and musical
instruments) and randomly mixed together, then after a day or so, tested
the subjects on these words. Because all the conditions were established
ahead of time, this was an acceptable experimental design. The results
showed what Jung had shown in the 1930s: that people retrieved like
with like. This seemed to imply that the words were being categorized
together in memory.

Although this idea may not seem earth-shaking, it was quite revolutionary to psychologists who believed that memories were arbitrarily
connected to one another, as taught by the English Associationists and
the behavioristic learning psychologists. That memories should actually
be *classified* in some organized scheme profoundly challenged their views.
Unlike Sperling's visual buffer memory and Miller's short-term memory,
long-term memory seemed to be profoundly influenced by organizational
considerations.

By 1965, it appeared that there were three kinds of memory: sensory
memories, such as the visual buffer, which could hold about 12 items;
short-term memory, which could hold seven, plus or minus two, items
(if people were allowed to rehearse the items silently to themselves); and
long-term memory, a mysterious entity that held the bulk of what we
ordinarily call memory, and which seemed to be sensitive to organizational effects. Often these three types of memory were encoded in a linear
model, as it were, end-to-end: First, sensory information entered a sensory buffer; then some of the items in the buffer were selected to go into
short-term memory, where seven of them could be rehearsed, until finally, they could enter long-term memory. This linear model was perhaps
naïve, but it was clearly cognitive — nobody expected actually to *see* these
memories in the flesh — and it did account for a great many observations.

Because the linear model was so clearly cognitive, perhaps we should
ignore what was wrong with it. But the cognitive revolution did not really
stop in 1965; it has continued in one way or another and is still continuing today. It is true that by 1965, the *metatheory* of scientific psychology
had already changed to include unobservable constructs as a routine matter. But while we will focus on the years 1955 to 1965, it would be a pity
to neglect more recent developments.

What was wrong with the linear model, with the idea of information flowing from sensory to short-term to long-term memory? For one thing, it was self-contradictory. There is a problem with the very idea of an "item" in memory. What would constitute an "item"? In Sperling's 3 × 4 visual display there are some 12 "items," but a backwards "t" would not show the same effects on a subject as a normal "t", because of its unfamiliarity. Similarly, in short-term memory, the sequence "1776, 1492, 1914, 1942" would be remembered easily, whereas the same numbers presented backwards would be very difficult to remember. Obviously, what constitutes an "item" depends on familiarity — but familiarity implies that something was experienced before, perhaps many times, and over a long time; thus, familiarity itself depends on long-term memory. The way in which information is handled in a visual buffer or in short-term memory depends, in itself, on long-term memory. Therefore it cannot be true that information flows only one way, from sensory buffers to short-term memory to long-term memory, because long-term memory is needed *in the first place* to define the items in the buffer memories.

Thus the linear model did not last very long. For the first time in the history of the new cognitive psychology, some purely theoretical influences were helping to change the thinking of some psychologists (*e.g.*, *cf.* the first and second editions of Norman, 1967 and 1976).

Artificial Intelligence researchers had at first attempted to set up computer systems able to recognize auditory, visual, and linguistic inputs in ways rather similar to the linear model; but they quickly realized that there were far too many ambiguities in the input to permit a deterministic flow of information. Thus, the sentence, "Time flies like an arrow," was interpreted by a computer as meaning "A certain kind of a fly, called a 'time fly,' has a liking for arrows." This may seem like a unusually silly interpretation, but the same interpretation is perfectly all right in a sentence such as, "Fruit flies like a banana," because fruit flies *are* a certain category of fly that have a liking for bananas. So the difficulty was not that the computer constructed a totally implausible interpretation of the sentence, but, rather, that it did not have enough contextual knowledge to resolve the genuine ambiguities in the sentence. Ambiguities abound in ordinary language. When human beings have the right contextual knowledge, we resolve such ambiguities very quickly. But without context, we encounter the same difficulties that hobbled the early computer models of language comprehension.

Artificial Intelligence workers soon recognized that any sentence requires abstract, prior knowledge in order to be understood. Comprehending "Time flies like an arrow" requires prior knowledge about metaphors, about the fleetingness of time, about flying and its similarities to other speedy forms of motion, and it requires information about the speaker and his or her purposes, the social and semantic context, and so on. Any linguistic input requires "top-down" information, which is derived from many kinds of abstract knowledge, as well as "bottom-up" information, which is derived from the input itself (Winograd, 1972). When this need for contextual information became widely understood, a great deal of work in Artificial Intelligence began to focus on specifying contextual knowledge in more and more detail.

Psychologists who were in touch with these developments now realized that they had made the same mistake in interpreting their experimental results. Information available to the senses also is frequently ambiguous, and it, too, requires prior knowledge to be decoded. "Long-term memory" was needed to deal with the material in "short-term memory" (*e.g.*, Norman, 1976). The upshot was that it made much more sense to interpret short-term memory as a special aspect of long-term memory, a buffer that not only introduces materials into long-term memory, but also reflects long-term memory. We might say that short-term memory is what happens to long-term memory when it is unable to organize information in the most compact way. When chunks of memory are separated from the context that normally gives them meaning, the relationships between the items is lost. But if the relationships between the seven items in short-term memory are restored, the items stop behaving as separate units, and start acting as a single item. Thus it seems that short-term memory is just a special case of long-term memory. The buffer memories are just a "front end" for the normal, very large, and highly organized repository of our knowledge.

This realization signalled a new era in the methodology of scientific psychology. For the first time there was a fruitful confluence between empirical psychology and theoretical work.

Other Aspects of Mental Representation

During the 1950s, '60s, and '70s, a great many other experiments were being performed on the general topic of mental representations. The issue of *imagery* was rediscovered, and shown to be testable after all, after some 50 years of rejection. Work by Paivio (1971) and Cooper and Shepard (1973) showed that precise, reliable experiments could be performed with mental images, and that the resulting data were clean and simple. There are several curious historical addenda to this. Consider, for example, the commonsense idea that an image is *conscious*, in fact, that an image is a conscious representation of something. During the 1960s and '70s, in the midst of much research on imagery, this rather obvious idea could not be stated by experimental psychologists, because the word "conscious" was still under the ban. This curious gap has continued to lead to considerable confusion to this day (Baars, in press).

But is the expression "conscious representation" not redundant? Aren't all representations conscious? The answer is clearly no — my memory of yesterday's breakfast presumably exists even before I retrieve it, and it becomes conscious only when it is retrieved. Indeed, the Russian physiologist E. N. Sokolov (1963) had already made some elegant arguments for the existence of unconscious representations for those repetitive stimuli to which we have become habituated (the things we have gotten used to). Certain findings about attention also suggest that unconscious representation and information processing could take place (below). The fact is, however, that these realizations did not become generally accepted until the late 1970s.

Although Artificial Intelligence workers had been dealing with highly abstract, complex, and active representational systems since the 1950s, psychologists in general were not ready to accept the idea of abstract mental representation. Some remarkable work by John Bransford and Jeffrey Franks, two graduate students at the University of Minnesota, helped to convince many skeptics of the need to postulate more powerful kinds of knowledge representation.

Bransford and Franks conducted experiments in which they presented several simple stories in a series of sentences, without asking their subjects to memorize the sentences. They simply asked a short question about each sentence, to make sure that its meaning was understood. Afterward, people were presented with completely new sentences and asked which ones they had heard before. Invariably, if the meaning of a new sentence was consistent with the meaning of an old sentence, the subject reported having heard it before. Yet subjects were quite able to detect the novelty of even very similar-sounding sentences, *if* those sentences had a slightly different meaning. Recognition ratings for the new sentences were a linear function of the number of semantic propositions contained in the sentences (Bransford & Franks, 1971; Bransford, 1979).

These experiments are quite natural, because they simply ask the subjects to do what they normally would — that is, try to understand the sentences. But the results have had far-reaching consequences. They have compelled a deeper psychological theory than was hitherto permitted. The memory for "gist" — some sort of meaning representation — is obviously quite a bit better than the memory for actual sentences. Follow-up work showed that subjects also confused with the original sentences those new sentences which expressed immediate inferences from the original meanings (Bransford, 1979). The implication is that we construct semantic representations from the direct meaning conveyed by the sentences.

In the mid-1950s, it was still common to ridicule the notion of mental representation. Twenty years later, the issue became the core of the new psychology. Over several decades, psychologists were forced, by clear empirical results, to adopt a highly abstract theoretical language. Instead of chains of stimuli and responses, they found it necessary to speak of abstract semantic representations that encode not just the meaning of individual words, but an inferential, deeply interpreted representation of the world. In its theoretical sophistication the new perspective was light-years beyond stimulis–response theory.

It now appeared that human beings in general represent their world much as scientists do — in abstract theoretical terms. The abstract theories are highly active: People perform numerous symbolic inferences with them. Mental representations seem to be economical and effective, and they require fast-acting, automatic symbolic processes to make them work. The human nervous system, far from being a passive bundle of connections between stimuli and responses, begins more and more to resemble an enormous, highly sophisticated, active, intelligent, and flexible mechanism.

The Issues of Attention and Consciousness

Consciousness was of course the great bone of contention between 19th-century psychology and the behaviorists. Wundt and James believed that psychology *was* the study of conscious mental contents, and Watson and his followers often denied the very existence of consciousness. The analysis of "attention" was said to be the great accomplishment of 19th-century psychology, and surprisingly, the concept of attention did not entirely disappear during the behavioristic era. At least in the 1950s, American behaviorists began to speak again of stimulus-selection mechanisms, such as Pavlov's "orientation reaction" and the "observing response," whereby animals turn their sensory receptors toward a source of stimulation. But even this was an utterly impoverished version of what had been known about consciousness and attention in the 19th century.

Even though 19th-century psychology defined itself as the study of the contents of consciousness, it was handicapped in dealing with consciousness itself because it *presupposed* consciousness. On the very first page of his book, *An Introduction to Psychology* (1912/1973), Wundt remarks on this fact:

If psychologists are asked, what the business of psychology is, they generally make some such answer as follows, if they belong to the empirical school: that this science has to investigate the facts of consciousness. . . .

Now although this definition seems quite perfect, it is really *to some extent a vicious circle. For if we ask further, what is this consciousness which psychology investigates? the answer will be "It consists of the sum total of facts of which we are conscious."* (p. 1, italics added)

In this sense, psychologists such as Wundt and James were prevented from really seeing the issue of consciousness as a *problem* for scientific investigation. In part, this difficulty was due to their unwillingness to recognize the existence of unconscious processes; one cannot discuss an entity without considering the absence of that entity. But even Freud, who was certainly willing to infer the properties of unconscious processes, had little to say about consciousness *as such*. Thus, in *An Outline of Psychoanalysis* (1940) he writes:

The starting point for this investigation is provided by a fact without parallel, which defies all explanation or description — the fact of consciousness. Nevertheless, if anyone speaks of consciousness, we know immediately and from our most personal experience what is meant by it. (p. 34)

Like many 19th-century thinkers, Freud was greatly impressed by the existence of unconscious factors, but had little to say about conscious processes. Perhaps they seemed too obvious.

Behaviorism broke the vicious circle regarding consciousness, only to deny its existence altogether. Watson viewed consciousness as nothing but "the soul of theology," and given that theology was clearly unscientific, so was consciousness.

All the same, behaviorists did break the conceptual logjam imposed by the assumptions of 19th-century psychology. Tolman wrote a speculative paper on consciousness in 1927. But it was Clark Hull who put into words something that was unclear to the psychologists of the 19th century — namely, that consciousness might actually be *a problem* demanding a psychological explanation. As he wrote in 1937:

. . . to recognize the existence of a phenomenon (i.e. consciousness) is not the same thing as insisting upon its basic, i.e. logical, priority. Instead of furnishing a means for the solution of problems, consciousness appears to be itself a problem needing solution. (p. 29)

This remark represents a high point in behavioristic thought. Had he been allowed to think freely about this problem, Hull might have proposed an interesting theory of consciousness. But of couse in his day, the narrow limits on psychological theorizing kept him from fully using his theoretical imagination. Thus Wundt and James could not discuss consciousness because it was presupposed in everything they did, and behaviorists could not talk about consciousness because to do so required metatheoretical permission to postulate unobservable constructs. Only today is it possible to avoid both of these presuppositional traps.

Consciousness is a pervasive psychological issue. Commonsense psychology takes it for granted that people are conscious of anything they sense in the world around them, that dreams, images and hallucinations are conscious, and that we ordinarily exercise conscious control over our actions. On the other hand, everyday psychology also assumes that sleep and coma imply the absence of consciousness, that we lose consciousness of repetitive events as we get used to them, and that when we become very skilled at some routine action we tend to lose consciousness of it as well. Common sense, then, views consciousness as constrained in a number of ways.

Even during the behavioristic era it was possible in some cases to find behavioral correlates for the things commonsense psychology describes in terms of conscious experience. For example, the fact that people lose awareness of constant or predictable stimulation was studied behaviorally as a decrement in the "orientation reaction" first analyzed by Pavlov (1927/1960). A dog will prick up its ears and look at a source of stimulation, and a number of physiological changes will take place in its body as it does so (*e.g.*, Berlyne, 1960). But as the stimulus is repeated, the dog will no longer point its receptors to the source of stimulation, and the psychological concomitants of the orienting reaction will cease as well. This is a behavioral way to describe habituation of awareness, without recourse to concepts such as attention and consciousness.

But some things cannot easily be described in such behavioral terms, and the prohibition against the idea of consciousness can create an awkward theoretical handicap. A notable case was Jerome Bruner's attempt, in the 1950s, to test the psychodynamic notion of repression by means of a "perceptual defense" concept (Bruner & Postman, 1947; Erdelyi, 1974). Repression is defined as a defense against a potentially conscious thought, but of course this vocabulary was not acceptable within experimental psychology in the 1950s. Rather, Bruner was forced to speak in terms of *perceptual* defense. Instead of consciousness, one was compelled to speak of perception (some behaviorists even considered this term to be mentalistic and, hence, unscientific). Bruner and Postman (1947) were able to show that briefly exposed taboo words were reported less often than neutral words, and interpreted this as evidence for the idea that people defended against the perception of these words. Bruner was a cognitive psychologist from the very beginning, and his work on perceptual defense was really an attempt to trigger an early cognitive revolution, one that would also do justice to psychodynamic concepts. As it turned out, however, although many hundreds of experiments were published on perceptual defense, the idea was criticized and lost credibility (see Erdelyi, 1974; Bruner, 1984).

There were several reasons for Bruner's failure to start a cognitive revolution. Perhaps the most telling was the inability of psychologists of the time to give a coherent account of a process that can *recognize* taboo words, and yet *prevent* the taboo words from being perceived. It made no sense to believe in this "Judas eye" — to think that a word could be detected and yet not perceived; but this is of course an idea that gives modern theoreticians no difficulty in principle. Words may be represented and processed in the nervous system long before they become conscious. But at the time, it made no sense to speak of "unconscious representation" of the taboo words, which would prevent them from becoming conscious. The distinction between conscious and unconscious representation could not be maintained, and as a result, the notion of "perceptual defense" was rejected as incoherent. Indeed, the same objection was often made to Freud's notion of repression. This rather sad episode in the history of psychology illustrates again that the effect of behaviorism was often to make perfectly good theoretical proposals incoherent and incomprehensible. Behaviorists did not even feel the need to argue against such ideas, because they seemed to make no sense, and a nonsensical idea cannot be tested empirically. In this way, some of the most interesting hypotheses in psychology simply went untested.

Psychologists began to rediscover consciousness and attention in the 1950s, when a group in England led by E. Colin Cherry (1953) and Donald E. Broadbent (1958, 1971) began to investigate the effects of listening to two spoken messages at once. In the 19th century it was common to speak of "the unity of consciousness," a phrase by which one meant that people can only experience one interpretation of a stimulus at a time. One way to show this unity is by giving people two streams of information, especially two streams of continuous speech. To be sure that the subjects are actually attending to the speech, they are asked to repeat one stream of speech even while they hear it. With practice, people become very good at this "shadowing" task, and are able to follow the input with a delay of a few tenths of a second; but under these circumstances people can only follow one stream of speech at a time. With this technique, it became possible to investigate consciousness and attention experimentally, though the *word* "consciousness," of course, was not used for several more decades. Much like the work on short-term memory, the findings were interesting, but ultimately led to a difficult paradox.

Broadbent initially proposed that the selectivity of attention occurred because the subject was filtering out unwanted information (1958). Thus, one could shadow only one stream of speech, because any other source of stimulation was being filtered out. Electronic filters were well understood at that time, and it seemed plausible that one simply "turned down the volume" in the ear that was receiving the unwanted speech. By 1958, however, this filter hypothesis had been elegantly disproved by two Cambridge undergraduates, who simply alternated two streams of speech between their subjects' two ears several times a second. Even under such circumstances, people continued to monitor only one message, and they still were unable to report the "nonattended" speech (Gray & Wedderburn, 1960). Thus it could not be true that one filters out the speech in one ear. Furthermore, in order to recognize the rapidly switching stream of speech as *the same one* even though it was coming into different ears, the subjects had to be sensitive to the *content* of the speech — the words' syntax and meaning. Otherwise the attended stream of speech would be confused with the nonattended speech. But if such decisions were being made on the basis of content, then how could one be filtering out the content?

Some time later it was shown that even the nonattended stream of speech had observable effects. For example, if the attended stream of speech contained an ambiguous sentence ("I am going to sit near the *bank*"), and simultaneous with the word *bank* the nonattended channel contained the word "water," the subject would tend to interpret "bank" as "river bank"; but if the nonattended channel instead contained the word "money," the subject's interpretation would tend to shift to "financial bank" (MacKay, 1973). Thus Broadbent's early proposal that the nonattended stream of speech was being filtered out was contradicted: The meaning of "water" or "money" had to be available unconsciously, so that the conscious word "bank" could be interpreted. But if unconscious information is processed just as conscious information is, what is the real difference between conscious and unconscious events? Broadbent had proposed that filtering out unwanted material helps to save processing capacity for more important information; but if all input is in fact analyzed, no work is saved. Again, a promising research direction seemed to lead to paradox.

The same kind of paradox was encountered in the study of short-term memory, where it seemed at first that sensory input is analyzed bottom-up. That is, we were presumed to analyze speech by examining first the sound, then the phonemes and morphemes, then words and syntax, and finally the meaning of the input. But work on short-term memory, as well as Artificial Intelligence theory, showed that this could not be true; that, in fact, one needed to use prior high-level knowledge in order to process even the lowest level of input. Top-down processes were needed as much as bottom-up ones. Thus, the filter theory of attention, which assumed that one could shut out the *sound* of nonattended messages, was bound to fail. Even the lowest level of input analysis may require high-level top-down processes. This realization explained, at least in part, why unconscious words seem to affect the semantic interpretation of conscious input, and also why it is possible to switch two streams of information rapidly between the two ears, without the subject's losing track of the attended message.

Clearly a great deal about consciousness and attention remained to be understood. But it was not until the late 1970s that psychologists were even willing to resurrect the word "consciousness" from its premature grave, and to address the issues it raised in an experimentally precise and theroetically creative way (*e.g.*, Mandler, 1975; Shallice, 1972, 1978; Baars, 1983a, in press). This is currently perhaps the most important theoretical issue in cognitive psychology, one whose outcome is by no means clear.

The Problem of Serial Order

Behavior takes place over time, and the components of behavior must be ordered. During the behavioristic period, only one theoretical mechanism was invoked to handle this serial aspect of behavior—namely the *chain* of stimuli and responses. An external stimulus was understood to evoke a response, which itself had stimulus properties, which were connected to the next response with its own stimulus properties, and so on. This, in essence, is Hull's theory, which was the most sophisticated attempt made to deal with this problem (1937). But in 1951, Karl Lashley pointed out some fundamental inadequacies of this conception. A chain of stimuli and responses cannot explain, for example, the cases where elements in the chain appear to "leapfrog" over each other. To make his point, Lashley cites the case of spoonerisms—"our dear old Queen" being transposed into "our queer old Dean."

There are numerous situations where parts of a sequential action appear to be leapfrogging. Take the case of active and passive sentences. "The boy chased the cat" is a near-paraphrase of "The cat was chased by the boy." In order to recognize the similarity of these sentences, one must be able to transpose the order of "boy" and "cat," and this capacity would require more than just a chain of word-responses. Wilhelm Wundt had made this very point when he noted that Latin grammar allows the order of words to change quite freely without changing the meaning of a sentence (Blumenthal, 1970).

The fact that chaining theories cannot explain leapfrogging elements can be made clear to a child: Picture a train going into a tunnel, with a locomotive, a passenger train, and a caboose. But at the other end of the tunnel, the train comes out in reverse order: The caboose comes first, followed by the passenger car, and finally the locomotive. What could have happened inside the tunnel? Well, maybe there is a parallel switching track or maybe a giant crane was used to exchange the caboose and the locomotive. But whatever mechanism we imagine, it must involve *more than a single* railroad track. In the same way, one must imagine more than a serial chain of elements in order to explain the exchange of phonemes in a spoonerism, or the ability people have to transform active to passive sentences. This realization forces one to abandon the sole theoretical mechanism that behavioristic theoreticians, such as Hull, were able to use.

Noam Chomsky first achieved fame with his monograph, *Syntactic Structures* (1957), in which he used the mathematical theory of automata to prove formally that the class of chaining theories (technically called Markov processes) cannot in principle represent even the simplest kind of grammar that is needed to represent the linguistic competence of human beings. (The simplest grammar that can describe some important aspects of sentence structure is called a "finite-state" or "tree-structure" grammar. It is effectively the same formalism that most people learn in elementary school by "diagramming sentences.") Chomsky went on to prove further that any grammar able to represent such things as the similarity between active and passive sentences would have to be even more powerful than a tree-structure grammar. This powerful but minimally necessary grammar he called a Transformational Grammar.

In many ways Chomsky's argument was a formal equivalent of the informal argument given by Lashley (1951) and by Wundt in the previous century (Blumenthal, 1970). There is a class of symbolic strings called "mirror-image strings," in which the first half of the string is a mirror-image of the second half. Thus ab, abba, baab, abbbba, and aabbaa are mirror-image strings, whereas aabb and baa are not. Anybody can learn to recognize mirror-image strings very quickly, and almost anyone can suggest a formal procedure to test whether a string is a mirror-image string. But it can be proved mathematically that such a string cannot be represented in a general form by a chain grammar (Markov Process). Thus, even so trivial a learning task as recognizing a mirror-image string cannot be represented by a Markov process. Hull's chaining theory was proved unable to account for linguistic competence, or for any other ability of similar complexity. This proof was later generalized to cover all chain theories of serial-order behavior (Bever, Fodor, & Garrett, 1968).

Chomsky's work caught on slowly, but once it became widely understood it had very great impact. Its effect must be understood in terms of the enormous resistance to complex theory shown by behavioristic psychologists. Behaviorists were intent on producing extremely parsimonious theories, theories that did not postulate any more elements than were strictly necessary. Chomsky's formal proofs made it clear that these parsimonious theories *could never, in principle, explain what they were intended to explain*. The theories lacked adequacy. Thus psychologists were forced to postulate more complex theories than before.

This development had a curious outcome, because it was not long before it was proven mathematically that Chomsky's proposed Transformational Grammar was formally equivalent to a Turing Machine (Turing, 1950). But a Turing Machine can compute *any* function whatsoever. Thus a Transformational Grammar, which is the *minimum* necessary grammar to account for language, is formally equivalent to the *maximally* powerful kind of theory. Very soon after Chomsky's work, computer scientists working in Artificial Intelligence began to develop grammars other than Transformational Grammar, but these too, were invariably equivalent to Turing Machines. Indeed, there seems to be no viable system that can model some significant part of human behavior that is less powerful than the most powerful mathematical system. What all this means is that *the mathematical theory of automata can suggest no kind of parsimony for any system able to account for some significant part of human behavior*. All theories must be mathematically maximum theories.

One can suggest other aspects of theoretical parsimony, such as computational efficiency, fast-processing speed, and limited memory load, but these properties cannot be handled by the theory of automata. In order to place constraints on the set of possible psychological theories, psychologists would have to look elsewhere than pure mathematics.

The Problem of Inferring Process and Structure

Increasingly the question was raised: Under what conditions can one infer the existence of invisible, but theoretically necessary, constructs? Chomsky had suggested that language cannot be understood except by reference to *rules*. Indeed, according to Chomsky, the sentences of a language are generated by rules in much the way algebraic formulas are generated by the basic elements and operations of algebra. But rules are abstract entities — they are symbolic representations that can account for very large sets of observable events. And for the speakers of a language, of course, the rules are not conscious. Sets of rules make up a structure, a relatively stable knowledge representation. But structure is not enough to make knowledge work. Rules must actively operate on incoming information, on information in memory, and on plans for controlling actions. These requirements raise the issue of *process* as well as *structure*. An adequate cognitive psychology must be able to infer both process and structure.

Structure was usually inferred by what might be called *equivalence operations*. People will treat two superficially different events as part of one unified structure: Two different orientations of the same physical object (for example, a chair) are treated perceptually as just two aspects of the same "thing"; two paraphrases of a sentence are often confused with each other in memory, as are two similar-sounding syllables, or two acoustically different versions of the same phoneme. These equivalence classes can be represented theoretically as a single structure, so that at an abstract level, the two sentences that are confused in memory may be represented in one structure.

This view of mental structure corresponds directly to what people for ages have called "knowledge." The Indo-European roots of the word "knowledge" go back to the very earliest known languages, with roughly the same meaning; so the idea of knowledge is at least 4000 years old. Very often we can infer that people know something by presenting material in one form and testing their knowledge in a different form. College examinations may present paraphrases of the original material, to test whether students can remember the abstract content of the sentences they hear as well as the sentences themselves. If this equivalence class exists, one can infer knowledge. In a way, then, cognitive psychologists assess knowledge in the same way everyday psychology does.

Finding evidence for mental *processes* is a good deal trickier. The main source of evidence for inferring process has come from measurements of reaction time in fairly simple tasks. In the 19th century the Dutch psychologist Donders (1868) suggested a way of measuring the duration of mental processes by interposing " . . . into the process of the physiological time some new components of mental action" (p. 418). Donders knew, for example, that the time needed to respond to a single predictable stimulus (called *simple* reaction time) was always shorter than the time needed to respond differentially to one of two possible stimuli (*choice* reaction time). For example, he showed that the time needed to react to an electric shock delivered to *either* the right or left leg was longer than the time needed to react to a shock that would invariably be given to only one leg. The time difference between these conditions was 66 milliseconds, and Donders interpreted this time difference as the time required to choose between the two possible responses in the choice reaction time task. But notice that some of this time might be needed to choose between the two *stimuli* (left or right shock) rather than between the two *responses* (saying "left" or "right"). To distinguish between these two interpretations, Donders added a *third* experimental condition, in which several stimuli were presented but only *one* had to be responded to (the so-called "c-reaction"). He proposed that:

(1) Stimulus Discrimination = c-Reaction Time – Simple Reaction Time
    Time

and

(2) Response Choice Time = Choice Reaction Time – c-Reaction Time

Thus he could separate, by inference, the time needed to select the right stimulus from the time needed to select the right response. These values he found to be 36 and 47 milliseconds, respectively, in a verbal reaction time task.

Donders's clever solution to the problem of inferring processing time was based on some debatable assumptions. Even in the 19th century some psychologists argued that other explanations for Donders's results were possible. For instance, in simple reaction time (where only one response is possible), subjects might be better prepared to make the response than in a choice reaction time task. The difference between simple and choice reaction time is not just that a "stage" has been added — there is a qualitative difference as well. Moreover, Donders assumed that all mental processes must be discrete and serial. This may sometimes be so, but there is much reason to think that some processes are gradual, interactive, and parallel.

Interest in the use of reaction time tasks for inferring the duration of mental processes received a great boost as a result of the cognitive shift (*e.g.*, Sternberg, 1966; Posner, 1978). In 1969, Sternberg proposed a new approach to the inference problem, the "additive factors method," based on a statistical technique called analysis of variance. Using analysis of variance, one can discern the effect of several independent variables on some dependent measure such as reaction time. It also provides a way of deciding whether two or more variables interact in their effect, or whether the individual effects are only additive. Sternberg proposed applying the same logic to the study of reaction time. His method is not based on adding or deleting stages of processing, but on the possibility of *selectively influencing* the duration of different stages (Ashby & Townsend, 1980).

In his first demonstration of the technique, Sternberg manipulated three variables in a choice reaction time task: First, the quality of the stimulus was either degraded or normal. Second, the number of stimulus–response alternatives was varied. And finally, the compatibility between stimuli and responses was varied between high and low compatibility. The results indicated that stimulus quality and stimulus–response compatibility both had additive effects on reaction time, but that these two variables interacted in a nonadditive way with the third, the number of stimulus–response alternatives. These results were interpreted to mean that there were, indeed, two separate processing stages. The first, or *stimulus encoding* stage, was affected by the quality of the stimulus and by the number of alternative stimuli that had to be evaluated. The second stage, consisting of *translation* and *response organization*, was affected by stimulus–response compatibility, and also by the number of alternative responses available.

Sternberg's additive-factors logic has been widely applied, and other methods have also been proposed. A large and active research literature has sprung up. But is the goal of it all — a reliable method for inferring the details of human information processing — really within our reach? It may be too early to tell.

Cognitive Science: The Rise of a Theoretical Psychology

Perhaps the most exciting recent development growing out of the cognitive revolution is a new trend toward integrating all the major disciplines concerned with studying the nature of knowledge. This new interdisciplinary field has been called "cognitive science," and it includes cognitive psychology, linguistics, philosophy, Artificial Intelligence, and the neurosciences. These fields are indeed developing a set of common concerns, and even, to some extent, a common language. This new, integrative trend is most encouraging — no longer is it necessary for psychologists to prove their scientific standing by rejecting philosophy or neurophysiology as irrelevant to their concerns. Rather, there is a wide appreciation of commonalities in the problems encountered by philosophers, psychologists, linguists, Artificial Intelligence workers, and neuroscientists. Indeed, at a theoretical level, these problems often seem to be identical.

Artifical Intelligence provides the theoretical core of cognitive science, because it gives us a theoretical language that permits us to be precise about cognitive issues. I have briefly mentioned the study of Artificial Intelligence, but only in passing. Given the widespread suspicion of theory in experimental psychology, for many years only a few scientific psychologists took Artificial Intelligence work seriously. It appeared to be entirely theoretical and nonempirical. It was not until the 1970s that a significant group of psychologists began to look seriously at this field (Norman, 1976; Anderson & Bower, 1973; Anderson, 1980). The rise of cognitive science signals a change in the rejection of theory among psychologists, and the reasons for this new receptivity are worth discussing.

Psychologists have been involved with the development of computer languages from quite an early point (see the interview with Herbert Simon, Chapter 7). Allan Newell and Herbert Simon, who considered themselves to be psychological scientists, helped develop some of the first higher-level computer language, and were apparently the first to articulate the very important idea of recursiveness in high-level computer languages (Newell & Simon, 1972). They and other pioneers in the 1950s developed the first simulations of intelligent human functions, including short-term memory, problem solving, chess playing, and logical theorem proving (see Newell & Simon, 1972; Feigenbaum & Feldman, 1963; Schank & Colby, 1973). Such simulations performed several functions: They showed that computers can do some things that are considered signs of intelligence when performed by human beings; and further, they suggested a possible theory of the way in which human beings do the same task. Thus, a simulation of chess playing can serve as a theory of how humans play chess — in this case, a largely incorrect theory. Finally, any other theory of chess playing, language comprehension, or emotional conflict could be encoded in a computer program if it were made sufficiently explicit. Thus, computer programs provide a natural theoretical language for stating psychological hypotheses in a very explicit way. And any theory that cannot be made explicit enough to run on a computer is *ipso facto* a faulty theory.

This last point is of enormous importance for psychology. Historically, scientific development is severely hampered without a theoretical language that can naturally model the subject matter of the science. If Newton had done nothing more than invent the infinitesimal calculus, which is a natural language for modeling the movement of objects in space, his place in the history of physics would have been assured. Psychology has never had a language able to express *in a natural way* the facts we observe. That language now seems to exist, and if this were the only contribution made by Artificial Intelligence, its place in the history of psychology would be assured.

Psychologists have often tried to apply to their subject the kinds of mathematics that proved so successful in the physical sciences, with generally poor results. Early in the 19th century, the physicist J. F. Herbart tried to apply algebra and even calculus to model the way in which thoughts rise to consciousness, but this attempt was essentially metaphorical (Miller, 1964). There was no way to quantify the strength of a thought with any precision. Similarly, in this century, Hull attempted to use algebraic formulas in an essentially metaphoric fashion; and Kurt Lewin tried to apply ideas from mathematical topology, using vectors to indicate the strength of a goal, a bounded region to represent the "life space," and so on (see Miller, 1964). By the 1950s, a more sophisticated and modest group of mathematical psychologists appeared, who applied more appropriate kinds of mathematics to certain limited psychological problems: probability theory, decision theory, and signal detection theory. Some of this work has been quite valuable, and yet, all of these mathematical applications still assume that the kinds of mathematics that work in physics and chemistry will fit the requirements of psychology.

In particular, it is assumed that *quantification* is important for representing psychological phenomena. It is quite possible, however, to get mathematical precision without quantification — for example, in symbolic logic, Boolean algebra, topology, and, perhaps most important for psychology, in the theory of automata and a related field called recursive function theory. There are many reasons to believe that some kinds of nonquantitative mathematics are more important for psychology than standard algebra. For example, Chomsky's theory of linguistics is based entirely on automaton theory. In linguistics, one deals most naturally with a string of symbols, and quantitative questions about these symbols are irrelevant. What is important about a sentence is not how loudly it is spoken, nor even how long it is; what is important is its meaning, its syntactic structure, the words it contains, and the like.

There are some remarkably simple ideas that make it possible to model language, semantics, and other kinds of qualitative representations of the world in a natural way. I have mentioned Chomsky's work on grammar, which used tree-structures and Transformational Grammar. In effect, a Transformational Grammar is a mathematical system that allows tree-structures to be transformed into other tree-structures. With this property, the Transformational Grammar becomes equivalent to a Turing Machine (see p. 177) — that is, it can then be shown formally to be capable of computing any mathematical function. Transformational

Grammar is one language that is capable of expressing an important set of facts about natural language that cannot be expressed by a less powerful system. But there are other languages of equal computational power, many of which are more convenient than Chomsky's grammar for performing certain symbolic operations. These languages were developed in the 1950s and '60s, based on a mathematical theory about tree-structures called "recursive function theory." The most popular computer language based on this theory is called LISP (for List Processing language).

The basic idea of LISP is very simple. A tree can have any number of branches, and the labeled intersection of each branch is called a node. LISP provides a set of commands able to trace along the branches of a tree to find the nodes, and the labels at these intersections can direct the program either to another node or to another tree. Thus, the syntax of a sentence can be modeled in LISP, just as it is in the "sentence diagrams" that most people learn in elementary school. But trees can be related to other trees, and this capacity raises the formal power of LISP to that of a Transformational Grammar (equivalent to a Turing Machine).

Suppose now, that we want somehow to represent the meaning of a sentence in such a way that we can model the effects found by memory psychologists. If we wish to represent the meaning of the word "buy," it is clear that we must relate it to a number of similar meanings: For example, there is reciprocity between the words "buy" and "sell," which can be shown in a LISP format. Similarly, we would want to relate the word "buy" to the words "buyer," "seller," and "medium of exchange," and to a subjective assessment of value by the buyer and seller, and so on. In a natural way, a very dense network of relationships begins to emerge between all these components, which can be symbolized by labels on a complex set of tree-structures. Such semantic networks are quite effective in representing meaning structures so that a computer containing the semantic network can answer questions about the subject of buying and selling, generate semantically equivalent paraphrases, relate one part of a discourse to another, retrieve relevant facts, make inferences from the facts given, obey commands stated in ordinary language, solve certain problems, and even generate some analogies.

This is really the proof of the pudding, of course. One can make a plausible case that a language such as LISP is a natural way to encode human knowledge, but this argument will not convince many people unless one can show its effectiveness in particular cases. That has been done abundantly. LISP has been used to model parts of human knowledge in a variety of domains, to parse and generate sentences, recognize speech, play chess and other games, simulate the behavior of a paranoid patient in a mental hospital, generate pictures, and control the movement of a robot (Boden, 1977). All this does not mean that LISP is the ultimate language for the representation of psychological facts, but it does mean that it is far more effective than any previous theoretical medium. And of course, LISP is not at all a *quantitative* language. LISP makes it easy to represent sentences, but hard to represent algebraic equations. Yet it is entirely precise from a mathematical point of view.

Psychologists have found it difficult to deal with a mathematically precise but nonquantifiable theoretical language. All experimental proof-procedures available to psychologists were aimed at testing quantitative hypotheses. Further, any system that simulates an intelligent human ability must be enormously complex and interactive. In fact, it is a behaviorist's nightmare: Artificial Intelligence theories contain thousands of theoretical entities, all interacting with each other at enormous speed. There simply were no experimental methods for assessing the empirical implications of such a complex system, but it seemed that nothing less complex and symbolic would do the job of simulating interesting human functions. Thus, empirical psychologists were caught in a bind: The minimum system needed to model the process of understanding natural language is enormously complex, far beyond the proof-procedures available; and yet something at this level of complexity was needed to do the job. (Neurophysiologists are probably not so distressed by this, given that the nervous system has a comparable awesome level of complexity.) In this situation, it is perhaps surprising that psychologists were receptive to Artificial Intelligence work at all.

Not all cognitive psychologists even today are receptive to Artificial Intelligence (*e.g.*, Neisser, 1963b). Even those who are not, still profit from the "breathing space" created by the computer for psychological theorizing. The capabilities of computers makes it easier to propose all kinds of theories. Of all cognitive psychologists, perhaps the most uncomfortable with Artificial Intelligence are the strongest empiricists: those who still maintain the suspicion of theory inherited from behaviorism. They will continue to insist on direct empirical proof, and this is of course all to the good. There is widespread misunderstanding of this "computational metaphor" for psychology, as well as some intense disagreement from those who are familiar with it (Weizenbaum, 1976; Neisser, 1963b). Psychologists are often said to believe that people are like computers, but this is a crude way of stating the case. There are, in fact, a number of useful levels of the computational metaphor, some more conservative than others.

First, and most conservatively, there is the claim that any precise psychological theory can be modeled on a computer. This is almost certainly true. The modern digital computer has its limitations, of course: It is only a very fast, serial device for executing entirely explicit, discrete instructions. Thus, it would seem unable to represent situations that require parallel operations, or analog (as opposed to digital) operations, or those that are imprecise. But all of these limitations can be overcome. Digital computers can simulate analog processes to any desired degree of precision. The serial operating systems of these computers can also simulate parallel processes, and in recent years a great deal of very important work has been done with parallel "distributed" systems, which are networks of ordinary computers. And, finally, the representations maintained by computers do not even have to be entirely explicit: They may be probabilistic or make use of a logic called "fuzzy set theory" (Zadeh, 1975). In sum, there is no reason at this point to believe that computers have *principled* limitations in representing interesting psychological facts.

A stronger, less conservative, claim about the computational metaphor for psychology is that *computers and humans are both information processors*. (This claim is not inherent in the previous point that computers can represent interesting things about people — computers can also represent interesting things about houses, but no one claims that houses are information processors.) We have previously cited some reasons to think that the human nervous system works to process information — that it is not sensitive to physical energy as such, but only to information; that it tends to treat different physical events as identical if they are abstractly the same, and so on.

Perhaps the strongest version of the computational metaphor claims that when computers are confronted with tasks similar to those that humans must solve, they are driven to the same kinds of solutions. In analyzing speech, computers must use both top-down and bottom-up processes, just as people apparently are obliged to do. In input and output, both computers and people require buffer memories in order to relate events arriving at different times. A number of such similarities have been found, but no one is likely to take them for granted without investigating the human side of the analogy with great care.

Any of these reasons are adequate justification for the psychological interest in Artificial Intelligence. This is a very significant development in the history of psychology, but it raises some troubling questions as well. As a young science, psychology has not yet had to face the possibility that psychological knowledge might be misused. If psychological theory achieves some genuine level of adequacy at some point in the future, this possibility will have to be faced.

Behavioristic Responses to the Cognitive Revolution

There has been surprisingly little in the way of controversy in the cognitive revolution. No doubt many behaviorists felt opposed to the new approach, as the interviews in Chapter 3 indicate, but not much of this opposition appeared in print. As I mentioned, the single great public controversy took place as a result of Noam Chomsky's negative review of B. F. Skinner's book *Verbal Behavior* (1957). In his autobiography (1976, 1979), Skinner tells us how this attempt to provide a detailed behavioristic account of language was to be the ultimate achievement of his life's work, a project on which he had worked for almost two decades before it was ready to appear in print. In view of his original training as a serious writer of "psychological" short stories, we may guess that Skinner's attempt to explain language in terms of operant conditioning had a great personal as well as scientific significance.

Skinner considered language to be essentially a chain of responses emitted by a speaker when the environment called them forth. His theory holds that children learn language by a process of trial-and-error conditioning, facilitated by the community of speakers surrounding the child. To some extent, verbal responses would be differentially reinforced by adults, so that "correct" utterances would gain the child attention, hugs, and other reinforcing stimuli. As these utterances were reinforced, they would tend to grow in frequency.

I have already indicated that by the time Skinner's book was published in 1957, the world had already changed. Noam Chomsky, then a young and still obscure linguist at MIT, was in the process of gaining a reputation for a new and disturbing approach to language, which claimed to prove that all contemporary theories of language were grossly inadequate to explain even the simplest and most obvious facts. Thus, when Skinner's book was published, it became grist for Chomsky's mill. Asked to review *Verbal Behavior* for the influential journal *Language*, Chomsky attacked Skinner's theory with the kind of vigor and theoretical perspicacity that has seemed to be a specialty in linguistics (Chomsky, 1959). In effect, he argued, Skinner's work had nothing to do with language, because Skinner knew nothing about language as such. Skinner treated language simply as another instance of the kind of behavior that could be observed and manipulated in animal experiments. But language was demonstrably *rule-governed* and *generative* (in that an infinite number of new sentences could be generated from the grammar of a language), and to understand language one had to postulate the existence of a powerful theoretical construct, a Transformational Grammar, which was sensitive to the regularities *underlying* the immediate observable "surface" facts of language. Any sentence in a language and, indeed, any natural language as a whole, was only a phenotypic instance of an underlying genotype, just as any organism is only a particular realization of an underlying genetic plan. Indeed, Chomsky argued, there is much reason to think that our capacity for language is not learned in any simple sense, but that it is part of our biological inheritance. Needless to say, according to Chomsky, Skinner's theory failed in all respects to account for these facts. Even further, no imaginable behavioristic theory could handle such facts, for much the same reasons that Skinner's theory failed: Behavioristic theory was averse to postulating rules, because rules are abstractions, and behaviorism was committed to the analysis of concrete, observable things. Generativity of responses was not acceptable to behaviorists, because responses were thought to be paired with stimuli through a process of conditioning. The deep rule-structure underlying surface sentences could not be observed directly and, hence, was considered to be unscientific. In almost every respect, Chomsky's arguments contradicted the behaviorism of Watson, Skinner, and Hull. His facts were not collected in the laboratory using precise experimental designs and operational definitions, but came simply from everyone's knowledge of their native language. Moreover, the idea that language capacity could be largely inherited ran counter to the behavioristic emphasis on environmentalism.

Chomsky's review of Skinner's *Verbal Behavior* had great impact among linguists and psychologists, far more so than the work it attacked. At just about this time, a new field called "psycholinguistics" was taking shape — a field created to study language by combining the efforts of psychologists and linguists in one coherent domain. Although psycholinguistics began behavioristically, it was open to new ideas, and soon cognitive thinkers were taking over. Psycholinguistics provided the first ground for collaboration between Chomsky and perhaps the single most influential figure in the cognitive revolution, George A. Miller. Miller, whose interview appears in the next chapter, propagated Chomsky's views among scientific psychologists. In a joint paper, Chomsky and Miller (1958) showed that it was impossible for people to acquire by conditioning all the sentences they could speak and understand — indeed, people appeared able to understand more sentences than there are seconds in a lifetime! Clearly these sentences could not be learned one by one, whether by conditioning or by any other means. People must have a relatively small set of rules that enables them to put together many different sentences.

Skinner never replied to Chomsky in print, although the two did meet in public debate on several occasions. In any case, they had little to say to each other (see their interviews, Chapters 3 and 7, respectively). Their theories were so different, the kinds of evidence they considered had so few common elements, and their methods were so alien to each other, that genuine communication appeared to be impossible. In fact, their attempts to communicate illustrates graphically one of Thomas Kuhn's claims about scientific revolutions: that even with the best intentions, adherents of different paradigms are not able to reason out their differences — they simply talk past each other.

Some of Skinner's followers answered Chomsky in print (*e.g.*, McCorquodale, 1970; Salzinger, 1970). Some years later, Skinner himself wrote an interesting article called "Why I Am Not a Cognitive Psychologist" (1977) which I discussed earlier. These replies came too late to be effective. By this time — the late '50s and early '60s — the cognitive point of view had already emerged in many different places, for many different reasons, not all of them inspired by Chomsky. Indeed, one of the striking aspects of the cognitive revolution was this sudden emergence of common insights among people who were socially and geographically far removed from one another. When water turns to ice, crystal formation begins in many places at once, and the transition to the solid state is quite sudden. We cannot point to one place in the liquid as *the* starting point of the phase-change from liquid to solid — the phenomenon is quite literally a function of the whole. There is an appealing analogy between the cognitive shift and such a change of phase in a physical liquid.

There have been occasional attempts to bridge the gap between behavioristic and cognitive points of view, but these attempts at integration have not been very persuasive. Some psychologists tried to develop an intermediate position, but were ultimately driven to believe either one or the other, and it soon appeared that most of the active researchers in human psychology were moving to a stronger and stronger cognitive position. That trend has continued for several decades, and at this writing it has not yet stopped.

The Liberal–Conservative Continuum: Five Cognitive Psychologists

Five individuals may be said to typify the new psychology. All five can be called cognitive psychologists, but they differ greatly in the degree to which they accept cognitive premises. From the most to the least conservative, they include the following: *Charles E. Osgood* attempted to adapt Hullian behavior theory to the question of linguistic meaning in the 1950s, and has held firmly to this position ever since. *James J. Jenkins* began with a major research program designed to test an intermediate theory of language learning, appropriately called "mediational theory". Finding his empirical results disappointing, he moved toward a more Chomskyan point of view. *George A. Miller* called himself a "good behaviorist" in a book published in 1951, but soon afterwards took the lead in guiding other psychologists toward an increasingly cognitive position. *Jerome S. Bruner* was clearly too impatient to wait for others to catch up, and as a result probably touched on more interesting issues in his career than any number of other psychologists, at the cost of some loss of influence. And finally, *Herbert A. Simon* started outside of psychology proper, and began doing work in Artificial Intelligence 20 years before it became popular; he has since seen the field move more and more in his direction.

Osgood was deeply concerned from a very young age with the issue of meaning in language (1975). As a good experimentalist, he saw the question of linguistic meaning as essentially a problem of measurement. If scientific psychology was to address the issue of meaning in a respectable way, it would have to be operationalized, brought into the laboratory, and best of all, quantified. This is, of course, the familiar emphasis on quantification derived from the physical sciences, and it does not appear that Osgood considered that meaning might not be *naturally* quantifiable in the usual sense of the word, or that one could be mathematically explicit about meaning without using numbers. But in the 1940s and '50s, few people considered this possibility seriously (but see Brunswik, 1946). Within the limits so defined, Osgood's work was remarkable: He did, indeed, manage to develop a well-specified measure of something much like meaning, but not the kind of meaning we speak of when we say "the meaning of this word or sentence" — rather, Osgood's work seems to deal with *connotative meaning*.

Before Osgood's work, behavioristic psychologists interested in the question of meaning were much concerned with a phenomenon called "semantic generalization" (Razran, 1961). Generalization refers to the process whereby a conditioned response can be made to occur to a stimulus that is similar to, but not identical with, the original stimulus. Thus, a 1000-cycle tone can be made to elicit salivation, and as a result, a 990-cycle tone will also elicit some salivation. The trouble was that stimulus generalization didn't seem to apply to language learning. If one conditioned a response in an adult to a word such as "vase," one did not get generalization to a similar-sounding word such as "maze" or "haze," but rather, to a *synonym* of the first word—for example, "urn." But if the synonym had no physical similarity to the original word, how could a theory of conditioning account for the generalization? Adults seemed to treat two stimuli as equivalent, even though they had no physical similarity!

Osgood (1953) suggested that there must be some underlying similarity, but because he could not freely postulate the existence of abstract representations, he was forced to adopt the solution that Hull had proposed to the problem of goal-representation (Chapter 2): There had to be some small response (much like Hull's fractional anticipatory goal response) that had stimulus-properties (so other responses could be conditioned to it), which was evoked by both of the physically different synonyms. Thus, underlying the physically different synonyms there was a single, physical, potentially measurable entity. In a clear analogy to Hull, Osgood called this invisible but potentially observable response an r_m—a fractional meaning response. Notice that the r_m is invisible, and in that sense it resembles the theoretical constructs of full-fledged cognitive psychology. This kind of theory is called a "mediational" theory because invisible stimuli and responses are postulated to meditate between visible stimuli and responses. Once that postulate is accomplished, one can apply the standard laws of conditioning to show how semantic generalization (and many other phenomena) could work.

But how is one to tie down the r_m to some measurable experimental operation? Here Osgood made a brilliant and perhaps lasting contribution. It was already known that people rate words in a consistent way when using a seven-point scale whose end-points are labeled by virtually any pair of polar adjectives. For example, a word such as "love" is consistently rated as more "soft" than "hard," more "high" than "low," more "slow" than "fast," and so on. Because many of the scales produce the same ratings for any number of words, one can collapse the redundant scales into three dimensions that capture most of the information contained in them. As discussed earlier, the three dimensions are (1) potency, (2) activity, and (3) evaluation. In a book entitled *The Measurement of Meaning* (1957), Osgood, Suci, and Tannenbaum showed that the same three dimensions may be found in many different cultures—indeed, Osgood's work with the dimensions of meaning has probably seen more crosscultural validation than any other research performed by an experimental psychologist.

This was a major empirical achievement. But it was not so clear whether Osgood's work exhausted the meaning of meaning, or whether there were other, legitimate senses of "meaning" that could not be treated in this way. After all, in the three-dimensional space defined by Osgood's three major components of meaning, a word such as "nurse" might occupy almost the same point as a word such as "kindness," "pilot," or "schoolteacher." Yet these words seem to differ in terms of some other kind of meaning than the one measured by Osgood and his colleagues. Further, Osgood's theory of meaning as an r_m was not received kindly by cognitive psychologists when they began to turn their attention to it (Fodor, 1965). Ultimately, other psychologists began to borrow formalisms from Artificial Intelligence, which could express these other aspects of meaning in a more adequate fashion (Norman & Rumelhart, 1975).

Yet the three dimensions of Osgood's system do express something about the meaning of words. As I pointed out in Chapter 2, Osgood's three dimensions are perfectly paralleled by the three dimensions of conscious experience discovered by Wilhelm Wundt (1912/1973) in the 19th century: Wundt's pleasure and pain, strain and relaxation, and excitation and quiescence correspond respectively to Osgood's evaluation, potency, and activity. Here is another exquisite historical irony—that a strict behaviorist could rediscover the same phenomenon first found by the much-criticized introspectionists, but not with all the massive armamentarium of modern science: strict experimental designs, careful subject selection, elaborate statistical techniques, and crosscultural validation. We may take this apparent coincidence as a favorable sign: Perhaps it means that different psychologists, using very different methods, may still discover the same world. Even so, it seems more accurate to call Osgood's kind of meaning something like "connotative meaning"—some residue of feeling and attitude that is held in common in our evaluation of nurses, pilots, and schoolteachers.

Today, Osgood's work represents the old guard in psychological research on language function, both in its faults and virtues. His results are precise, clearly operationalized, replicable, and robust. But his theory, by modern standards, is much too parsimonious and insulated from the normal linguistic processes that people engage in. On the other hand, that theory can be seen as a step in the direction of representational theories, which state baldly that there exists some abstract level of representation in human psychology, a level that need not be directly observed, but helps to make sense out of a host of phenomena that cannot otherwise be understood (*e.g.*, Miller & Johnson-Laird, 1976).

As a conscientious experimentalist, Charles Osgood could not permit himself such theoretical freedom in the 1950s. People who exercised such freedom at the time were simply not considered to be scientific, and indeed, some had to pay the price of exclusion from the community of "serious" psychologists for this very reason.

James J. Jenkins is also very much an experimental psychologist, though his career differs from Osgood in interesting ways (see interview in Chapter 5). Jenkins attempted to perform a rather heroic series of experimental tests of the mediational theory of meaning and syntax. His interview describes these experiences well, and the reader is referred to it for details. Jenkins's attempt to test mediation theory failed in certain critical ways. In the face of this failure, Jenkins was able to stand back from the standard behavioristic framework, and reexamine the issues from the ground up. In his ability to keep changing with the field and discover a fruitful *modus vivendi* with the new point of view, Jenkins's work was remarkable. Yet his research remained essentially experimental, and, thus, in the rough conservative–liberal dimension, he belongs somewhere between Osgood and a somewhat more theoretical psychologist, George A. Miller.

Miller's work has been mentioned already in connection with the linguist Chomsky, who triggered a cognitive revolution in linguistics at roughly the same time that the cognitive revolution took place in psychology. Miller began as a psychophysicist at Harvard with a strong mathematical background. On three different occasions he imported into experimental psychology a quasimathematical framework for the consideration of other psychologists, and three times psychologists accepted his point of view. The first imported framework was *information theory*, a mathematical theory developed during the Second World War to describe the carrying capacity of communication channels such as telephone lines (Miller, 1964). Although this theory was and is of fundamental importance to computer scientists and psychologists, it seemed to have little to do with the kinds of problems faced by experimental psychologists. In particular, the mathematical definition of "information" seemed to circumvent the whole issue of representation — information was defined as a choice made between alternatives in some existing representation in a message-receiver, as a consequence of the same choice signalled by the sender of the message. Insofar as the message caused the receiver to make the same choice, information could be said to have been transmitted.

But how was one to represent the alternatives to be chosen in the first place, especially when those alternatives approached the kind of complexity needed to represent real human concerns? This question was simply not dealt with. Thus, information theory seemed to beg the question of knowledge representation. Nevertheless, in the theoretically impoverished environment of the 1950s, it was a step forward for psychologists to learn something about information theory.

Next, Miller discovered Noam Chomsky. Although he was a linguist, Chomsky's criticisms of the kind of theoretical mechanisms used in behavioristic linguistics also applied to behavioristic psychology. Further, psychologists found some experimental evidence in favor of Chomskyan ideas, though the experiments were only suggestive. As a result of Miller's espousal of Chomsky's ideas, language psychologists began to study whole *sentences* — prior to this, they had focused only on single words, and on the connections between words. But if language was to be understood in terms of a set of rules able to generate sentences, then sentences were clearly the proper units of study. It was not long before Chomsky's theory passed from the scene as a viable psychological theory of language, but here again, the very act of thinking about a genuine theory which did not apologize for itself, had a favorable impact: In the process of considering and rejecting such theories, psychologists were becoming much more theoretically sophisticated.

Miller had led the field toward information theory and Chomsky's Transformational Grammar, but he was a bit late in arriving at the next major step — the use of full-fledged computational theories. Others were there before he moved "Toward a Third Metaphor for Psycholinguistics" (1974), in which the perception, production, and acquisition of language was viewed in terms of symbolic information processing. This is still the dominant metaphor in the psychology of language, and it seems likely to last for some time. The computational metaphor is very theoretical, and even in this third metaphor, Miller was able to make an original contribution (*e.g.*, Miller & Johnson-Laird, 1976). But the kind of leadership that he supplied to psychologists before — essentially the courage to consider abstract mathematical systems that might have some relevance to psychology — was no longer needed. From being the major theoretical leader in the field, Miller had by 1974 become one of many leaders.

Miller's career contrasts with the career of his friend and colleague, Jerome S̈. Bruner, who is well known outside of psychology proper, especially in the field of education. Bruner is a man of great charm and brilliance, as are many of the others disucssed here, and has made major contributions in many different parts of psychology. Yet his influence has been surprisingly attenuated, especially in the most rigorous circles in experimental psychology. The impression one gets is that Bruner simply did not have the patience to wait for the rest of the field to catch up. Always 10 years ahead of the community, he was not recognized and relied on in the way Miller was. Conversely, one suspects that George Miller may have sometimes adopted a point of view in which he did not really believe, simply in order to stay in touch with the rest of the experimental community. This is admittedly speculative, but some of this book's interview participants hint at something along these lines.

The most "radical" cognitive psychologist discussed here is Herbert A. Simon. By present standards, his radicalism is well within the bounds of modern cognitive thinking, but for most of his career, although the psychological community was moving in his direction, it moved very slowly, and he was considered an outsider until rather recently. Herbert Simon is currently the only cognitive scientist who has won the Nobel Prize — or rather, he is the only Nobel Laureate who considers himself a cognitive scientist. (There is no Nobel Prize in psychology, of course. Simon received the prize for his work on the economics of the firm, which he considers to be cognitive science, although the Nobel committee probably conceived of it as pure economics.)

Because he was not trained in the behavioristic point of view, Simon never felt theoretically constrained by it. He was familiar with formalisms in other sciences, and when the opportunity presented itself he felt free to participate, in collaboration with Allen Newell and others, in the development of the key ideas now used with great success in Artificial Intelligence. Thus he has helped to make major contributions in economics, computer science, and cognitive science. But for most of his career, Simon was clearly not considered to be a psychologist by most psychologists. (For this reason, I present the interview with Herbert A. Simon in my chapter on "Nucleators," people who created nuclei of psychological interest outside the self-defined boundaries of psychology at the time, and whose work forced those boundaries to expand.)

Thus we have a continuum from Osgood, who made a strong attempt to apply Hullian behaviorism to a cognitive problem; to Jenkins, who found that the mediational theory would not work, and was able to move to a new theoretical perspective; to Miller, who introduced psychologists to three new theoretical approaches, staying always close enough to the field to be understood, but far enough ahead to be followed; to Bruner, who made a number of remarkable contributions, but was too far ahead to be fully trusted by many psychologists; and to Simon, clearly an outsider who made his major contributions in the guise of economics and computer science, when in fact he saw his work very much as theoretical cognitive science.

Organization of the Cognitive Interviews:
Adapters, Persuaders, and Nucleators

All of our cognitive interview participants can be placed on this continuum of theoretically conservative versus liberal thinkers. In the following chapters, however, their interviews are grouped in a slightly different way. Chapter 5 contains interviews with *Adapters*, those psychologists who were able to adapt to the revolutionary change in psychology — from a strong professional commitment to behaviorism to an equally strong commitment to cognitive psychology: George A. Miller, Marvin Levine, George Mandler, and James J. Jenkins.

Chapter 6 is about *Persuaders*, cognitivists who were never behaviorists, and who view their role as a matter of persuading the rest of the field to give up an inadequate approach. Whereas the Adapters may have had to face a crisis of personal change, the Persuaders confronted an indifferent or perhaps hostile scientific community, and they had to maintain their independent perspective regardless of the resulting intellectual and social pressures. This group of interviewees consists of Ernest R. Hilgard, Ulric Neisser, Walter B. Weimer, and Michael Wapner. With the cognitive shift in psychology, the Persuaders have not been satisfied to accept membership in the cognitive community. Rather, they have continued to evolve new perspectives, and now present the cognitive community with a set of challenging new ideas. They have not ceased in their attempt to persuade the psychological community of the need for change — they have only shifted their ground.

The third and last group of cognitivists I call the *Nucleators* (Chapter 7). The word "nucleator" is borrowed from physics, where it signifies a particle that serves as a nucleus for a cluster of new particles, much as small dust particles in the atmosphere can trigger the formation of ice-crystals to produce snowflakes. By analogy, a scientific Nucleator serves as a nucleus for scientific activity outside the boundaries of the conventional scientifc community. These individuals came of age intellectually before the cognitive shift, outside of what was then considered to be psychology. They came from engineering (Donald A. Norman), from mathematical linguistics (Noam Chomsky), philosophy (Jerrold A. Fodor), or, in the case of Herbert A. Simon, from a combination of economics, political science, and computer science. According to Kuhn (1962), it is common for outsiders to have a disproportionate impact at a time of scientific revolution, and it is not surprising that these individuals have been extraordinarily influential. Some psychologists may not consider Fodor, Chomsky, and Simon to be "true" psychologists, but it is interesting to note that in their own thinking, all these individuals considered themselves to be "doing psychology" from very early on. Sometimes it is unclear whether it is Mohammed who comes to the mountain of psychology, or *vice versa*. But there is no doubt that these Nucleators have enormously enriched scientific psychology by the gifts they have brought from their respective fields.

5

The Adapters:
Psychologists Who Changed
with the Revolution

Our first group of cognitive psychologists started their professional lives as behaviorists and changed their perspective along with the mainstream of the research community. George A. Miller, Marvin Levine, James J. Jenkins, and George Mandler all began by considering themselves as behaviorists, although we can always detect some nonbehavioristic influences in their graduate training. Each performed state-of-the-art work for some time during the cognitive shift, and each represents an important theme in the shift.

George A. Miller indeed represents not one but several significant themes: the early role of mathematical psychology and information theory; the rediscovery of short-term memory; the influence of Noam Chomsky in demonstrating that behavioristic theories of language were inadequate *in principle* (see Chapter 7); early influences from computer simulation studies along the line of Simon and Newell; and more recent work on advanced topics in cognitive psychology, including a computational theory of language and perception (with Philip Johnson-Laird), studies in metaphor, and studies of word meaning. Miller has led significantly in all of these areas, making an extraordinary range of contributions. In spite of his continuing leadership, Miller's work has been relatively free from controversy; indeed, his prestige has been so well established that his involvement in a new problem has often served to signal other psychologists that some previously taboo topic was now safe for respectable researchers.

Marvin Levine is probably the most behavioristic of the cognitive psychologists represented here. In fact, his work has been consistently acceptable to both behaviorists and cognitive psychologists. His early work focused on mathematical modeling of problem solving in a discrimination-learning task (see the interview with Howard H. Kendler, Chapter 3). Levine's principal theoretical construct — the "hypothesis," as defined by a subject's choice on blank trials in the discrimination task — is closely tied to observables, and leads to precise quantitative predictions.

James J. Jenkins received graduate training in industrial psychology but developed an interest in basic topics such as language learning. In collaboration with others, Jenkins performed exhaustive studies of the *mediational* approach to verbal learning — an approach that acknowledged the need for some unobservable constructs in understanding language, but treated these constructs as internalized stimuli and responses. When this program failed after the most thorough testing, Jenkins decided to abandon it, and developed an interest in the Chomskyan approach to language. More recently Jenkins has joined in a profound challenge to associationism in human learning, developed by his students John Bransford and Jeffrey Franks. His own research interests have moved to speech perception, especially from the "ecological" point of view of James J. Gibson.

Finally, George Mandler has maintained two separate research programs, one in memory and the other in emotion. Mandler was trained at Yale at the height of Hullian behaviorism, but early in the cognitive shift he began to advocate an *organizational* account of memory in contrast to the associationism favored by more conservative psychologists. In a sense, his is a Gestalt approach to memory: Instead of dealing with connections between associated elements, it emphasizes the role of larger organized wholes. In his work on emotion, Mandler has emphasized the role of cognitive factors in emotional experience. Mandler also has profound interests in the history of psychology.

Obviously we cannot make a hard-and-fast distinction between the psychologists I have labeled the "Adapters," presented in this chapter, and the "Persuaders" and "Nucleators" presented in the next two chapters. Each cognitive psychologist interviewed in these pages has played all of these roles at some time. Nevertheless, the interviews in this chapter may best represent the process by which many psychologists adapted to the new perspective: the step-by-step experimental contributions that together snowballed into the cognitive shift.

George A. Miller: Leadership in the Cognitive Shift

There is little doubt that George A. Miller (b. 1920) has been the single most effective leader in the emergence of cognitive psychology. Although a number of psychologists played leadership roles in the cognitive groundswell beginning in the mid-1950s, Miller's influence was felt at several critical turning points. Miller began his career as a behavioristic psychologist studying psychoacoustics and received his doctorate in 1946 for work on the intelligibility of speech in noise. In this work it was natural to use statistical models that specified the dependency of each word in a sentence on the previous word (Markov models). These Markov models, in turn, led him to a consideration of information theory as a basic theoretical tool for psychology (Shannon & Weaver, 1949). About this same time Miller also rescued a fundamental fact of immediate memory from undeserved obscurity — namely, the limitation on the number of unrelated "items" — letters, numbers, words, and the like — that can be kept in mind at one time. This limit, he proposed, is seven, plus or minus two, and his paper, "The Magical Number Seven, Plus or Minus Two" (1956), is one of the most entertaining as well as one of the most significant landmarks in the cognitive shift.

Chomsky (1957) had been able to show formally that Markov models had limitations that would forever prohibit them from representing any human activity as complex as language. Miller was one of the few psychologists to recognize the force of this theoretical argument early on, and he did much to make it understandable to other psychologists (e.g., Chomsky & Miller, 1958). In the 1960s, Miller's elegant lecture on the psychological implications of Chomsky's grammar, given at many major universities, became famous. Indeed, Miller's work made clear the psychological relevance of linguistic concepts in both syntax and phonology. It was difficult to test Chomsky's Transformational Grammar experimentally, however, because it was still in the process of theoretical development. Hence, Miller moved in several directions: toward computational models of language and perception (Miller & Johnson-Laird, 1976), toward the study of metaphor, and toward empirical studies of word meanings. Consistently in his career Miller has been in the forefront of major innovations without getting out of touch with mainstream psychology.

What were the ingredients of Miller's effectiveness as a leader in the emergence of cognitive psychology? Leadership in psychology, as elsewhere in life, is a complex commodity. In Miller's case it includes a variety of factors. His background in "respectable research" in the Harvard laboratory of S. S. Stevens certainly created a solid foundation, as did his empirical contributions and his mathematical skill. These created appropriate credentials, while exposing Miller to the most intellectually stimulating crossroads in America, the scholarly community in Cambridge, Massachussetts, centered about Harvard and MIT. His career demonstrates, throughout, the importance of being in the right place thinking the right thoughts at the right time. Many of his personal characteristics were no doubt helpful: his notably lucid writing style, his capacity for presenting novel arguments with humor and drama, his consummate lecture style, his personal charm and ability to maintain relationships with other actors in the "invisible college" that was creating cognitive psychology in the '50s and '60s.

In some other lifetime George A. Miller might have become a good politician, in the best sense of that word. He continually showed an awareness of long-term possibilities, but was able to translate this concern in ways that psychologists with shorter perspectives could understand and respect. Leadership in psychology, as in other areas in life, is often the art of the possible. A very important ingredient of Miller's leadership was his acute sense of timing: knowing when the psychological community might be receptive to a new idea. In this sense, Miller exercised more effective influence than his brilliant peers Jerome S. Bruner and Herbert A. Simon, who pursued their interests far ahead of the more conservative segments of the psychological community.

Finally, Miller was able to exercise a good deal of what can only be called personal magnetism. No doubt at some point he might have developed a "school" along the lines of B. F. Skinner and S. S. Stevens, but he lacked the inclination to do so; he was too intensely self-critical, as he tells us in the interview, and his own perspective never stopped evolving.

George A. Miller has been the recipient of numerous honors, including election to the National Academy of Sciences in 1962, and the presidency of the American Psychological Association in 1969. He has received the Distinguished Scientific Contribution Award of the American Psychological Association, and the Howard Crosby Warren Medal from the Society of Experimental Psychologists. Miller is currently James S. McDonnell Distinguished University Professor of Psychology at Princeton University.

Interview with George A. Miller

Q: How did you get started in psychology?

A: As an undergraduate at the University of Alabama I was a joint major in English and Speech. Like most people who haven't decided what they want to do, I got into several things: English, theater, speech correction, and debating. From studying speech correction it seemed to me that all the interesting things were in psychology. After the bachelor's in 1940 I took a master's degree in speech at the University of Alabama. A man named Donald Ramsdell offered me a job in the Alabama psychology department; I had been sitting in on some of his seminars because I thought that a lot of the interesting questions in speech pathology came down to clinical psychology. I had a wife and a kid to support, so Ramsdell put together three teaching assistantships to make an instructorship in Introductory Psychology for $1,000 a year. I had taken no psychology courses at this time, so I spent the summer before I started teaching, madly reading introductory psychology texts. I had 16 sections of Introductory Psychology to teach each week. I hope that what I told those kids was right, because after 16 times through it I started to believe it myself.

Ramsdell encouraged me to go on in psychology, and in 1942 he sent me off to summer school at Harvard. I wanted to study clinical psychology, but I spent that summer taking advanced experimental from Boring and Beebe-Center, and history from Boring. That was when I met Wendell Garner — yes, Wendell; that was before they nicknamed him Tex after Vice President Garner, who was from Texas. We were both first year graduate students and we roomed together that summer. We were both pretty good, and we competed to see who could memorize Woodworth's text (1938) the fastest.

At the end of the summer I went back to Alabama for another year as instructor, but Tex stayed on and continued to impress all the physiological and experimental people with his brilliance. Since they thought of Tex and me together, his successes made it very easy for me when I returned to continue my graduate work the next year. I can't remember ever deciding to reject clinical psychology in favor of experimental, but I moved in that direction because it was so easy to do.

And, too, because of the war. As a speech therapist at Alabama I had learned enough about vocal communication to make myself useful to Smitty (S. S.) Stevens at the Psychoacoustic Laboratory. Smitty hired me to work on voice communication systems for the military, and Cliff Morgan managed to get me a presidential deferment. My special project was the design of optimal signals for spot jamming of speech. It was a top secret project for the Signal Corps, and I learned a great deal about electronics and acoustics during the two years I spent on it. I think I still had some idea about returning to clinical some time in the future, but that wasn't possible while the war was going on.

Let me tell you a funny story about that. When the war ended, Smitty persuaded the department that Tex and I didn't need to do a thesis, because we had already demonstrated our ability to do research. So they accepted the technical reports of our military research as our theses. That was very nice of them, but it had a funny consequence. At my PhD oral only two people were cleared to read my thesis! So the faculty had to question me very discreetly. Instead of jamming, we talked about the effects of noise on intelligibility, which meant that I had to turn all my data upside down. What I had been thinking of as "good jamming" then became "bad interference," and what was "bad jamming" became "good listening." You can imagine how it went. They asked a cautious question, and then there was a long pause while I turned the answer upside down in my head. It must have sounded phony as hell! The social and clinical psychologists — Allport, Murray, White, Bruner, who were now my enemies — probably thought I hadn't written a thesis at all. At the end I left feeling I had done very poorly.

I went and sat in E. G. Boring's outer office and waited for the verdict, and the time dragged on and on. I got panicky — I assumed they were having a violent fight about me. It must have been 45 minutes before Boring came bouncing in. "Oh," he said, surprised to see me, "Congratulations!" Jerry Bruner told me later that they had passed me immediately and then had gone on to a department meeting about some details of the split between psychology and social relations. But it was the most miserable 45 minutes I can remember.

Q: How did the split of the Harvard Psychology Department into Social Relations and Psychology affect you?

A: Quite deeply, but we were not really enemies. I think Tex and I were the last two PhDs awarded by the old Department of Psychology, before the split. But my sponsor, Smitty Stevens, was a very strong personality — you either loved him or hated him, but you couldn't ignore him. And he and Gordon Allport simply couldn't stand each other. So Gordon joined with Talcott Parsons and Clyde Kluckhohn to create a new department, the Department of Social Relations, where he expected everything to be nice and pleasant. Since I was affiliated with Smitty, I was part of the old department, and all the clinical, social, personality, and educational types were on the other side. Not enemies, really, but rivals.

I hated it. Not only because the split ended any ideas I might have had about becoming a clinician, but because I was really interested in communication, which is a social process if there ever was one. Because I took an experimental approach to communication, Harvard isolated me from my natural allies. I once asked Gordon Allport why he didn't consider me a social psychologist, since I studied social interactions. He looked surprised and said very simply, "Because you don't know any social psychology." And he had arranged it so I wasn't likely to learn any.

At the time, the split was defended in terms of the shared interests in psychology, sociology, and anthropology, but I have always believed that it would never have happened if Boring and Stevens had not been the kind of people they were. Difficult people, with strong opinions. It didn't happen anywhere else, and when the principals had all retired, Social Relations was quietly disbanded. It was all the result of a conflict of personalities.

The difficulty of working with Smitty continued after the split. When B. F. Skinner joined the Department — in 1948, I think — he and Smitty had just as much trouble getting along as Allport and Smitty had. In fact, the rump department — that was what Boring called it — quickly became polarized between Stevens and Skinner, between psychophysics and operant conditioning. The rivalry was intense. My continuing interest in human communication made it difficult for me to subscribe loyally to either side.

Q: At the time you were going to graduate school, how was behaviorism perceived by psychologists?

A: It was perceived as the point of origin for scientific psychology in the United States. The chairmen of all the important departments would tell you that they were behaviorists. Membership in the elite Society of Experimental Psychology was limited to people of behavioristic persuasion; the election to the National Academy of Sciences was limited either to behaviorists or to physiological psychologists, who were respectable on other grounds. The power, the honors, the authority, the textbooks, the money, everything in psychology was owned by the behavioristic school. Those who didn't give a damn, in clinical or social psychology, went off and did their own thing. But those of us who wanted to be scientific psychologists couldn't really oppose it. You just wouldn't get a job.

Once you got a job, you could begin to complain about it. But not until some people who were established began to say out loud and in public, "I don't find this a satisfying way to understand the things I am interested in," could you throw this thing off.

I would say up into the mid-'50s that that was the situation. It was the controlling picture in psychology — certainly when I was a graduate student in the early '40s, and through my young manhood. By the '50s you could sort of see that there were other things, and by the mid-'50s you really decided that behaviorism wasn't going to work out. I mean, if you've gone already to a criterion of 50 successive failures, how much further do you have to go before you're persuaded that it isn't going to work?

Q: How did you see the neobehaviorism of Hull and Spence at this time?

A: Well, Hull's *Principles of Behavior* (1943) came out while I was a graduate student at Harvard. Jim Egan, Leo Postman, Tex Garner, and I used to meet to discuss psychology; we had to educate each other, because all the big people had gone off to save the world. Jim Egan was an Iowa-based behaviorist who was very interested in Hull, and when the book came out he made us read it. I was interested in the mathematics, and I quickly became convinced that Hull didn't know his ass from third base as far as mathematics was concerned. I think there was one sentence in there, about page 10, that made it very difficult for me to continue. He has an equation with e^{-it} in it. Now that looks familiar to me, because as an acoustician, I knew that "$-i$" is the square root of -1, and "t" is time; that's a spinner. Then I read Hull's footnote: "e" is a mathematical constant which for the purposes of this book we shall assume to be 10! And "t" is the number of trials, and "i" isn't the square root of -1. I thought it violated the standard mathematical conventions in a ridiculous way.

Jim Egan believed in the Hull program, I think, and was eager to get through the war to work on it. Tex Garner said, Jesus Christ, if we ever ran out of ideas, look at all the things we could test! And I would say, Tex! The purpose of theory is to make experimentation unnecessary! What are you doing? What kind of theory is it that makes all of these experiments necessary? So we disagreed. I didn't think much of Hull. I'd gone back to his mathematico-deductive theory of rote learning (Hull, Hovland, Ross, Perkins, & Fitch, 1940), and I saw that one of the axioms was that there exists a memory drum. You kind of wonder about the depth of thinking that's gone into that.

Q: There exists a memory drum?

A: Well, that was a basic axiom. "Memory drums exist." Well, look at it some time! It's absurd.

What was it like in those days? Well, there was a general faith that psychology could become a science, and that it would do so by observation of behavior. You didn't have to believe that mind didn't exist; you only had to say that if it did exist, there's not much I can do about it.

Q: This would be the position of operationists such as E. G. Boring and S. S. Stevens?

A: Yes.

Q: You own work seems to have been remarkably unaffected by the dominant influence of neobehaviorism.

A: Look, you couldn't be unaffected by it. If you stayed home and didn't talk to anybody you might be unaffected. But if you'd go to a meeting people would tell you, "You're wrong: This is how it is." It influenced me more in my attempts to do verbal learning — I learned early on that I didn't want to do animal conditioning. If you didn't work with animals, you were not as much caught in the neobehavioristic outlook. At Alabama I had kept rats in my office and developed asthma as a result. Animal hair still upsets me. It was one of the very best things that ever happened to me, because it meant I had to work with humans, who I'm apparently not allergic to. Now, a lot of people who get allergic to pigeon dust or animal hair just put on masks and go ahead and suffer. That was not my way.

There was a tradition of human research from Ebbinghaus through Thorndike, McGeoch, and Irion down to Melton, Postman, Underwood, Martin, and many of those people, like Hull, tried to interpret all the verbal learning data in terms of Pavlovian conditioning or operant conditioning. But they still had a body of solid empirical data. I didn't give up on verbal learning until it became apparent to me that it had absolutely no relevance for what goes on in classrooms. I later learned to talk about this in terms of Tulving's distinction between semantic and episodic memory (1972). What you want to get across in the classroom is semantic learning — that is, it's a matter of learning rules rather than concrete experiences as such — but what we were always doing to people in verbal learning experiments was episodic. And our results for episodic learning just did not generalize to semantic learning, which was disappointing.

When looked at critically, Hullian attempts to reduce verbal learning to classical conditioning were clearly absurd. Trace conditioning is hard enough to set up in an animal, and the idea that you had all these conditioned traces that were causing all kinds of overlapping inhibitions — it just seemed utterly implausible.

My thinking was influenced by computers perhaps earlier than most people's. Even while I felt that I should be behavioristic, I was willing to play around with these other ideas. The generation before me felt that you couldn't use a term without having a physical instantiation of it. And on that criterion, we now have physical instantiations, by means of computers, of fabulous things! Things that they had never dreamed of. So, just accepting that as your license to talk, sure, you could talk about memory, syntactic rules, plans, schemata, and the like. We didn't believe that computers were giant brains, but we could see the similarities. McCulloch and Pitts (1943) down at MIT were pointing out the similarities in the late '40s. Norbert Wiener (1961) had done several things that I was interested in. All that was very much a part of my world, so I didn't feel the need to be quite as constrained as the neobehaviorists.

Q: Why do you think psychologists have been so attracted to behaviorism?

A: Look, people motivate themselves in different ways. Ann Roe studied psychologists years ago, and found that whereas famous biologists all liked their fathers, famous psychologists all had problems about their fathers. They were out competing with them, destroying them, or whatever the Freudian nonsense is. I think it's true. I think people who went into psychology in my day were by and large rebels against figures of authority. The behaviorists were very much in rebellion against the structuralists like Titchener and the Chicago functionalists. This sense of overthrowing what has always been accepted, and thus freeing yourself of having to learn history is so important in behaviorism.

Herb Jenkins once explained to me the attraction of Skinnerian psychology to a graduate student. He said, "You know, you can learn Skinnerian psychology very quickly: The first day you're there, you learn that statistics is no damn good. Bang! like that. I don't have to worry about *that*. The next day you learn physiological psychology is no damn good. Bang! just like that. You don't have to worry about it. The third day you learn that the history of psychology is no damn good. Bang! just like that, you've handled that. You go down any road until you come to Fred Skinner, and *that's* where psychology starts. It's really like that!"

Q: How did you begin to make the transition from a behavioristic point of view?

A: I began being more and more statistical. I began taking these objective measures, and it seemed to me that what you really had was not behavior, but the records of behavior. And those were the things I was trying to understand. This was like Skinner. Skinner never looked at a pigeon; he looked at the trace on the cumulative recorder. Who cared whether the pigeon was pressing the bar with his bill or his tail!

Fred Frick and I published a couple of amusing articles—retrospectively amusing—trying to apply information theory to Skinnerian things, which we called "statistical behavioristics" (Miller & Frick, 1949; Frick & Miller, 1951). I haven't looked at those in years. We were trying very hard to reach out to the Skinner end of the laboratory world. It seemed to me that all the problems of psychology were down there—they weren't in the cochlea, for heaven's sake.

Q: Problems such as motivation?

A: Yes. Why would psychology be interesting, if not to find out why people do what they do? Skinner's work was much closer to those problems than Smitty Stevens's was.

About 1950 or so I went off to MIT and got involved in air defense again. All of my early development was supported by military money, until the Vietnam thing made it just absolutely impossible for anybody with a conscience to continue. And so I quit then and haven't had a dime of military money since.

So we began to use statistical techniques to analyze sequences of responses. To me, the analysis of a bunch of bar-presses that came out of a box and the analysis of a bunch of key-presses from a keyboard were on the same continuum. That was what I was trying to understand.

Q: So already you were talking about the process of selection from a finite set of messages, along the lines of information theory.

A: That's what Shannon taught me was important (Shannon & Weaver, 1949). It's hard for young people now to see why that would have been so important, but it was. I remember experiments that we studied carefully, experiments on the perception of form, where you would take some visual form down to perceptual threshold by lowering the illumination or by shrinking it in size. And the notion was that circles, let's say, are easier to perceive than triangles. Well, different people got different results, so there was a problem. If you look back at the way those studies were run, they never said explicitly to the subjects, "You have to recognize which of the following five forms it is"; it was always, "What *form* are you seeing?" It could have been Minerva arising out of the sea, as far as the observers knew.

Q: The experimenters were acting as if they were testing *any* arbitrary form.

A: Yes, but of course after a while the subjects knew perfectly well what forms they were using, and began to expect only those forms. This changes the results you get. There were lots of experiments that did not specify in advance the set of alternative stimuli and responses that were available to the subject: sloppy, slushy stuff. One thing that information theory and mathematical psychology did — it made it obvious that you had to specify those aspects of the experimental situation. The experimental situation is different from free, God-given behavior in just that way. Otherwise you couldn't make any sense of the results.

I was deeply involved in the statistical properties of sequences of symbols and written messages when I encountered Chomsky in 1954, who looked at it and said, "That will never converge on English." It never occurred to me that it would, or indeed should! So here was a new way of thinking about it. What do you mean? He came out with this idea that he has since used to conquer the world, which is that a theory of the generation of messages should generate all and only the grammatical sentences in a language and not simply make one set of messages more probable than another.

Noam Chomsky was my assistant about 1957 at a summer seminar on mathematical psychology at Stanford — as I recall these things now, I wonder, *this* guy was working for *me*? A publication on so-called *Finite-State Languages* came out of that (Chomsky & Miller, 1958). I was very interested in the mathematical aspects of what he was talking about, something that since then Chomsky seems to have lost interest in.

As I thought about Chomsky's arguments, it occurred to me that if you try to learn English using purely statistical approximations to English — by learning transitional probabilities between words — then when you look at the size of the set of sentences 20 words long, it turns out that you have to learn an astronomical number of connections in order to generate just exactly the set of English sentences and no others. I think it works out that the average number of possible transitions following any word in a sentence is on the order of 10 — that is, at any point in a sentence there is an average of about 10 words that can follow that word. So, in sentences about 20 words long — which is not very long, that's about the average length of sentences in the *Reader's Digest* — that would lead to 10 to the 20th power number of sentences. And there are less than 10 to the 10th seconds in a century.

So if you imagine that you have been learning one transitional probability per second since you were born, you would not have had enough time to learn more than a tiny fraction of all the sentences you can in fact produce and understand. Somebody figured that given the age of the universe there would still not be enough time to learn all those connections between words. At that point I was pretty well persuaded that no sort of statistical theory would ever generate what we wanted.

What Noam gave me was a new goal: not just to state the statistics of messages, which is still a useful thing to do if you're running a telephone system. But no, we're looking for a theory of the message generator. And that is not a statistical thing; in spite of the way I have wandered in this conversation, I am *not* generating successive words by some random process.

Chomsky opened up a whole new set of possibilities for me. And the first thing to do was to steal a problem from Edward Sapir, who talked about the "psychological reality" of linguistic concepts. Now Sapir meant phonological concepts, but I set out to test the psychological reality of Noam's syntactic concepts. He's since disavowed this whole thing, but at the time he thought it was an interesting thing to do. Later he said, "Nobody would do anything that stupid! That's not what I was talking about. I was talking about competence, not performance." But at that time it wasn't all so clear. So we tried it. We were all at Stanford together; we told the class to go home and look at their kids, and bring back the mistakes that their kids made, because we assumed that that would cast some light on which of the phrase-structure rules they had learned. They all came back and said that they had listened for a long time and they couldn't catch the kids making any mistakes. They didn't say anything very complicated, but what they said was all right! The kids only made mistakes if they ventured into something new.

Those were very exciting days. I had several students who did interesting work trying to test the psychological reality of these ideas. And in retrospect it does turn out that phrase structure has a psychological reality. At the time we thought that transformations did, too, but the book by Fodor, Bever, and Garrett (1974) makes a strong case that we were wrong. And also the theory of Transformational Grammar has changed. Negation is no longer a syntactic transformation — it's something that is inserted in the base component. The interrogative is still a Wh-fronting transformation all right, but even the passive, which was the third one we used, is not introduced by a transformation. But we were working before Chomsky's 1965 book; so, as we were trying to test the psychological reality of syntax, the syntactic theory we were testing was moving out from under us.

Q: I believe that you were more responsible than any other person for introducing Chomsky's work to American psychology.

A: I think so, I think so. I knew Noam before any other psychologists knew him, and tried very hard to get that style of doing science known among psychologists.

Q: And there was some skepticism, I suppose.

A: Still is, still is. Sure. Noam's a tough cookie. Once he was given some recognition, he could handle it all himself. He didn't need me any more.

My opinion is that Noam helped to broaden our definition of scientific psychology. And so he has been an important psychologist. There is now a way of establishing generalizations and developing them that was not available to us before. And there is a set of substantive claims about language, about human beings, that focus more in Chomsky's work than anywhere else. And that's important. Whether it's true or false. My God, if being right was necessary for being important, we wouldn't have many important psychologists! The fact that he's a master polemicist, that he's far off on the left, a sort of political Trotskyite, that he's alienated many Jews by his position on Zionism, all that has nothing to do with his value as a psychologist in my eyes.

Q: In the introduction to your 1951 book, you called yourself a "good behaviorist." At what point did you find your own perspective changing?

A: I said, "The argument goes as far down the behavioristic path as one can clearly see the way." I guess I realized that I would never be a good behaviorist somewhere between '55 and '58. By 1960, when Jerry

Bruner and I founded the Center for Cognitive Studies at Harvard, I was finally willing to march under the banner of cognitivism.

In reaching back for the word "cognition," I don't think anyone was intentionally excluding "volition" or "conation" or "emotion" (Hilgard, 1980b). I think they were just reaching back for common sense. In using the word "cognition" we were setting ourselves off from behaviorism. We wanted something that was *mental*—but "mental psychology" seemed terribly redundant. "Commonsense psychology" would have suggested some sort of anthropological investigation, and "folk psychology" would have suggested Wundt's social psychology. What word do you use to label this set of views? We chose "cognition."

But "cognition" was meant in a very broad sense. When Jerry Bruner and I started the Center for Cognitive Studies at Harvard, did we mean to exclude anything that a computer can't do? Emotion, will, motivation? No, of course not.

Q: And in terms of the experimental psychology as a whole, what would you put as a rough time for the shift?

A: I don't see any break—any saltus—in a rather gradual shift. More people started programs in psycholinguistics and Artificial Intelligence; cognitive social psychology was getting more popular—it was just gradually happening.

Q: Would you use words like "revolution" to talk about the change?

A: I wouldn't use words like "revolution." To me, it's not like that. A lot of people were living in this house for a long time, and then some people built a house next door, and pretty soon, a lot of people moved from one house to the other. And the original house is still occupied—there are not as many people hoping to be happy there as there used to be—but they're still there. Maybe someday it'll be totally unoccupied. But was it a revolution? No, it was an accretion. If you want to talk in those terms, I think I agree with my philosophical friends who speak of the cognitive emergence as a return to commonsense psychology (Stich, 1983). I think most of us were united by opposition to behaviorism, not by any clear notion that there was a correct alternative theory to it. We just knew that we weren't going to understand what we were interested in *that* way.

Different people went in different directions, and if there was anything "common," it was the old "commonsense" about the way people are, how the mind works, that there *is* a mind; that memory, expectations, beliefs, emotions, all those words refer to something real, and that it's our job as psychologists to find out what it is.

Q: You've mentioned one day in September 1956 as a significant date in the emergence of cognitive psychology.

A: It was a meeting of the Special Group on Information Theory of the IEEE at MIT, where we actually had Noam Chomsky's preliminary paper, before *Syntactic Structures* (1957) came out; my first publication on the magical number seven; one of the first publications of the General Problem Solver by Newell and Simon. All of that happened in 1956. That rather unusual meeting seemed to me to signal something interesting.

Some people say the Hixon Symposium in 1948 was the seminal event. I don't agree, but it was symptomatic; the fact that you could have a meeting like that at that time meant something. People were discovering one another. At MIT I remember hearing Allen Newell say, after hearing Chomsky's paper, "That's just what we are doing when we do so-and-so"; Herb Simon replied, "Well, maybe."

Q: Your own work seems remarkably free of the behavioristic constraints that limited most psychological research in the late '40s and '50s.

A: I guess it was. If I'd gone to Iowa for graduate school, things would have been different. A lot of lucky things happened to me.

Q: Do you think that your college background in literature and theater may have helped to broaden your perspective as well?

A: It was more a matter of being haunted by that background — of experiencing the psychology we were developing as inadequate to deal with the things I'd learned in literature and drama.

Q: When you began to take a decidedly cognitive tack, how did more conservative psychologists react?

A: Well, I remember conversations with people who would say, "You don't really *believe* this, do you?" And I would think, "What do you mean, I don't believe it; do you think I'm lying to you? What kind of a faker do you think I am? Really." "But a person like you, George Miller, known to have done good scientific work . . . "

Q: This would be a response when you would introduce Chomsky's work, for example?

A: Yes.

Q: Do you think that being at Harvard and MIT made a difference? I have the impression that in psychology, the Cambridge area was much broader in outlook than the rest of the country.

A: It was much more cosmopolitan than most other places. I suppose that New York City was also a great crossroads for the immigrants who were coming in.

But the times were changing. The computers catalyzed things that would have happened more slowly anyhow. Computers give us an existence-proof of the complexity that is possible in information-processing systems. This made us all feel a lot freer.

There were other influences, of course. Carl Hovland had a very important role in my development in freeing me to think about thinking, and in generalizing the realms to which information measurement could be applied. Other social psychologists such as Leon Festinger and Fritz Heider had a lot of input toward the emergence of cognitive psychology. Social psychologists had never sold themselves down the behavioristic river the way the experimentalists had. They were still interested in people, and would stoop to any way to learn more about them. If it was behaviorism, fine; if it wasn't, well, that was fine too! In my thinking Heider was a great source of sanity; Heinz Werner was a great source of sanity; Bruner, coming from social psychology; and Festinger, talking about cognitive dissonance. That's one of the ways that the word "cognition" got revived.

Psychologists in Europe had not bought in on behaviorism — with the possible exception of Russia, where they had a behaviorist disease of their own. I had a Fulbright professorship at Oxford in '63–'64, and shortly after I got there, Larry Weisskrantz invited me to come over to give a talk at Cambridge. So I gave the talk I was then giving in the States: The first half hour I lambasted hell out of the behaviorists, you know, and the second half hour I said how I thought it should be done. And afterwards Larry came up to me and said, "George, that was a very interesting talk; but tell me, what was all that about behaviorism?" I thought, "What?" He said, "You know, there are only three behaviorists in England, and none of them were here today!"

After that I finally stopped giving my lecture about behaviorism. I don't think I've waxed this eloquent about it in 15 years. I stopped criticizing the behaviorists — who God knows are hard-working, upstanding people, trying to understand what they can. I don't criticize them anymore. They do their thing, I'll do my thing. Maybe we'll converge if we both have the truth.

Q: Perhaps one of the first clear signs of a cognitive shift was the book by yourself, Eugene Galanter, and Karl Pribram called *Plans and the Structure of Behavior* (1960). What was the history of that book?

A: In 1958 Carl Hovland and Herb Simon and I organized a meeting together at the RAND Corporation in Santa Monica. The Social Science Research Council funded a set of meetings including Cliff Shaw, Allen Newell, Ed Feigenbaum, Roger Shepard (who was my post-doc at Harvard at that time), and we did some computer simulation together. The next year I spent at the Stanford Center for Advanced Study in the Behavioral Sciences, and Eugene Galanter and Karl Pribram were there. And I'd come along with all this material from this summer seminar. We began meeting together, and our discussions got rather interesting, so we decided we should record them; and the first thing we knew we'd written a book. We showed it to Newell and Simon, who hated it. So I rewrote it, toned it down, and put some scholarship into it, and it is now the book *Plans and the Structure of Behavior* (1960).

Newell and Simon felt that we had stolen their ideas and not gotten them right. It was a very emotional thing. Since then I've discovered the good thing about Herb is that he can be shouting at you one minute, and the next minute have a drink with you. You just don't back off with Herb Simon—otherwise he'll bully the hell out of you. His aspect is different from any other person's I ever knew. I had to put the scholarship into the book, so they would no longer claim that those were their ideas. As far as I was concerned they were old familiar ideas; the fact that they had thought of it for themselves didn't mean that nobody ever thought of it before.

Q: Was there any direct influence from Norbert Wiener and cybernetics (1961)?

A: Well, Norbert was around, and we read his books, and we all were impressed with things like the Turing test and the Rosenblueth–Wiener–Bigelow paper on feedback systems that set their own goals (1943). Those things had quite a freeing effect. It took me a long time to realize that to say that the brain is a Turing Machine was not just a Jim-peachy-dandy thing to say—that seemed to mean that there could be *some* theory: You could create some Universal Turing Machine that would work just like the brain! Wasn't that a powerful thing to say? And one day somebody said, "Yeah, that's very powerful, that's like saying, 'If you had a theory of the brain, you could write it in ink!'" "Oh, you're right—that's about all it does say." But at the time these things seemed very powerful. Anything I can understand, I can write a theory for.

Q: Certainly, compared with Markov models, that *is* a very liberting realization.

A: Oh, yes, yes! That frees up that early modeling enormously. Of course, it is clear now that the Markov model was not only very constrained, but that it had the wrong constraints; finding the right constraints on Turing Machines is exactly what we are trying to do now.

When I came back from that year (1959 to 1960) at the Stanford

Center for Advanced Study, I thought that the Center was really marvelous, and that bringing together people of different backgrounds was great. I wanted to go to Stanford — that seemed to be where things were happening. At Harvard, the split between the Departments of Social Relations and Psychology was terrible. Bruner was unhappy in the Department of Social Relations and was trying to get back into "real" psychology; I was in Psychology, and my communication interests were all social in nature. And so we got together and tried to create a Camridge-based version of the Stanford Center for Advanced Study in the Behavioral Sciences. At that time, McGeorge Bundy was dean of the College of Arts and Sciences at Harvard, and we decided to ask Bundy whether or not we could have a center where we could invite people to stay for some period of time. He reached into his bottom righthand drawer and pulled out a house that the James family had originally lived in . . .

Q: That's a wonderful coincidence.

A: Yes, it seemed just right. And with a grant from John Gardner, then president of the Carnegie Foundation of New York, we remodeled the thing. We had about eight rooms that we moved into: the new Harvard Center for Cognitive Studies.

All the time we were trying to get something new started, there were three major figures that Bruner and I kept in mind who gave us faith that it was possible to do good psychology without being behavioristic. One was Sir Fredric Bartlett; in 1955 there was a summer conference at Cambridge University where I got to know Bartlett, and I respected him greatly. Another major figure was Jean Piaget; Piaget visited us several times, so I got to know him. And the third was A. R. Luria, in the Soviet Union, who under the inspiration of Vygotsky had somehow held out against all of the Pavlovian types. We admired and had ties to those three men, each in their different ways. We felt they gave us continuity back to Americans whom we respected, like James, Dewey, Woodworth, Thorndike, psychologists before the Watson crystallization of psychology. Back to the old functionalist school.

By the time we were self-consciously breaking free from the behavioristic patterns, all these influences had their effect: the existence of sensible people in social psychology and of great and inspiring figures in Europe were extremely important in giving us the courage to go ahead.

Q: Was there any influence from psychoanalysis?

A: Well, we were all sort of dissatisfied customers. But, no, I don't think so. I read *The Interpretation of Dreams* (Freud, 1900/1953), and Chapter 7 of that book is to me one of *the* great essays in cognitive psychology. But that is recognition after the fact: It didn't seem to influence us at the time. I had gone to Harvard to become a clinical psychologist, and there's no teetotaler like a reformed drunk. That was shut out of my life. In terms of influence on me when I came to Harvard, I could make the connection with Harry Stack Sullivan more than with Freud. I was one of the early researchers in this country in Rorschach technique, and I was around Henry Murray's clinic when they were developing the Thematic Apperception Test.

When you looked at studies of the child for evidence for the value of psychoanalytic theory, that was pretty discouraging, and quite properly so, I think. But I can still remember taking Henry Murray's course in personality and clinical psychology, and going to his seminars whenever I could. Some things he said made a big impression on me. He was very antibehavioristic in those days, and made me aware that there were counterarguments to behaviorism. For instance, you describe a person lifting a spoon to his mouth, and Harry would say, "That description doesn't tell you anything about what they're doing: Are they feeding themselves? Is it nurturance? Or is there poison in the spoon, and are they killing themselves? From the behavioral description alone you have no idea of what's really going on, until you know what the need system is." I believed that; I just didn't know what to do with it.

I think psychoanalysis influenced Bruner more than it influenced me. He published two or three papers, I think, as a result of his careful reading of Freud. In that literature I was more interested in and influenced by Otto Fenichel, I guess, than by Freud. Fenichel was the only real scholar I seemed able to find it those days in that literature. Of course Freud wrote beautifully and was fun to read. But he kept changing, and you had to remember whether you were reading the early Freud, middle Freud, late Freud, Freud answering Jung, you know. It's dangerous to try to understand Freud unless you understand a *lot* of Freud. I never felt I really had any insight into it.

Only in retrospect can I see the relevance. It's a little bit like reading a book and thinking, "God, what awful trash!" and you mark it with exclamation points: "Terrible, terrible book!" Twenty years later you come back to it, pick it up off the shelf and start to read it: "Gee, this is pretty good, isn't it? Why wasn't I ready to understand what this person was trying to say?"

Q: Psycholinguistic studies of the "psychological reality" of syntax went through something of a shock after Chomsky's 1965 book changed syntactic theory fundamentally, thereby pulling the theoretical rug out from under many researchers. Did this affect your work as well?

A: About '65–'66 I had given up on syntax—in that area, the theory changed too rapidly. I decided that in spite of all I had said about sentences being more important to study than lists of words, I was going to go back and look at words. I thought that there was still something to be done there. And so I began my interest in lexical memory at that point, and that's what I have been doing work in ever since.

By 1967 I got fed up with being at Harvard and moved to Rockefeller. At Rockefeller there aren't departments, there are just professors who have laboratories. I opened a kiddie lab at Rockefeller, and for 3 years studied the cognitive development of 3-year-olds—a very chastening experience. I'd always had around me people who were interested in kids, but I'd never done it myself. So I decided it can't be very hard. It was terrible. I just couldn't think like a 3-year-old. They really outsmarted me. And I finally gave up. I wrote a little book about it (Miller, 1977). Then Rockefeller got a new president who didn't seem to be sympathetic to psychology, so I came here to Princeton, and began to get actively interested in vocabulary development again.

Beginning in 1970 I spent three years at the Institute for Advanced Study at Princeton. Philip Johnson-Laird was there the second year, and we got to arguing about some work I had done on verbs of motion. Our book *Language and Perception* (Miller & Johnson-Laird, 1976) grew out of that. We saw it initially as an attempt to see how far you could go with an empiricist notion of how language is learned. Could you discover that part of the language which has to be taken as given? It's a little bit like writing a compiler for a new computer language. You can write almost all of it in the higher-level language, except for a small part which translates that language into machine language. That's the way we thought of English, that is, there is all of this elaborate stuff, except for one small part which translates it for the brain; we were trying to figure out whether we could get at what that one small part was—to what extent it depended on empiricist experience with the things named and the actions named for the child.

Q: It's a kind of "bootstrapping" idea of how language is learned, then?

A: That's what we had in mind. Well, the book got to be too long; nobody has ever read it. It has lots of interesting ideas in it, some of which we've since developed. It was good. Phil's a good person to work with. Afterwards he decided he would try to test our ideas, incorporating them into computer programs. I decided I would try to test some of them by seeing how some of these things developed in children.

Neither one of us was much interested in doing experiments, although we had both come from experimental psychology. Because it seemed to us that a lot of good people were doing those experiments already, and they weren't teaching us a whole hell of a lot that we didn't already know; if we didn't know it already, we didn't believe it!

Q: Did you feel that experimental psychologists were asking the wrong questions about that problem?

A: In a sense. There are some questions you can't ask with an experiment. Some of my friends — and I won't name names — would not believe that people have two arms and two legs unless you could do an experiment proving it.

Q: Since the mid-'60s you have focused on lexical memory and vocabulary development.

A: Yes. I'm interested in dictionaries now, really. I think dictionaries have been misused in the school system. When you tell a kid who asks you what a word means, "Look it up in the dictionary and write a sentence using it," it's the worst thing you can do. That'll guarantee he'll never ask *you* a question again. Jim Deese reported this back in about 1967 in his presidential address to the Eastern Psychological Association (Deese, 1967). He reported that a teacher who had seventh grade kids look up the word "chaste" in a dictionary found that the kids produced sentences-like "The amoeba is a chaste animal," "Even after much use, the plates were still chaste," or "The milk was chaste." They were all things that you could justify by looking at the definition and taking it literally. "Chaste" is defined as "pure" or "simple in design."

Last spring, Patti Gildea and I went out and collected our own data from the schools about children writing sentences from dictionary definitions. If the kid knows the word in advance, then the results are pretty good. If he doesn't know the word in advance, his chances of learning anything from the dictionary are just zilch. I sort of have it tagged now as the "Mrs. Jones stimulated the soup" phenomenon. Because if you look at the definition of "stimulate," it says "to stir up."

The first step is to show that what they are doing in the schools under the heading of "teaching dictionary skills" is a waste of time. The second step is to ask, Well, what *should* they be doing? And you know perfectly well that kids learn from context. And you learn through context. You hear the word, and you say, "I don't know quite what it is, but if I hear it again, maybe I can begin to figure out what it means."

I imagine a person who is in this state of being interested — he's heard "eleemosynary" or something — and while he is waiting for it to happen again, he meets a lexicographer who says, "Oh, I've got 50 occurrences of that, I've got them on cards. Here, let me help you, you don't have to wait for the word to be said again. In fact, I'll help you even more than that, I'll give you my *precis* of this pile of occurrences: I call it a *definition*." What I would like to try is a pedagogical dictionary that concentrates on instances of use. There are so many words that I know how to use perfectly well, but which I don't know how to define. There are some experiments by educational psychologists who have shown that giving three or four examples of using words in context will help a kid more than giving definitions. If you want to know what a "barbarian" is, well here are 3 sentences using it: Now write your own sentence using the word. It works.

Q: Obviously, some sentences give more information about the word than others.

A: That's what we're doing this year; we want to be able to recognize the characteristics of a pedagogically good context. To say, "The aardvark is good" will not tell you anything about aardvarks. It'll just tell you it's a noun — that's about all. It turns out that dictionaries have made enormous assumptions about the psychology of language users. Not much attention has been given by lexicographers to the criteria of sentences illustrating use, and that's what we want to look at.

The thing that worries me about the contextual method, though, is that when kids in everyday life learn words from context they learn them in total situations, not just the verbal context. They see it, they hear it, they smell it, they taste it, whatever's going on at the time the word is used. So next year, I want to use interactive video; you could have lots of pictures on the screen of people using the word in appropriate contexts. That's where I'm going now.

Q: Over your career, your work seems to have become more and more theoretical.

A: I really began with the assumption that scientific psychology was possible, and that you could put order into the field in the same way physicists put order into their field — by mathematics. That's why I came here to Princeton and studied mathematics with Von Neumann, and with Willy Feller and John Tukey. Then I learned that anything you can do with an equation you can do with a computer, plus a lot more. So computer programs begin to look like the language in which you should formulate your theory. But the farther I go with that, the more limitations I see.

There are things that I deeply believe are true which I don't know how to capture in programs. It isn't so much a matter of finding that mathematics is wrong, or that computer programs are wrong — none of them seems adequate to say what we've got to say.

But I think that you've got to earn the right to say that. You've got to work through the tools that are available to you at a given level. So I've tried all of that, and I've really earned the right to do something a little freer now.

Q: Some people maintain that the critical difference between behaviorism and cognitive psychology is the willingness of cognitive people to postulate theoretical constructs that go beyond the observed behavior.

A: I think that describes a lot of cognitive people, but it's a little unfair to the behaviorists. Lashley thought he was a good behaviorist, and he speculated quite freely about how the brain accomplished what it did. Not all behaviorists were as stupid as John Broadus Watson — a lot of them were very intelligent men. Edwin B. Holt, for instance, speculated quite freely about the causes of behavior. Tolman called himself a purposive behaviorist. God knows I would love to claim Tolman as a cognitive psychologist, but he considered himself to be a behaviorist. Guthrie made some very bold and simplifying speculations about learning.

It's only Fred Skinner, who somehow, through his leadership, his charisma, and his willingness to defend absurd positions, has put a stamp on behaviorism in a way that makes people say that behaviorists were antitheoretical. I don't think they were. I think they were enormously optimistic about how simple the theory would be. But not until Skinner did anyone have the notion that you wouldn't have to have theory.

I take Skinner as my definition point for behaviorism, because he was my colleague at Harvard for so many years, and I know his system so well. It's easy for me to fall into that. But you wouldn't say that Hull was atheoretical.

Q: In a sense, one could say that even Hull was antitheoretical, because of his insistence that all of his constructs were not really constructs at all, but were potentially observable muscle and glandular responses; because of his physicalistic reductionism, in other words. He apparently felt that theoretical constructs were not really inferred entities, but abbreviations for a lot of observable behavior. In that sense, Hull was not really *free* to postulate theoretical constructs. Certainly Hull would balk at anything like mental representations.

A: But isn't that a theory? The fact that it is inadequate or even absurd doesn't mean that it is not a theory. Perhaps our problem here is with what it is a theory *of*. I think behaviorists confused the evidence with the subject matter of psychology, but that doesn't mean they were antitheoretical. Hull thought he had a theory, and so did most of the other behaviorists. I see having a theory and feeling free to introduce new theoretical concepts as different things.

Q: Do you think that experimental psychologists tend to be relatively atheoretical even today?

A: If you could have an atheoretical psychology, there'd be a lot of customers. But some of the preference for less theoretical ways of stating things is just a good scientific impulse. Occam's Razor tells us not to go to the more complicated hypotheses until we've exhausted the simpler ones. I think that's probably healthy. But that doesn't mean that no theory is needed — that was the claim Skinner made (1957).

Q: Do you think that the failure of Hullian theory was traumatic to many psychologists, and helped to discourage them from trying large-scale theory?

A: If you look at the history of psychology generally, then Donald Hebb (1949) is the last of the big-theory boys. There hasn't really been one since. Big theories used to be the accepted way to do psychology: It's what Wundt did, James, Freud, McDougall, Titchener, Pavlov, Watson. They had systems that explained everything. They got enormous depth by virture of accepting enormous vagueness. Hebb was the last of that breed. But I don't think that the end of that kind of theorizing and the end of behavioristic power should be confabulated. I think those were two different developments.

Now we're all down to minitheories. You take a little phenomenon and try to explain why a person moves his finger when he does, or something of this kind. If you can't explain a simple little phenomenon, then nobody has the courage to try these larger questions. And it worries me a little bit: because I don't think that we can go on this way without straightening out our house at some point and saying, "*These* are the domains that we want to build relatively coherent and encompassing theories about."

The question is, then, What are the constitutive problems that define the natural domain for psychology? In recent years I've taken "consciousness" to be the constitutive problem of psychology. I can tell you how interested I will be in something depending on how relevant it seems to be to the nature and function of conscious experience. Now you could take "intelligence" as your constitutive problem. Or you could take "will." But to me, consciousness seems to do it fairly well, though those others obviously stand as real possibilities.

But taking "memory" as the problem, or some other relatively limited domain — you're an expert in memory, I'm an expert in attention, he's an expert in language, and somebody else is an expert in vision, or in hearing — how are we going to tie all these things together? It's hard even within a single area, like trying to build a computer that can recognize speech by simulating human speech perception. First, you've got Fourier Transforms out at the ear, and then you've got the statistics of nerve impulses going up the auditory nerve; then you've got some stochastic nonsense going on in the auditory cortex; and then phrase-structure grammars going on somewhere; and then maybe logic for relating different sentences. Who in God's name can take five theories as separate as those and build a machine to do all of it in a coherent way? You spend more time trying to interface these different ways of processing information than you do on the individual components. It's almost theoretical chaos.

Q: So you see a theoretical problem today in working with multiple minitheories?

A: How do you interface them? If the theory you have at one level of information processing is totally different from the theory at another level, how do you put them together? Even if they are at different levels, say "machine language" versus FORTRAN, how do you translate between them? We don't have any of those translating programs.

Q: You've suggested that there are at least three natural constitutive problems for psychology: intelligence, will, and consciousness. By "will" you mean the classic ideas of volition?

A: Yes.

Q: It seems to me that volition has been rather neglected in cognitive psychology. You wrote about it in *Plans and the Structure of Behavior* (Miller, Galanter, & Pribram, 1960).

A: We talked a little bit about it there, and I think there are a couple of pages about it in Miller and Johnson-Laird (1976). It keeps coming back to me as a critically important thing. Kurt Lewin obviously thought it was important, and he was right. I think will is terribly important; I just don't have anything worthwhile to say about it. Just because it's important doesn't mean you can do anything with it. As I used to say to my students, I can foul up any one of your experiments by an act of will. Now why doesn't that make "will" more important than the stuff *you're* studying? And the students would struggle with that for a while.

In particular, I tend to believe that there is a will, that people can be held responsible for their actions; and whether that view comes from ignorance of how the brain actually works or not, it's still true that you can't run a society without it. And so, whether it's conventional or innate, we'd better understand how it works.

As regards consciousness, I find the computer thing interesting, because it seems to me that if you can program a computer to do it, that means you don't need consciousness to do it. So, to that extent, I have narrowed down the need for consciousness.

Q: Would you argue that consciousness is not a computational event?

A: I don't know. I don't know what it is. But as well as I can understand how computers work, I see no need to paint *some* of the processes red and say *those* are conscious, and all the rest of them black and say *those* are unconscious. I mean, that gives me no more insight into how the information processing is achieved. Phenomena like the Sternberg short-term memory scanning experiment (Sternberg, 1966) show that short-term memory cannot be the same as consciousness—because it takes time to consciously read out of short-term memory to see if the digit was there or not. But still you get people like Herb Simon—I love the man, in spite of the disagreements we've had—talking about the short-term store as if it were the same as conscious awareness (Ericsson & Simon, 1980). If you want to say that people don't remember anything that they weren't conscious of before, Ericsson and Simon put that in different words, saying that nothing is put into long-term memory unless it has gone through short-term memory. But to me those two claims do not seem equivalent.

Q: Your career history has been rather unusual in the sense that you have continued to move through several different perspectives without finally alighting on one true way to do psychology; so there has been a lot of movement, at least from 1950 onward.

A: I moved even faster before 1950. One thing that worries me as I get older is the danger of becoming like some of my elderly colleagues who seem to nurse their problems, as if they felt that if they ever solved them they wouldn't know what to do. Suppose I knew the answer to this question, what would I do? It's a great fear of mine that I might get into a situation where I would have a problem that I didn't want to solve, because if I solved it I'd have to retire.

Q: Do you have a way of characterizing the difference between yourself and some other psychologists?

A: Just this general observation. Psychologists are rebels. You get your motivation where you can. If your motivation is to show that everybody else has been an idiot up to now, then obviously the best person to show has been an idiot is yourself.

Q: Clearly not everybody in psychology has taken *that* particular tack.

A: No, obviously not. But very often I think that I have understood what people in some area were saying, and I have published and worked in that area, and then later outgrown it. And then I attacked it. I was attacking myself as much as anyone else. Saying, "God I was stupid. Now I think I see better what we should have been doing."

So, yes: I assume in a good Popperian way that anything I'm saying is eventually going to turn out to be wrong—it's just that some things take longer to falsify than others. But they're all wrong somewhere or other. It took a long time to prove Newton wrong, so that was a good theory. But eventually even that was proven wrong. So I'm pretty sure that any substantive claim I make with any confidence today will eventually turn out to be false. And I just hope that I find out why it's false before other people do—that's all.

Marvin Levine: An Evolutionary View of the Cognitive Shift

Marvin Levine (b. 1928) received his undergraduate education at Columbia University, and continued at Harvard, where he worked as a research assistant for both B. F. Skinner and George A. Miller. He completed his graduate work at the University of Wisconsin in 1959, with a dissertation supervised by Harry F. Harlow.

There are interesting similarities between Levine's career and Howard Kendler's (Chapter 3). Although Levine considers himself a cognitive psychologist and Kendler considers himself a neobehaviorist, one suspects their areas of agreement are greater than any disagreement they might have. Both were exposed to a variety of viewpoints in their graduate training, both see the behavioral–cognitive shift as evolutionary rather than revolutionary, both have contributed significantly to the study of discrimination learning, and both have received acceptance from behavioral as well as cognitive psychologists. Perhaps Levine is rather more theoretical than Kendler, especially because he proposed a highly successful representational construct—the notion of specific, operationalizable "hypotheses" in the discrimination task.

By his own account (Levine, 1976), Levine was very much influenced by the *experience* of doing a discrimination learning task. In such a task one is asked to choose between two figures that might differ in several dimensions of variation, such as size, shape, color, and orientation. The task is to choose one or the other figure in each trial, and usually one is told whether the choice was "correct" immediately afterwards. Over a number of trials, one attempts to find the dimension of variation that is always "reinforced" (considered correct). As Levine and Fingerman

(1974) have remarked, the task of simultaneous discrimination learning is "almost irreducible in its simplicity" (p. 720). Yet the task permits psychologists to vary the number of relevant and irrelevant dimensions, the frequency of reinforcement, and the like.

The problem, as Levine saw it, was to take one's experience of testing several different hypotheses until the correct one was obtained, and to find *objective* evidence for this experience. Behavioral conditioning theorists assumed on the basis of numerous experiments with animals that learning of the correct response was gradually reinforced, because one could observe over a group of subjects, a gradual increase in the correct answers. Bower and Trabasso (1963), however, had already pointed out that the gradual increase in correct answers occurred only when responses were averaged over many subjects. That is, each individual subject showed a discontinuous learning curve, but because different subjects learned at different points, the group curve appeared to be gradual. This was consistent with the subjective experience reported by subjects and psychologists alike during the task — of testing clear hypotheses about the different possible answers, until one hit upon a successful hypothesis. Levine's problem was to develop "some way to probe for and detect the learner's hypothesis at any point in the learning task" (1976, p. 124).

His solution was to insert a series of *blank trials* (trials without feedback) into the task, on the assumption that without feedback, subjects would stay with their original hypothesis (an assumption that was tested independently). Their choices on the blank trials presumably indicated their hypotheses. But why not simply *ask* the subjects about their hypotheses? Levine (1976) answers that

We were still trying to persuade the conditioning theorist that his theory about S's [the subjects's] choice-responses was wrong . . . his view was that S's statements, having reference to personal, unobservable events, were irrelevant, and worse, unscientific. The only legitimate data, the only data to be theorized about, were S's choice responses. I felt, therefore, that the most influential probe would be based on S's choices during the task. (p. 124)

The resulting data fit almost perfectly an elegant and simple theory developed by Levine (1959, 1966): He had assumed that subjects sampled from a domain of possible hypotheses, staying with each apparently successful hypothesis until it was disconfirmed, and only then switching hypotheses. The simplicity, persuasiveness, and theoretical success of the model made it difficult to disagree with. Levine's work is almost a paradigmatic example of the ways in which early cognitive psychologists were able to persuade their skeptical colleagues that representational constructs (such as "hypotheses") were indeed reasonable and scientifically respectable.

Interview with Marvin Levine

Q: I'd like to start by asking how you got involved in psychology.

A: In 1947 I was an undergraduate at Columbia and an all-round, nondescript bright student. I was doing B + or A − work in everything. I started as a math major, in fact, but I saw more and more that my interests were shifting and that I wasn't quite good enough to be a real mathematician. Once I started to get into the advanced courses, competing with the young stars in the New York area — well, I wasn't in that league. But more than that, I began to realize that things to do with people fascinated me. I hadn't quite thought about it as a basis for a career or a profession, but I just began to notice that. And there was talk about the new scientific psychology program being instituted at Columbia. Keller and Schoenfeld (followers of B. F. Skinner) were essentially taking over the undergraduate program. There was a certain excitement about that that I had felt even on the fringes, and I suddenly saw psychology being a focus for all my interests in philosophy, art, and music, as well as math and physics. Keller and Schoenfeld organized the undergraduate courses around Skinner's ideas.

When Keller and Schoenfeld took over, introductory psychology was based on their book, which was then being written, (Keller & Schoenfeld, 1950). It was what later came to be referred to as "Skinner for Beginners." The viewpoint in that program was that Pavlov was a figure of historical importance, and Thorndike was really a forerunner who did operant conditioning in a clumsy way, and then Skinner came along and straightened out the whole field. You get tremendous concentration on Skinner. The second year was a laboratory sequence in generalization, discrimination, and motivation, and it was more of the same. So I received a very special conception that Skinner was the leading psychologist in America and that he was the vanguard of scientific psychology. At the end of my third year, Keller came to me and asked, would I want to go to Harvard for graduate work as Skinner's assistant? I explained that I didn't have enough credits to graduate. And he said, "Well, just go to summer school and we'll waive the rest of the credits that you need." That's the way it went. So, knowing little about American psychology, or psychology in general, and thinking that Skinner's orientation was the only one, I went to Harvard for two years. I worked with Skinner for a year, and realized that I had nothing more to learn about his viewpoint. I also learned about the breadth of psychology.

George Miller had just then come back from a year at the Princeton Institute for Advanced Studies. I asked him if I could work with him, and he accepted me. There I started working on problems of language that he was interested in, looking at language as a stochastic process. We did about seven months' worth of work together, after which I left Harvard. I obtained a masters' degree and left, went to work, and was drafted. During that period I learned about the psychology department at the University of Wisconsin. I met a few graduate students who had been there and who were very enthusiastic about the place, and I read the work of Harlow and others. I liked the program. And so, unlike the way I went to Harvard, where I was naïve and was pushed into going, in the case of Wisconsin I made a more sophisticated decision.

Q: What was it about Harlow that seemed to be intriguing?

A: Well, of course I knew about the learning-set work (Harlow, 1949).

Q: Which is?

A: What happens when you give an animal not just a single problem but a long series of similar problems. You may remember that Harlow showed that the problem-learning process changes, from the very slow, conditioning-like learning in the early problems, to a very rapid, almost "insightful" learning in the very late problems. That was with monkeys. Harlow had a monkey laboratory and at that point he had published work in learning sets, which I was impressed with. He'd published work on curiosity, which is today little known unless you're in the field of motivation; but at that time, his paper on curiosity had a considerable impact for a number of reasons. For one thing, it broke completely out of the Hullian drive-reduction mold. I don't know whether young people remember about drive reduction, but that was Hull's notion of the basis for reinforcement. That conception had dominated the field for about 10 years.

Q: And Harlow's point of view was what?

A: That there were intrinsic incentives that attracted the animal, incentives that had nothing to do with drives based on deprivation or hunger. In one study, for example, he demonstrated that animals in an enclosed room would press panels to look out at various objects. Things that moved and lit up were more attractive than things that were related to biological drives. They would rather look at an electric train going around and flashing its light than at bananas and raisins. He combined the curiosity work with manipulation, and showed that the monkeys just like to manipulate things, and that by manipulating, they learn. They formed discriminations just based on their interest in manipulating things.

I learned about this while I was in the Army, about 1954. I also learned that Harlow was starting an infant monkey project. So Harlow was breaking out of what I felt were the restrictions of the S–R approach that you found in the work with rats and pigeons. A lot had to do with the organism he was working with — a monkey — partly because it sits up and looks at you directly, and partly because it does fairly complex things that you can interpret as being complex.

Q: Like what?

A: Well, like being curious, being playful, being attracted to the odd object. It's hard to think of a pigeon being playful. It just wouldn't naturally occur to you to investigate playfulness if you had studied only a pigeon. With a pigeon, you just put him in a box, close the box, and push the buttons to start the automatic apparatus.

Monkeys make eye contact. I began to wonder what would happen if I wore dark glasses (one time I came in with a mask). Or, why does a monkey become shy if you look directly at him? I subsequently learned that people that have been doing field research with monkeys have documented this phenomenon.

Bill Mason visited an island in the Carribean where there were a number of troops of monkeys. There was an anthropologist living on the island who had gotten to know the monkeys in a fairly intimate way, and who had been accepted by them so that the monkeys would function in their ordinary ways in his presence. When Bill came, the monkeys showed the typical avoidance response to strangers. Bill described how he was sitting on the beach with the anthropologist and there were no monkeys around. The fellow warned him that it would take time before any would come near him, that there was, in fact, a large troop at the edge of the beach. Then a couple of males from the group started approaching them. The anthropologist instructed Bill not to look at these males, because eye contact would threaten them and scare them away. He had to sit with his profile to these animals and look at them out of the corner of his eye to see them approach him. Being with the monkeys suggests these kinds of problems that you wouldn't have gotten with these idealized laboratory animals that had been used previously.

There may be another more subtle property to it. Harlow reached his maximum fame with "surrogate motherhood" (Harlow & Suomi, 1970). The story of that again reverts to the virtue of shifting from rat to monkey. They used to diaper infant monkeys. They would put the animal out on these steel veterinarian tables, you've seen them in the vets' offices, shiny steel table tops that are easy to clean up. The infant monkey would scream and kick and claw until it would get the diaper. The monkey would grab the diaper cloth and would calm down. It settled right down, much like a child. You see, another aspect of working with the monkey is that there's something about a generalization of our human responses to children to these monkeys. You begin to think in more human terms than you would in working with a rat or a pigeon. Harlow looked at that phenomenon and suggested that maybe that's the nature of love. And that's how the contact–comfort work all got started. Contact comfort with the surrogate mother was essentially a reinforcer that Harlow compared to love. He just put that nice terrycloth around the wire doll, resulting in the classic pictures of the little monkey hugging the doll.

You know, in the shift from conditioning to cognitive theory, Harlow is an important transitional figure. Although he didn't have a cognitive theory of his own, he was certainly dissatisfied with conditioning theory. He tried in one project after another to transcend the restricted outlook of conditioning theory. All his research — learning-to-learn, curiosity, love, other interpersonal dynamics — all have this character of breaking the old bounds.

Q: Did he have a strong theoretical orientation?

A: Well, he tried to develop a theoretical orientation in the conventional way, starting with learning theory. However, he moved from that into the social-interaction work, starting with the love research. The direction of his career since that time has been toward social interaction, and to the extent that he is a theorist, he has a theory of social interactions.

Q: You worked for Harlow then?

A: Oh yes. I received my PhD from Wisconsin, working most of my three years there in Harlow's lab.

Q: And where did you go afterwards?

A: Remember that I had started out as a math major in college. I ended up as a math minor, which means I had five semesters of mathematics. In those days, the late 1950s, mathematical theory was developing in the field of learning, led by William Estes, Bush, and Mosteller, and several other people. The monkey researchers, who were performing wonderful experiments in the field of learning, were basically nonmathematical. It almost was a perfect correlation: If you worked with monkeys, you didn't use mathematics. Here I come into this monkey laboratory, you see. I had had three semesters of calculus or something, so Harlow sat me down and made me his lab theorist. I had a privileged position there. I was free to think over a variety of problems. Harlow had written an extremely penetrating paper on systematic responses in the monkey, which he called "error-factor theory." In fact, to the extent that Harlow was a theorist in the field of learning, it centered around error-factor theory.

Q: "Errors" are defined by the discrimination learning task?

A: Exactly right. Error-factor theory grows out of discrimination learning.

Q: In a certain sense, from the viewpoint of the animal, to make an "error" may be in fact a perfectly rational and correct thing to do, whereas from the viewpoint of the task it may be the incorrect thing.

A: If you're going to talk freely about the viewpoint of the animal, I'll say that from the viewpoint of the animal, an error was an error most of the time. When an animal was correct, he got raisins. And he wanted raisins, there was no question about that. When there was an error, you could even see irritation. That's another thing about monkeys, they grumble. You can see irritation. He'll take the object and he'll hit it.

So the animal is looking to maximize getting raisins. When he didn't get raisins, in Harlow's interpretation, an error factor was interfering. An error factor would be like a preference. Consider position-preference: This means that for some reason the animal just sits on the righthand side and pushes the righthand object. If the raisin was always hidden under one of the particular objects, say a cylinder as opposed to a block, the objects would be randomly located on the right or on the left and the animal would be correct only 50% of the time. But this animal would take the raisin when the correct object was on the righthand side and grumble when it wasn't. That would be an error factor.

Now, an error factor that may *not* be an error factor from the viewpoint of the animal is stimulus-preference. Sometimes the animal liked the wrong object. Now, start out with two brand-new objects: Harlow used what he called "junk objects." So the two objects might be an orange juice can and a blackboard eraser. The raisin is under one of these, and the animal has to learn which one it's under; it changes positions from trial to trial in a discrimination fashion.

In a learning-set experiment, if an animal has had 500 problems, he's extremely good. That is, he'll go to an object, and if it's the wrong object, he'll never go to it again. Starting with the second trial, he'll always go for the correct object. He can be given a brand-new pair of objects, unrelated to any of the preceding. You randomly put a raisin under one of these, the correct object for that problem, and again you see the same thing. If the animal is right, he will always go for the correct object; if he's wrong on trial one, starting on trial two he'll always go to the correct object. That's after 500 problems. Now you give him problem 501. He's been performing at asymptote for the last 50 problems, and suddenly he makes an error on every trial. The objects for problem 501 might be a toy soldier and a block of wood, and the raisin is under the block of wood. In starting out, the monkey goes for the toy soldier and he's wrong. Okay, that's trial one. On trial two he goes for the toy soldier. On trial three he goes for the toy soldier. What's going on? The animal has a stimulus-preference. That's a case where from the monkey's standpoint, it may not be an error. He's decided he likes the toy soldier: He wants to see more of it, handle it, and keep it as long as they're not going to take it away from him. But that would be an error factor from the *experimenter's* standpoint. You have a number of these error factors.

All of Harlow's students, whenever they did a learning-set experiment, studied every problem to look for error factors. What they found was a real hodgepodge. In every new experiment. people thought they saw different systematic patterns of response; they found new error factors, or they took old ones and measured them in new ways. That small domain of research and analysis was becoming chaotic.

I took for myself the problem of bringing order into that field. I wanted to develop a theory of error factors; a theory of systematic response patterns that would permit you to look at a large number of patterns simultaneously, and to estimate their relative strengths. I wanted a theory that would permit you to say, for example, that 50% of the errors are caused by position-preference, 20% by stimulus-preference, and so forth. The existing analysis didn't permit that. They could just essentially document that these patterns were occurring. I wanted to derive this analysis from a set of basic principles of animal functioning. That became my PhD thesis; I worked on that for about 2 years, pretty much as a hobby. When you start with a theoretical question like that, if it doesn't work, you've got nothing. As a result, I could not treat the search for a theory as a hobby while I did my course work and my research. After what seemed like a fruitless two years, I suddenly solved the critical problems.

Q: And what was it that you came out with?

A: Well, a theory of systematic responding in the learning-set experiment. I had to make some changes from Harlow's way of looking at it. I had to look not only at systematic patterns that produced errors, but at systematic patterns that produced correct responding as well. If you're going to look at systematic patterns that produce correct responding, you're now talking about a larger class of systematic patterns. The literature had a precedent for that, and that was Krechevsky's hypothesis work: He called his larger class "hypotheses" (Krechevsky, 1932). So I started talking about hypothesis behavior in monkeys, and, as I say, the theory clicked. I found a way of axiomatically stating the description of the underlying processes, and these axioms led to a measurement technique with which I could estimate the strength of the various response patterns, both correct and incorrect. And so systematic responding became the subject of my intellectual focus at Wisconsin. It provided me with a PhD thesis, which was almost immediately published in *Psychological Review* (Levine, 1959).

In my last year at Wisconsin, an important event happened: I stumbled upon an experiment on responding by human adults in a two-choice test. The author had found systematic patterns of responses, and analyzed them from the standpoint of Hullian theory. Essentially the author shrugged his shoulders, concluded that Hullian theory doesn't account for the data, and left it at that. Reading his experiment, I wondered whether there were determinants of the systematic patterns in this experiment that would account for the results — whether my theory couldn't be modified to account for these data. I applied that kind of analysis, and it worked. It wasn't such a big deal, except that it encouraged me to think about applying my little theory to humans. In doing that, a subtle change crept into my thinking. In the monkey, the hypothesis was the pattern of response itself. In the adult human, the hypothesis was not one-to-one with the pattern itself. Instead, the hypothesis was the subject's prediction of what was going to happen in the sequence of events. This prediction was manifested in the pattern of responses. Thus, the hypothesis was a prediction, a state of the *subject*, which was manifested in a unique pattern of responses.

Q: Is the difference that the human can state the hypothesis?

A: No, not at all. I dealt only with systematic response patterns. In later years I had my subjects state hypotheses, but in those days never. And for good reason. There were excellent reasons why I avoided talking to my human subjects. I made no apologies about that.

Q: I assume that monkeys have expectations about future events: Would such expectations not be the same as an hypothesis?

A: Well, it turns out that the things Krechevsky was calling "hypotheses" and the things Harlow was calling "error factors" had nothing to do with the other construct that was coming out in cognitive theory that was called "expectations."

Q: Which was from Tolman's work?

A: Which was from Tolman. And remember, Krechevsky was a student of Tolman's; he received his PhD with Tolman. Krechevsky, I think, liked to consider patterns of responses — that is, "hypotheses" — as synonymous with "expectations." I know that Tolman referred to Krechevsky's hypothesis work as part of the cognitive orientation. In my opinion, with good hindsight, having worked with adult humans, and having seen the kind of theory we need there, and also having worked with monkeys, and having seen what kind of theory we need for them, response patterns in rats and monkeys reflected something more mechanistic than expectations. Harlow stayed more neutral when he called a response pattern an "error factor" than Krechevsky did when he called it an "hypothesis."

Q: What is the difference, as far as you're concerned, between an "expectation" and an "hypothesis"?

A: Well, let's not for the moment use rigorous behavioral operational definitions; let's talk in everyday terms. For the human, each concept, hypothesis, or expectation implies a prediction about how events will proceed. An hypothesis can be verified or falsified. In the monkey, however, an hypothesis is simply the determinant of a systematic pattern of response, for example, a position-preference or a stimulus-preference. These have nothing to do with any prediction by the animal. Thus, a monkey with a stimulus-preference will go to the wrong object, will make an error again and again. The adult human on the other hand, recognizes that his hypothesis is not verified. He expects something else to be the basis for the solution to his problem. He changes his hypothesis, his prediction, and his mode of responding. He rarely makes the same error twice.

Q: So the hypothesis is always in the context of a problem to be solved, in which the feedback is taken as information toward the solution of that problem?

A: Essentially yes, although there are interesting uses of the term "hypothesis" in language comprehension and in perception. That's very fluid right now, but it was standard 20 years ago that the term "hypothesis" was used primarily in a problem-solving situation.

Q: You were doing a kind of cognitive psychology in a world that was very behaviorally oriented. Were there any problems with that? For example, have you talked to Skinner about your work?

A: I have not spoken to Skinner about my work, and I don't know that he is familiar with it. Personally, I think he would be very interested and accepting of it. I certainly have an intellectual debt to Skinner: He is a first-rate experimentalist, very concerned with taking a theoretical construct and making it manifest directly in behavior. The theoretical construct for him was "learning," or "response strength." He plausibly interpreted response strength as rate of responding. Thus, he didn't have to calculate anything that the animal was doing. He just looked at the rate of responding. In other words, he explicated the theoretical construct so that you could see it in the behavior directly. That is, in effect, what I did as well.

I took this notion of "hypothesis" and found a way to make each hypothesis one-to-one with a unique response pattern. By looking at response patterns, therefore, I could know a human subject's hypothesis, that is, his prediction in that problem situation. Like Skinner, you see, I, too, explicated a theoretical concept directly in behavior. I could now experimentally investigate the dynamics of hypothesis-testing. Did people always keep a hypothesis when it was confirmed? Did they always reject a disconfirmed hypothesis? How many hypotheses could they simultaneously monitor? It was like opening a small window on the mind.

Q: This brings me back to my question about the behavioristic context. Here you are, starting to do this cognitive research, opening "a window on the mind" with humans, in a field dominated by conditioning theorists working with rats and pigeons. Why was your work accepted?

A: An interesting development was taking place within conditioning theory. You're absolutely correct that in the '30s and '40s, rats and, later, pigeons, were the proper subjects. The researchers were not interested in these specific organisms, however. Skinner, for example, was not studying the behavioral features of the albino rat in order to know specifically about rats. Everyone professed to be interested in the human. The rat was just a little man whose environment you could perfectly control, and who did not have the complications of a long, unknown history. But everyone felt that there was promise in this approach, because it would reveal fundamental laws about *human* behavior.

Well, in the 1950s, conditioning theorists began to feel that that promissory note was coming due. They began to apply the theory to adult human behavior. For example, Skinner was publishing his books on *Verbal Behavior* (1957) and *Science and Human Behavior* (1953); Bill Estes, the then leader of mathematical conditioning theory, started testing the theory with college students. Therefore, the fact that I was working with humans was not a problem. In part, even the tasks that I used were similar to those used by the mathematical conditioning theorists. We had college students learning in two-alternative discrimination-learning tasks. The tasks weren't different from the ones that I described for the monkey.

Q: The tasks may have been the same, but you differed in theory. They saw the learning as a reinforcement process, whereas you were using a cognitive language.

A: The difference was not just in language. For them, the human was a passive learner. Reinforcement and extinctions gradually, slowly over trials, built up the strength of the correct response, and weakened the incorrect responses. For me, the human was active. He was testing out first one hypothesis, then another, until he hit on the correct hypothesis. I viewed the human in these tasks as an active problem solver, rather than as a passive conditioned learner.

Q: How, then, did your work come to have an influence on behaviorists in the field?

A: There are two or three reasons. One is personal. Let's go through that one quickly. When we last discussed my career, I was obtaining my PhD at Wisconsin and researching in Harlow's lab. The psychology department at Indiana University was then the home of Estes and Burke, and was the center of mathematical learning theory. Indiana announced a faculty opening for a new PhD, and Harlow, my advisor, felt that I would be an excellent candidate for that position and urged me to apply. I did and was hired. Consequently, for the next 6 years I came to know some of the leading people in learning theory. I even sat in on Estes's course for the graduate students. The faculty was later joined by Jim Greeno and Frank Restle, other leaders in this field. I therefore learned intimately the opposing point of view. I certainly developed a high regard for their theoretical rigor and learned some of their techniques. Furthermore, I could almost daily bring my research to everyone's attention. There was little chance of being neglected.

Q: You're saying that this personal contact was important?

A: Oh, yes. Although equally important were other things happening in the discipline, both in conditioning theory itself and in psychology generally. We're now talking about 1959 and the early '60s. When an adult human, a scientist, has the behavior of the adult human as his domain of scientific inquiry, something peculiar exists. It is a situation unlike that in any other field of science. The scientist and his subject can, so to speak, change places. Thus, I would say to my research assistant, "Why don't you run me in some of these problems?" When you take advantage of this unique, peculiar opportunity and run as a subject, you can see the process from the inside; you can see what is happening inside yourself as you're learning. You're very active on the inside.

Although this isn't a rigorous proof of anything, I think it partly explains some of the tentativeness the conditioning theorists started to have about passive, gradual-strengthening-of-responses in the adult human. Thus, Estes developed an all-or-none theory founded on sudden, one-trial conditioning (sounds like insight, right?), and Frank Restle (1962) shifted over to his own mathematical version of hypothesis-testing theory. As a result, my work, which, like theirs, both focused on response patterns and was cast mathematically, became interesting to them.

Also, there were softening influences in the field at large. The British and the physiologists were doing convincing research on attention. "Memory" was coming back as an important psychological concept.

Q: Hasn't "memory" always been a part of American psychology?

A: Yes. But that concept suffered under behaviorism, along with all references to internal states. For example, the most influential behaviorist books on learning, Skinner's *The Behavior of Organisms* (1938), Hull's *Principles of Behavior* (1943), and Kimble's *Conditioning and Learning* (1961), all omit the term "memory" from their indexes. They never mention it. Furthermore, theorists in the '40s and '50s were interpreting the data of forgetting in terms of extinction and Pavlovian inhibition. So, yes, it was important that in the 1960s memory was coming back in. The Petersons were also at Indiana at this time. They were doing their spectacular research on short-term memory (Peterson & Peterson, 1959), and were having their own kind of influence on the local conditioning theorists. There were other influences of this kind. Psycholinguistics was getting off the ground, people in Artificial Intelligence were talking about computers having strategies and memories. It started to become hard for the conditioning theorist, working with the adult human, to insist upon his behavioristic restrictions. Too much of value was happening elsewhere.

Q: So you see conditioning ideas fading away during the '60s?

A: That's a fair statement. At least, other things were coming to overshadow them. There is, however, an important durable influence of the behavioristic phase of American psychology.

Q: What is that?

A: Insistence on rigor. Make your experiments as clean as possible, make your theorizing as clear and as hard-headed as possible. In doing research on cognitive concepts, have your data as tightly connected to those concepts as possible. For example, I later started having subjects introspect and state their hypotheses in words. I called these statements "introtacts," with a nod toward Skinner. There was no ambiguity. The introtact data resembled exactly what we were obtaining from response patterns. That insistence on precision, on experiment-theory tightness, I think, characterizes cognitive psychology today. In no small measure it reflects the behaviorist influence. We now talk about internal processes, but always try to find a clear behavioral manifestation.

Q: It seems to me that all the earlier work in cognitive psychology was exactly of that kind. That is to say, it made observable certain things which were thought to be unobservable, such as imagery, memory, and in your case, hypotheses.

A: Well, I think the emphasis was on finding *compelling experimental methods.* And I think that a large part of the problem with the early prebehavioristic work in introspective "cognitive psychology" was that they did not have compelling experimental methods. For someone to say, "I see this picture and it is fading rapidly" was not terribly compelling, in the sense that, say, Sperling's (1960) work was compelling about the existence of an image.

Q: How do you see Sperling's work fit in with the idea of making the rapidly fading image observable?

A: Sperling was able to demonstrate that a subject had available a large store for immediate visual information, a larger store than people had heretofore presumed. By clever experimental techniques, he showed that that store of information dwindled rapidly with time. With very little in the way of arbitrary assumptions, he was able to derive a curve showing the decay in the size of the store of the visual information.

Q: So he would show an array of letters or numbers to a subject, and show that people could retrieve any member of that array, if they were appropriately cued after the array was already off the screen. But their ability to retrieve the rest of the array decayed very rapidly. And this would be considerably better than simply to report the same facts from introspection.

A: The data that existed 50 years ago would be some qualitative characterization of an experience that a person was having. And that was less compelling for at least two reasons. One is that that sort of data didn't square with people's notions of what constituted scientific data. Qualitative descriptions of inner experiences were different from the data of other scientific disciplines.

Another reason is that these descriptions produced the famous unresolvable controversies. For example, some people claimed they had imagery, and some people claimed they did not. One side insisted that those people who said they did not have imagery were not introspecting properly. There was this novel introspection technique—again, without parallel in the other sciences, which all by itself made it suspect—leading to irresolvable differences. Of course, that's all part of ancient history. I think that in the modern revolution, people such as myself and others working with cognitive processes are looking for excellent experimental techniques that would literally compel the interpretation. There was, little to argue about, for instance, when the Petersons spoke about short-term memory.

Q: Let me play devil's advocate: Why should psychology not do things differently from the other sciences?

A: You're asking for undergraduate lecture number 14. I think we have to go back to the world circa 1914. At the end of the 19th and the beginning of the 20th centuries we were seeing some really remarkable technological miracles. The technological revolution had been going on for some 200 years, but it was now very salient. Subways were being built, skyscrapers were going up, horseless carriages were suddenly appearing, diseases were being conquered. People then began to see, in a vivid way, remarkable fruit coming from the scientific method. The psychologists said, Look, if we're going to have comparable benefits from our science, we clearly must imitate the other sciences. Introspection was a case where the domain of inquiry—consciousness—was accessible only to a single person. This was clearly different from the relationship between the observer and the domain in other scientific fields. In the other fields, the domain was public. Many observers could simultaneously view, for example, an eclipse. In introspection, the domain itself was private. I'm responding to you, of course, in your role as devil's advocate. I'm explaining why, in the early '20s and '30s, it appeared legitimate to throw out consciousness and introspection. Today, the situation is different. I've already mentioned the fruitful use of one's own introspections as a source of hypotheses about theoretical processes. And then I described the modern "introtacts," the use of formal, carefully restricted introspections leading to neat data. I know — it's ironic, but I think we all owe that passion for rigor to the behaviorists. That continues to be a valuable, lasting influence.

James J. Jenkins: Beyond Methodolatry

In the previous two interviews George A. Miller and Marvin Levine described their experience of the cognitive shift as evolutionary. In contrast, the turning points for James J. Jenkins (b. 1923) were more discrete and clearly marked. Jenkins received his doctoral degree from the University of Minnesota in 1950, and in a short time became deeply involved in testing the behavioristic mediation theory of verbal learning. Mediation theory grew from Hull's claim that internal processes could be taken to be analogous to external stimulus–response (S–R) learning — that the same conditioning processes that can be observed externally could also take place between invisible stimuli and responses. Such a theory was evidently needed to account for language processes in human beings (see Chapter 4). Charles E. Osgood was particularly identified with this attempt to account for language and meaning behavioristically.

The most straightforward way to test mediation theory was by teaching people words that would function as "stimuli" and "responses," so that when shown word A (the stimulus), people would respond with a previously learned word B (the response). Next, one could teach a second pair of associated words B–C, and test to see if the subjects now found it easier to learn the association between word A and word C, even in B were never given. If this new association were facilitated, that is, if people found it easier to learn the A–C connection after having learned A–B and B–C, the facilitation of learning implies that the invisible element B helped to connect A to C. This "three-stage mediation paradigm" worked quite well (Jenkins, 1963), an encouraging initial result.

But it is further necessary to suppose that the invisible connections are able to *interact* with each other. In more recent language, it abstract terms must be able to deal with other abstract terms. To explain semantic generalization (the fact that responses conditioned to a word will generalize to its synonym) one had to suppose that the first word had an invisible meaning response (r_m) that was physically similar to the meaning response evoked by the synonym. Thus, there had to be a bridge between the two r_m's. This involved *four* mediation stages: Given A–C and B–C, then learning A–D should facilitate learning B–D. It was at this point that the empirical program to test mediation theory began to break down. In some heroically long and elaborate experiments, Jenkins and his co-workers failed to find the expected four-stage mediation (Jenkins, 1963). Thus a critical test of the best behavioristic theory of language seemed to fail.

The upshot of it all was well summarized by the title of Jenkins's 1974 Presidential Address to the Experimental Psychology Division of the American Psychological Association: "Remember that old theory of memory? Well, forget it!" Mediation theory seemed to provide a critical test of the adequacy of a behavioral account of language. When it failed, Jenkins began to question the entire behavioral approach.

Jenkins's subsequent work is remarkable in its flexibility and in Jenkins's willingness to depart from hallowed tradition to solve the puzzle of language. In particular, Jenkins was willing to abandon experimental methods that did not seem to work, for others that seemed more promising. This was professionally risky at a time when the "proper method" was taken to distinguish scientific from unscientific psychology. But in retrospect it seems clear that adherence to very limited experimental designs and techniques hindered more than helped progress. Jenkins was able to overcome such "methodolatry" over a period of time, but this was by no means easy.

In his subsequent career Jenkins was particularly active in encouraging other psychologists to consider the work of Chomsky, J. J. Gibson, and, of his own students, John Bransford and Jeffrey Franks. Each of these in his own way challenged the accepted findings and procedures in experimental psychology, and helped move the field generally in a more cognitive and ecologically valid direction.

Jenkins has occupied a number of prominent positions in experimental psychology, most recently Chairman of the Board of Governors of the Psychonomics Society, the main society of experimental psychologists.

Interview with James J. Jenkins

Q: How did you get started in psychology?

A: Oh my, that wakes ancient memories. I remember being terribly intrigued by Psychology One. I had a really good professor at a tiny college, who made the course stimulating and got us to read psychology. Then I went off to World War II and in the course of being a weatherman and finding that work distressing, I tried to decide whether I wanted to be a politician, an engineer, or a psychologist. I read a lot of politics and decided that was not what I wanted, and then I got hooked on the notion of combining my social-service drive with psychology, and "getting psychology to work for the common man" sort of thing. I was going to be a psychologist with a labor union and help in the great revolution of workers-run-factory.

The only place I ever heard of that had any work going on in this direction was Minnesota, so I applied to graduate school there. It's the only place I ever applied to. I didn't know that people were supposed to apply to more than one place, and when I didn't hear from them right away, I got on the train and went to Minneapolis, and said, "Well, are you guys going to take me or not?" I really didn't know anything.

So they took me, and gave me the then princely award of a 3/8 assistantship. That paid $900 for the academic year. So I was rich, and went to graduate school, and discovered, of course, that what psychologists did was not what I had supposed they did. I found that my social-service drive was not as high as I had supposed it was, and I became fascinated with research.

When I finished my PhD, which was in industrial psychology, I had two choices. I could stay at Minnesota and teach and do research, or I could go to General Motors. General Motors was paying three times as much, so it suited my martyrdom to stay at Minnesota, where there was freedom of research. And that's how I got into academic psychology, in 1950.

Q: How did you then start to work on the psychology of language?

A: We had done some work on mass communication and communication in industry, and the Social Science Research Council asked me, "Would you like to come and meet with a group that's going to study psychology and linguistics in Indiana?" I didn't have any summer plans — I'd starved every summer up to then — and so I said yes; and lo and behold, I was suddenly a psycholinguist. That summer I learned a lot about linguistics, and met interesting people: Charles Osgood, Eric Lenneberg, Joe Greenberg, Floyd Lounsbury, Jack Carroll, Susan Ervin, Tom Sebeok, and Sol Saporta. I took a course in grammar from Bernard Bloch, who was one of the gods who walked the earth in those days in linguistics, and got American linguistic structuralism right down the barrel.

Q: And did you believe it?

A: Well, I was astonished by it, because all the things that psychology hoped to be, these people said they were. Absolutely objective and absolutely reliable. It didn't make any difference who described the language, the descriptions were guaranteed to come out exactly the same. It was just an incredible set of pronouncements, and I was being the incredulous novice, taking notes like crazy about how wonderful linguistics was. I'm really glad that happened, because I suppose I never would have believed it if I hadn't been there. I still have the notes I took in Bloch's class, with his egregious assertions about what was possible, and how objective and formal the entire procedure was.

The linguistic paradigm — that awful word again — was thoroughly accepted. They had swallowed the old-fashioned operationalist philosophy of science from the '20s, and they believed they were doing it. And if everybody believes it, and nobody asks any questions, sure, that's what you're doing. The key was: Nobody was asking questions!

Q: And you started to have doubts about this?

A: Well, I was just thunderstruck by it, because, you know, as a psychologist I would ask, "What's the reliability of this description?" Some guy goes out and studies a language nobody else ever studies. He brings back a description of the language. What are the odds that it's right? That question was met with overwhelming scorn. "Why, of course it's right, because he used the right methods." It was justification through methods.

Q: Has anybody ever studied the reliability of linguistic descriptions?

A: Well, I think it's at least open to debate now. But in those days that was it. One person studied a language, and that was *his* language. Others didn't poach on his language. So it was the worst of all possible worlds: The method was assumed to be completely reliable, and the conventions of the field said nobody else had better go and test it. Linguistics was completely objective, behavioristic, positivistic, operational, and complete. Right? Well, of course, psychology wanted to be all those things. So our task was to supply the learning theory that was going to go along with this complete science of language.

Q: And that learning theory had to be a mediational theory (e.g., Osgood, 1953)?

A: Right. The mediational theory was really an attempt to build on the stimulus–response theory, to permit invisible things like internal stimuli and responses, but to be very explicit about these intervening variables. The hidden parts were all little s's and r's. If you look at the conferences in the late '50s (Cofer, 1961; Cofer & Musgrave, 1963), it's clear that even discussing intervening variables was regarded as radical. Invisible mediators were regarded as a departure from respectable psychology, and people like Leo Postman and Benton Underwood really fought that. They dragged their feet on mediators for a year and then finally convinced themselves by running some experiments in their own laboratories.

Q: Osgood's arguments for the existence of invisible stimuli and responses had to do with effects like semantic generalization — the fact that when a response was conditioned to a word, it would also occur to a synonym of that word, even though the synonym was a completely different physical stimulus. Since the meaning of the two words was the same, the conditioned response had to be connected to the meaning of the synonyms, and "meaning" was, of course, invisible. But what were your reasons for proposing a mediational theory?

A: Mostly transfer experiments. Suppose that you learn a list of paired associates, so that for every item A on the list you learn a paired item B. The A's are stimuli, and the B's are responses, according to our view at that time. Then you learn a B–C list in which B's are stimuli and C's are responses, and now the question is, will your learning with the B's help you to learn an A–C list, in which the B's are not presented? The results show convincingly that you learn an A–C list faster if you know some intervening mediating items. You implicitly chain from A's to B's and from B's to C's. In fact, the mediation hypothesis had been around for 200 years, but there was almost no experimental evidence to support the idea. And yet Osgood in his '53 book had to use it for all the higher mental processes.

So we finally engaged in this big program of experiments (Horton & Kjeldergaard, 1961), where we set up all eight possible three-stage mediation paradigms, and discovered that six of the eight yielded marked facilitation. This further disturbed people. The only kind of mediation they had been accepting up to that time was simple chains, A-B-C. And we showed that if two stimuli had a common response, then those two could be learned together more readily (A–B, C–B facilitates A–C). If two responses were common to the stimulus, then those two could be learned readily (B–A, B–C facilitates A–C). People weren't happy about that, because it made things more complicated than they'd hoped they would be, but the evidence for that was very good when we got through.

Q: So you feel a lot of satisfaction about that.

A: Oh, it was good stuff. The surprising thing is that these studies are what the animal people are doing right now: Mediation is very big in animal psychology.

Q: Really? That's fascinating, I didn't know that.

A: Well, yes, they're talking about "expectations" now, and "anticipations of outcome," and so on, and it's all the same old mediation paradigms. They have changed the language a little, but the work is exactly the same. Now it's called cognitive animal psychology.

Q: So you see history repeating itself, with animal psychologists going through the same train of thought that human experimentalists did some time ago. And presumably the reason is that good experimental psychologists are enormously reluctant to posit the existence of hidden constructs, such as expectations or, 20 years ago, internal stimuli and responses.

A: Yes. It's hard to believe how strong the resistance was. If you read some of those early conferences, there was a lot of defense against anything like this. The old guard had a lot of trouble with it, and I remember when Leo Postman finally ran a series of studies in which he found strong mediational effects, we were walking across the Berkeley campus and he said, "You know, the trouble is you never did those experiments properly. Now I've done them right, I believe them." That's the wonderful thing about experimentalists; they do believe in data as the ultimate argument.

The big disappointment was not that the phenomena weren't there or that the experiment didn't work, because the experiments were just gangbusters. We must have done 100 to 120 experiments, developing these ideas through word associations, natural language associations, and acquired laboratory associations. The thing that finally crushed us was that when we went to four-stage mediation (involving three learning stages and a test stage), which for a variety of reasons is essential to language, it turned out it didn't work out the way we thought it would. So you'd teach A–B, A–C, D–B, and then test D–C; the hypothesis was that A and D should function as equivalent stimuli. Because A–C is already learned, D–C should be easy. But it doesn't work that way: It's just too bad.

So about five of us ran a great huge hairy experiment. The research assistants were Phil Gough, Jim Greeno, Dave Hakes, and Erv Segal — a stellar cast! I think it took us a year and a half to run, and it had 16 conditions in it, trying to nail down the four-stage mediation thing. And the whole experiment blew; we didn't get a thing (Jenkins, 1963). You can make the four-stage paradigm work — but that isn't the point. To have it explain the acquisition of language it has to work *automatically*. And that's what we couldn't get. And, you know, if your machinery won't do what you think is necessary to do language, you sort of put yourself out of business. And so that was the great experimental debacle that softened me up. (*cf.* Jenkins & Palermo, 1964).

Then Chomsky pulled the rug out from under us. If you have a slot grammar of the kind that American structuralist linguistics tried to use, mediation theory is perfect for it. So we were very busy trying to provide the apparatus for a theory of linguistics that at that moment was being discredited. It's a very disappointing position to be in. I wrote a thing on psycholinguistics in 1966 (Jenkins, 1966), where I recounted some of that history, and pointed out that by the time we could supply the right kind of theory, the nature of what language was believed to be had changed (Chomsky, 1957, 1965). The whole theory was no longer appropriate. Very grim, very grim.

Q: You speak of the resistance to the mediation theory. Was there any problem in publishing the experiments?

A: Well, you always run into that. It depends on what period you're talking about. For example, the early mediation stuff was not regarded as interesting. It's not that editors and reviewers were against it—they just said it wasn't their kind of psychology. We sent one article to Arthur Melton at the *Journal of Experimental Psychology*, and he didn't even have it reviewed. He simply sent it back with a note, "This is of no interest to my readers." Lots of journals would simply not deal with us, or the referees would give us endless suggestions, "Why don't you do the following set of studies?" There are exceptions to that—I think that Leo Postman as editor of the *Journal of Verbal Learning and Verbal Behavior* was remarkable in his tolerance for dissident views. As a matter of fact, in the interest of encouraging new work, he probably let things through that were not nearly as methodologically sound as the traditional stuff.

The Bransford and Franks experiments came out in 1971 (see Bransford & Franks, 1971; Franks & Bransford, 1971), and we had a terrible time publishing them, because people kept asking for more and more evidence, and nobody really believed that the experiments worked. I remember Cofer writing me in great excitement, saying he'd replicated their language study and "My God, it worked!" And I thought, "Of course it worked, we've got 20 replications of it." But people just didn't believe it; they simply didn't believe the phenomena in those experiments. And now everyone thinks those results are trivial! But at the time, I think it's literally true that nobody in academic psychology predicted those findings.

I don't think that there is any end to resistance. I mean, if you're pushing the edges of the field, you're always up against some kind of resistance of that sort. You just hope for good editors, and you keep making your arguments and coming back over and over again.

Q: Do you sometimes think that psychologists became prematurely sophisticated in methodology, before it could really be used sensibly?

A: Oh yes! Yes, I believe that. They stopped looking at the world too early and tried to be scientists. I know this is an unpopular thing to say, but they got precision at the cost of validity. My favorite instance is a comparison of the early work in intelligence testing. Compare Spearman and Binet around the turn of the century: Spearman's 1904 papers on intelligence are really sophisticated in terms of measurement, and all off base with respect to content. Binet had weak methodology; didn't really care much about it; sort of formulated his methodology as he went along. He was just concerned with the validity of what he was doing, and he simply won hands down. Spearman was still trying to measure intelligence by having people judge shades of gray, and Binet had already unlocked the practical problem by building scales (see Jenkins & Peterson, 1961).

I think that kind of thing happened in psychology over and over again. People took what they thought was a manageable part of the field, and then tightened it all up without realizing how much they were constricting their theories and their view of the world. That's why it's always good to be around George Miller, because he always thinks psychology goes further than you do. He's always saying, "You know, we ought to have something to say about that problem or issue or idea." And I always think, "Is that psychology? Well, I guess it could be. We ought to think about that." Miller is very good at expanding people's points of view. He just keeps opening you up. He's had a lot of impact on me.

Q: What was your experience of the change of viewpoint?

A: I was at the Center for Advanced Study in the Behavioral Sciences at Stanford in '58–'59, the year that George Miller, Eugene Galanter, and Karl Pribram were writing *Plans and the Structure of Behavior* (1960). Osgood was there that year, and the center was full of linguists. It was a big psycholinguistics year, but they were mostly old-guard linguists. The only person there who knew anything about Chomsky was George Miller. The others never mentioned him.

That year enormously broadened my notions of what psychology was. Miller, Galanter, and Pribram (1960) were of course trying to push out the boundaries as far as they could go, and I thought that *Plans* was really a fascinating book. It's still a good book to shake people's heads up and get them out of the old tradition. (And more people are in the old tradition than we're willing to admit.)

In *Plans* they were trying to show over and over again that you had to come to grips with the idea of structure — a word that was anathema to psychologists of that period. Each chapter took a different kind of problem, and in each case the old approach of using simple associations was found to be deficient. For example, in the language chapter, Miller talks about how long it would take if you had to memorize all the 20-word sentences that you can probably handle in English.

Q: And it essentially takes you an infinite amount of time to memorize them?

A: Right. So he defeats the old methods of learning theory rather casually and handily, right off the bat. And once he got people set up for the notion that they've got to have some kind of structure, the question is what kind? Then he simply introduces the Chomskian theory, and says, "In the case of generative grammar, I furnish such a model."

Q: Why was George Miller believed when others were not? Chomsky himself, for example, must have persuaded very few psychologists.

A: Miller had earned his spurs in psychoacoustics, where he had done classic work. He was trained under S. S. Stevens at Harvard, and everybody had to agree that his work was pure and methodologically fine and all that; and George can do mathematics with the best of them, and that always impresses psychologists. So he was obviously a good guy, and when he started doing this crazy stuff in language, he brought legitimacy to it.

In 1965 I spent another year at the Center for Advanced Study in the Behavioral Sciences together with a very good group of people. Our intention was to study the cutting edge of psycholinguistics. Some of us were still thinking that we could push the mediation stuff then, because we simply didn't realize the full impact of Chomsky's work. Jerry Fodor and I had offices next door to each other, and we met every morning to talk about language. Then we met with Sol Saporta most afternoons to work on a book that we all wrote and never published. (A sketch of it was published; see Fodor, Jenkins, & Saporta, 1967.) The language group had Jerry Fodor, Sol Saporta, Wallace Lambert, Lyle Jones, and by absolute good luck, Franklin Cooper and Al Liberman from Haskins Labs in New Haven. Our research assistants were Don Foss and Ruth Day. Arthur Koestler, the novelist turned social scientist, was at the center that year, which was lots of fun. Bernard Bloch was there and Joseph Greenberg, among the linguists. Erik Erikson was there that year, too — it just kills me that we didn't get to interact with him more. Anyway, a top-notch group.

We sat down with *Syntactic Structures* (Chomsky, 1957) and Fodor and Saporta did a tutorial, sentence by sentence, through the book, trying to elaborate what the implications were. And that was just really fine — I mean you get people of this caliber together in a seminar, and they're obviously not afraid of one another. They ask the right questions and they're just so smart and so good.

Q: Chomsky shows in *Syntactic Structures* that any theory of language that assumes a chain of elements — a Markov process — cannot account for some very basic facts. Was that an important issue?

A: Yes, the whole business about demolishing Markov processes becomes a key part of the argument. Once you've done that, then the mediation models are out. Stimulus–response models are only a subclass of Markov models. In psychology, Markov-type models were extraordinarily popular — even after Miller and Chomsky published their refutations — they were sanctified by tradition. But English doesn't happen to be a language that can be generated by Markov models. Too bad. So that was really terribly good, it shook us all up and we all tried to work very hard on what things one could do differently.

It was a sort of schizophrenic period. Here we were busy on the one hand, defending the mediation studies, which were under attack in the psychological literature (see Jenkins, 1965; Jenkins & Foss, 1969), and on the other hand, admitting that regardless of the reality of the phenomena, mediation wasn't going to be useful in understanding language.

Q: You were one of a rather small number of psychologists who actually confronted these problems head-on. Why were you different in this respect?

A: Well, I guess the thing that has pushed me is that I have always cared about language. Doing the mediation experiments was not just playing the experimental game — we were doing them to get on toward understanding language. When it turned out we couldn't do language that way, I could have gone on and pursued the animal mediation work, for example. But I wasn't interested in mediation per se. I was interested in language.

For me, it's all about having a goal. If it turns out that the right kind of theory is outside of the paradigm, then you look outside of the paradigm. If you're not making any progress toward understanding the problem, you've got to change.

Al Liberman is a parallel instance. When he was working with speech in the 1940s, they were trying to build a reading machine for the blind, and he came into the research doing what a psychologist would do. He suggested that people couldn't follow the artificial sounds they were producing because the sounds were not differentiated enough — so he proposed to make the sounds more different from each other, increase the complexity. And when they did that, things got worse instead of better. At that point Liberman said, "Hey, this stuff doesn't work that way? How *does* it work?" When you are problem-oriented, you don't try to defend the psychological theory that isn't working for you.

Q: I assume you also know some psychologists who did not respond that way, who were unwilling or unable to adapt to the failure of the standard approach?

A: Oh, I think the woods are full of them. They go off and become deans, department heads, things like that. (I blush to confess that I have recently become a department head!) A lot of them just quit. I mean, there's nothing to keep a professor from just quitting research, right? He can keep busy, he's got a job, he's got students, and there's always a residue of people you can talk to who believe what you believe.

Q: But it must have been an unpleasant experience for those people.

A: I expect it's extraordinarily disappointing. Maybe I'm too eager to give up paradigms. I've never been in the position, I think, of trying to defend one that was dying. I've usually been in the position of saying, "My God, this doesn't work! We've gotta get something new."

There's a group that used to meet each year at a resort in California to talk about verbal behavior. In 1964–1965 I went to that meeting, and told them, "You know, we've got to work on generative behavior. We've got to work on rule-governed behavior." And everybody in the meeting jumped on me. I really was down. When you go to a group of your peers and everybody disapproves of you it's pretty hard. Charlie Cofer took me for a long walk down the seashore, and he said, "Buck up, it's OK. Remember when you were talking about mediation, all these people were saying 'You don't have to do all that work. We don't believe those theories. That's not the way to go.' Now they're doing mediation, and you're telling them it is not enough; they have to go to rules. Just hang in there, they'll catch up." Cofer always has a nice philosophical view of things. But I think that being problem-oriented is an awfully good thing for everybody, to keep you from getting stuck in a particular theoretical viewpoint or methodology.

Q: Perhaps one further challenge was for psychologists to realize that Chomsky's theory could not be directly translated into standard experimental psychology terms.

A: We had to learn that we couldn't just make a grammar into a set of psychological processes. That's been very hard for psychologists to learn. In an ideal world, you would want the linguistic distinctions to be psychologically real, right? But I don't see any reason to suppose that the formal apparatus that linguists use to generate the sentences of a language is at all like the psychological apparatus. I mean, the grammar is only a formal game to account for those phenomena.

Q: It's like traveling from city A to city B. The geographic relationship between the two cities is a "competence question," analogous to the linguistic work, but how you actually travel from A to B is a "process question." Psychologists usually have looked at process.

A: Yes, and the goals are different for the two kinds of theories. What might be simple in a grammar might turn out to be extraordinarily complex if you try to instantiate it in a psychological model. Classically, in linguistics, you segregate phonology, morphology, syntax, semantics and so on. But when you look at the acquisition of language, all of those levels are acquired simultaneously by the same organism, and the likelihood that they are embodied as separate processes is zero. It's just unthinkable that the organism would be sorting things into the same categories, as independent elements.

When Hildred Schuell and I worked on aphasia in the '50s and '60s, it came to me as a great bursting light that of course aphasia is basically one thing, that the special linguistic kinds of aphasia really have very little likelihood of existing (Schuell, Jenkins, & Jimenez-Pabon, 1964). I think they're mostly observational errors on the part of the clinician. But the brain isn't packaged that way, because language isn't acquired that way. The work that Schuell and I did says that the major factor in all kinds of aphasia is the loss of language, and overlaid on that, you find special emphases. But fundamentally you get just language loss. You can find an expressive aphasic who is said to have no receptive aphasia, but when you try some comprehension tests on him, it turns out he can't understand much at all. The literature says he is presenting symptoms of Broca's aphasia. It's only supposed to be an expressive deficit. These classical categories are really misleading. The underlying fact is that language doesn't come in compartments. That statement will probably get me into a lot of trouble, but it's true.

Q: Very interesting.

A: You don't care what kind of trouble I get into here, do you?

Q: No, I'm delighted. The more you say that sparks interest, the better. But to get back to the cognitive shift — what happened after your year at Stanford, reading *Syntactic Structures*?

A: The next stage transferred the impact to the people I knew best. I came back to Minnesota, and was asked to be director of the newly formed Center for Research in Human Learning. Late in the school year, we decided to have an active summer program, so we rallied our resources and called up the folks we knew. We invited them to Minnesota and promised we could give them a stimulating summer program. A lot of the participants were our PhDs from the last 10 years or so. The group included Horton and Kjeldergaard, Jim Martin, Chuck Clifton, Phil Gough, Don Foss, David Hakes, David Palermo, maybe Jim Greeno. Our outside instructors were Jerry Fodor, Walter Reitman, and David Premack. And one of the things, of course, that surprised us was that an awful lot of people who came had already made the move themselves toward a more cognitive way of operating.

It was a reunion and an attempt to reinforce the enthusiasm for the new view, to think about it and understand its implications. Fodor was presenting Chomsky, Reitman was doing computer simulations, and Premack came to offer something of a radical nature to the animal people. Premack and Fodor fought brilliantly all summer long, and it was very stimulating for everybody. Premack at the time was trying to hold down a more traditionalist point of view, although he has never been a traditionalist. And Reitman was bringing us a new view from the computer side, from Artificial Intelligence. All of that had a big impact on the people that attended, and it started a whole series of summer programs.

One summer we leaned really hard on perception. We brought Al Liberman to do speech perception, and both of the Gibsons, Eleanor and Jimmy. Jimmy Gibson, of course, was a radical in his own way. He had an enormous effect on everyone. Bob Shaw was our resident philosopher/psychologist, and he got converted to Gibsonism and went off to spend a year with Jimmy Gibson at Cornell. It was just a tremendously exciting time. The basic assumption was that things were boiling over, and of course there was going to be a lot of argumentation and debate, but a new day was coming. And of course, everybody toted around their little copy of Kuhn's *The Structure of Scientific Revolutions* (1962).

Q: So it was all in a friendly spirit.

A: Well, mostly so. There were some people whose toes got stepped on. Some of the local staff found the new Human Learning Center very hard to take, because the Center students were asking questions. They were not the usual questions about "that control group" or "what kind of statistics did you use"? They would ask questions like, "Why did you do that kind of research?" That's a very embarrassing question, you know.

Q: Clearly, Chomsky helped to define the problems in the old approach. But did he serve as a guide for the new approach also?

A: Without Chomsky it's not clear that we could have broken free from the old paradigm. It was a big help to say, "You know, there is more out there. You've got to give yourself more of a theoretical apparatus, and more machinery. Association isn't enough." Chomsky got people examining the presuppositions, and that's very freeing.

Q: But surely, Chomsky does not get into the problem of knowledge of the world, of semantics? Bransford and Franks's work, for example, is much more oriented to the abstract ideas used to understand the world, whereas Chomsky's abstract rules are used to generate the sentences of a language.

A: Actually, Chomsky did influence the Bransford–Franks work. Here is the history: Michael Posner and Stephen Keele (1968) showed that when you present viewers with random dot patterns that were generated from an underlying pattern, the subjects seem to abstract the prototypes. I learned about this at one of the California conferences, and I found that work so exciting that I could hardly sleep. I asked Posner to send me the stimuli so that I could run a replication right away. (Footnote about replications is: They're a damned good thing to do. Psychologists don't do enough of them.)

So Posner sent the stimuli, and by the time school was ready to start, we had the studies ready to run. Winifred Strange, who was a first-year assistant, ran the studies, and John Bransford and Jeff Franks were second-year students at the time. They were interested because I was excited about the research, and so they ran as subjects in the pilot studies. We were all impressed by two things. One, the experiment worked very well (see Strange, Keeney, Kessel, & Jenkins, 1970). First, you are trained on three sets of random dot patterns, and after delay, you are tested on many patterns, including the prototypes. You pick the prototypes, which you have never seen, as often as the actual patterns you have seen. Two, you didn't have any feeling that you *knew* the prototype. So the outcome of the experiment is nice and strong, but there is no intuitive conviction, no feeling that you really knew the prototype. So it lacked punch.

Bob Shaw suggested to his seminar that the problem was that there was only a *probabilistic* relation between the prototypes and the patterns that had been seen before. Every dot takes a random walk. There was no deterministic transformation, no set of rules that related the abstract prototype to the things you saw during acquisition. So John Bransford and Jeff Franks decided to set up something that was deterministic, some case where the underlying abstract prototype related to the stimuli in a totally rule-governed way.

John came down the hall one day and said, "I want to show you something." So I said, "Fine," and he put me in the experiment he and

Jeff had cooked up. He showed me 16 different geometrical figures, and asked me to draw the typical figure I had just seen. So I just sat there, and, of course, I generated the damned prototype that I hadn't seen! Then he said, "You've never seen it," and I said, "I can't believe that!" It had the intuitive conviction that the Posner–Keele experiment didn't have.

It worked on everyone. Don DeRosa, who was a postdoc that year, was absolutely certain: "I know I've seen that thing!" He grabbed the stimulus cards, and went through them, and, of course, it wasn't there. John asked me, "Do you think it's worth pursuing?" And I said, "Yeah, I think you've got something there." That was the beginning of the famous collaborative series of studies (Bransford & Franks, 1971; Franks & Bransford, 1971; Bransford, 1979).

So the transition here really comes about from probabilistic to deterministic rule-generation, and in that sense, it's a direct heritage of Chomsky's work in linguistics. Of course afterwards it was generalized to the ideas people build from sentences, and so on. All of the effects are very strong and convincing, and entirely at odds with the standard expectations that we had at the time about how people learn. So we loved the experiment and have done a lot with it in one way or another. We've got a new musical replication of it now (see Chew, Larkey, Soli, Blount, & Jenkins, 1982).

The next theoretical step was taken by Shaw and Wilson (1976). They showed that if you give people a generator group — in the mathematical sense, a set of elements able to generate the others — then you could get the Bransford–Franks kind of outcome. People will draw the prototype, or falsely recognize a new stimulus that is closer to the generator group than anything they actually experienced before. But if you give people the same number of instances where they do not form a generator group, you don't get the same results. Again here you have a generative system in the formal sense. If the subjects have sufficient examples to pick it up, they can also pick up the abstract structure.

Q: The idea of "picking up structure," of course, brings J. J. Gibson to mind. Where does his work come in here?

A: Well, Gibson comes in because he is looking for the structure that is perceived in the world. He is saying that the organism is adapted to perceive this structure. It has evolved to do that. In fact, the organism and the world evolved together. The psychologist's problem is to find out what the structural invariants are that the perceiver is picking up from the world. Bob Shaw has shown that a series of geometric transformations of a cardioid base will generate a set of faces, seen in profile, that appear to be of people of different ages. The "same" face will be seen, going from babyhood to childhood, adulthood, and old age. He guessed at the underlying mathematics, and showed that the cardioid transformation seems to provide us with the underlying structure we need in order to pick up the age of someone's face. You can see the enormous challenge of discovery—you've got to invent the hypothesis, the mathematical transformation that defines the generator set, before you can test whether people use it to perceive the world. Shaw used a lot of old biological work on the perception of faces. The whole idea of the cardioid as one plan for the growth of plant-leaves has been well known for years.

Q: So the cardioid transformation looks like one of Gibson's perceptual "invariants," which permits us to perceive someone's age. How are you pursuing this approach in your own work?

A: We've been terribly intrigued with the general problem of attempting to discover invariants. Our recent work is in speech perception. We're pushing very hard for the idea of dynamic invariants in speech. The classic case is that the same vowels spoken by men, women, and children sound the same perceptually. But acoustically, of course, the voices of children may be an octave or more away from the voice of a man, and the oral cavities are shaped differently. As a result, there are really not very many similarities when you look at the physical acoustics. What is it that remains the same?

The traditional viewpoint on vowels is that they are *steady-state openings* of the vocal tract, perceptually determined by the formant frequencies in the middle of a syllable. Our research in the last 10 years has shown that the vowel is better specified by the *dynamics* of the syllable over the whole course of the syllable, and most particularly by the beginning and end of the syllable (see Strange, Jenkins, & Johnson, 1983). The information at the onset and offset is more useful than the information in the middle of the syllable, exactly the opposite of what you would expect on the basis of traditional thinking. The same thing with musical instruments, of course. The information that tells you what instrument is playing is in the transitional phase—once the steady-state sets in, you've lost it. It's some kind of higher-order property, a dynamic property, but we haven't got it yet.

Q: And you believe, of course, that this supports your general notion of "contextualism," that all stimulation is relational, and bound to a particular context?

A: Yes. I've thought of doing a book on contextualism, but it's hard to make a book out of it that anybody would find readable. You just keep saying, "Well, everything depends," and people get a little tired of hearing that. So the best way to work with it is simply to show instances in one field after another, and let the instances do the work for you.

George Mandler: Cognition in Historical Perspective

George Mandler has been one of the most influential psychologists in the United States. As editor of the central journal *Psychological Review* (more recently with his wife, Jean M. Mandler), he had rather immediate impact on the direction taken by experimental psychology for almost a decade. In addition, Mandler has made significant contributions of his own to our understanding of memory, the study of emotion (his most recent book here is *Mind and Body* [1984]), and philosophical aspects of scientific psychology (in his book with William Kessen called *The Language of Psychology* [1959]).

In conversation, Professor Mandler seems to delight in sounding controversial and slightly shocking, but his ideas are obviously based on a great deal of thought. After being somewhat intimidated at first, one discovers that he welcomes other views and is willing to adjust to them. As a result, the conversation ceases to be a purely question-and-answer interaction and becomes, instead, a shared exploration of the issues. Professor Mandler has the gift of excitement about ideas and is capable of conveying his own excitement to others.

He evokes the atmosphere of behaviorism at Yale (the center of Hullian theory), where he took his PhD in 1953, and the subsequent transition, in which he played a leadership role comparable to Miller, Jenkins, and Levine (see interviews in this chapter). His excellent grasp of the historical circumstances that gave rise to various influential ideas gives a sense of immediacy to the story, and much of the interview is devoted to recounting the intricate mesh of events.

Some years after this interview, Mandler asked that it be accompanied by a *caveat*, which appears at the end of the interview. It stands as a useful caution, and applies to all other interviews in this book as well: The perspective of our participants is likely to change with time, and it is well known from psychological studies of memory that our memory of the past is strongly influenced by our current point of view. So, let the reader beware.

Currently George Mandler is professor of psychology and director of the Center for Human Information Processing (CHIP) at the University of California, San Diego.

Interview with George Mandler

Q: How did you get interested in psychology?

A: I was a late starter in psychology. I didn't start college until I was 22. I'm originally from Vienna, and I came to the United States in

1940; I was 15 then. I worked till I was 19, then I was drafted and was in the Army until I was 22. I went to college, and was a journalism and then a chemistry major. Then I took some psychology courses with one very, very good teacher, Bernie Mausner, and I got interested in the whole business. I thought of myself as a clinician. In 1949 I applied to graduate school. I had spent 1947 and '48 in Switzerland at the University of Basel, and generally was vaguely interested in psychology and philosophy. In 1949 I went to graduate school at Yale, as a clinician, and received a clinical PhD in 1953. By that time I was 29.

In those days, at Yale at least, nobody made any hard-and-fast distinction between clinical and nonclinical psychology. There were special requirements for a clinical degree, internship, and so on, but my thesis was not in clinical psychology. My thesis was in human learning, and what today we would call memory. I graduated with a clinical PhD but with broad interests. I had started to work on anxiety scales, and all my pre-PhD publications were in the clinical area. I went to Harvard in the Psychological Clinic. I continued that split until today; I've sort of gone back and forth between memory, cognition, and human learning on the one side and emotion on the other. It was nice to be in two fields, because when you get tired of the one you can do the other, and I finally got my emotion interests together. In August 1975 I published the *Mind and Emotion* book, and *Mind and Body* in 1984.

We were all behaviorists in 1950; and I certainly was a Hullian. Hull was still alive when I came to Yale. I didn't take any courses with him, but he was around and gave some lectures. That was "the future." Yale was the center of the universe, with possibly Iowa being the alternate world. That was where Kenneth Spence was, and the remnants of the Lewinians.

It's very funny to think back; we didn't have any conflicts in those days. My thesis was on response learning and response integration. "Cognition" was a dirty word for us. And it's important to remember *why* it was a dirty word and why a lot of people still don't understand what cognitive psychology in the 1970s is about, because they still have the old flavor of it. "Cognition" was a dirty word because cognitive psychologists were seen as fuzzy, hand-waving, imprecise people who really never did anything that was testable. That was the flavor of cognitive psychology.

Q: And then testability was the main problem?

A: Testability was a big deal! We even lived under the myth that Hullian theory was testable. We were very much under the influence of the logical positivists — the hypothetico-deductive system, testability, and meaning. Who were the cognitive psychologists? There was Jerry Bruner, a brilliant but undisciplined mind; and Snygg and Coombs (1949). You don't even know who Snygg and Coombs were. They wrote a book on the then cognitive psychology; but it had no theory. As for Tolman, you've got to talk to a Tolmanite. Tolman's theories, looking at them from Yale at that time, were vague and untestable.

I think the major problem in behaviorism was the *fear of theory*. I have a rather peculiar view of that. I think that what characterized American psychology and American science through the 19th century and into the 20th century was an antitheoretical point of view. I include Hull in this. Now what do I mean by that? I mean that one of the components of theory is the generation of useful *fictions*. That's what theories are about. Here was this great deductive theory that Hull had proposed, but when Hull generated fictions he was so afraid of generating real fictions, that his fictions had the *names* of observable events — little internal responses, and little stimuli. The fear of theory.

I think Skinner, the only brilliant man among the behaviorists, put it correctly — he doesn't like to have anything to do with fictions. That's the issue on which Skinner attacks theory. He attacks it on the issue of fictions, of making up entities.

Q: Right, but in particular, fear of making up reified entities? That is, attributing to the theoretical entities a concrete reality that they don't have?

A: Yes, but also fear of making up any entities. Because Skinner thinks eventually the resolution must come at the physiological level, and we have no business making up presumed physiological events. That fear of fictions has held back psychological theory, and that's what the liberation of the '50s and the '60s was all about.

Q: You call this liberation?

A: Yes. I think this is much more fun! I gave a talk a few months ago to a group of psychologists and philosophers, in which I said that one of the pleasant things about science is that it is fun and games. And the philosophers were very upset. I was attacked for being irresponsible and immoral, because science is a very important and serious business. How could I describe this as fun and games? Well, I think that is the difference between scientists and philosophers.

Q: Well, I'm sure that philosophers have fun and games too.

A: They take themselves terribly seriously.

Q: If science can be fun and games, are there rules by which the game is played?

A: The rules change. This whole business about defining science, and "What is science?" and all those introductory chapters in textbooks, "Why psychology is a science. We're a science, like everybody else, children!" I think that's bullshit.

Science is about reliable knowledge of the world. And then, once you say, "What do we mean by 'knowledge?' What do we mean by 'reliable?'" then some of the trappings of science appear. The scientist does it a little better because he is is a little more systematic.

Q: Do you feel that psychologists are defensive about being scientific?

A: Oh, terribly!

Q: And do you feel that was so 20 to 30 years ago, or has it changed?

A: I don't think it has changed. I think it's there all the way back to Wundt, too. Well, no, I think it has abated a little, because people are having a good time doing what they're doing, and they often don't give a damn whether anybody thinks it's science or not.

Q: Do you think that the newer viewpoint, cognitive psychology, is more pragmatic? That cognitive psychologists can afford to be freer about, say, the issue of subjective experience?

A: Sure. If it works, it works. We are pragmatic in that sense. I would, again, call it liberating. Whatever data you can use, you use. I've got an addendum to this, because I think that what modern cognitive psychology understands is what the German introspectionists never understood, and what the behaviorists got completely wrong. And that is, that no cognitive psychologist worth his salt today thinks of subjective experience as a *datum*. It's a construct. I've talked about that in *Mind and Emotion* (1975), and the old notion that private experience is a datum for science is just wrong. It's very useful as a construct.

Q: But is it a source of information?

A: It's a source of information in the sense that any theoretical construct that works is a source of information. *My* private experience is a datum for me as I make up my theory of the world. In constructing my own world, my experience is a datum. But science has as a major requirement its shared public aspect.

Q: You're saying that the behaviorists were wrong on this point?

A: They were both wrong and right. The behaviorists were right in saying that private experience can't be a direct datum, but they were wrong in rejecting all of it in any guise. The behaviorists didn't say, "OK, it's a construct, let's use it." They couldn't say *that* because they were so afraid of theoretical constructs that they didn't have that solution available. Psychology must talk *about* people. *Your* private experience is a theoretical construct to me. I have no direct access to your private experience. I do have direct access to your behavior. In that sense, I'm a behaviorist. In that sense, *everybody* is a behaviorist today.

Q: If the behaviorists agreed that science must necessarily be public, did this account for their attitude toward "attention" and other constructs that are not publicly observable?

A: Yes, probably. There is no "attention" in the behaviorist literature; except, of course, there is, because it is an important phenomenon that they couldn't ignore. It went by all sorts of names, such as "pure stimulus act."

Q: Do you have any ideas as to why behaviorism became such a dominant viewpoint in American psychology in the first place?

A: That's a question for the sociology of science. It has something to do with the American experience, with American sociocultural, political, and economic history. Science is part of culture and of society. I don't know why it happened, but I think if one were to look at other fields of knowledge in America, one would find similar developments; maybe not at the same time.

In the public eye, who was the great American scientist of the end of the century? It was Thomas Edison. But Thomas Edison really made no theoretical contributions. This does not deprecate him. Science in America was supposed to be real, and palpable, and produce results. And it didn't worry about theories about the whys and wherefores.

Q: But the shift to behaviorism was very rapid, wasn't it?

A: No, there's behaviorism in James, in Crozier (who was Skinner's teacher). There's behaviorism, the worst kind of behaviorism, in the functionalists. I think that like most human events, it was a gradual kind of thing. That doesn't mean that James was a behaviorist in the Watsonian sense; it just means that he showed movement in that direction.

Q: I take it you would agree that behaviorism, at least in the sense of 20 years ago, is no longer prevalent in American psychology?

A: What's "behaviorism"? There are all kinds of behaviorisms. It is still the dominant viewpoint in the emphasis on observable data in psychology. That has become so obvious that it's not discussed anymore. We observe the behavior of organisms. I think there are two things that we have given up: One of them is the *fear of fiction*, and the other is something that had nothing to do with behaviorism, but became part of the behaviorist viewpoint. It is *Anglo-Teutonic associationism*, and we've given that up. That, to me, is a real advantage of the cognitive viewpoint.

Q: And by "Anglo-Teutonic associationism" you mean . . . ?

A: A philosophical theory that jumped from Locke and Mill to Ebbinghaus and Wundt, and from Wundt to all the rest. Why Wundt, as an experimentalist, was an associationist is an interesting problem. If one were to predict what an experimental psychology would be doing in Germany at the end of the 19th century, one would say "Kant." That was the German philosophical tradition. And yet, *we're* more Kantian in modern cognitive psychology than Wundt ever was.

Q: In what sense?

A: Oh, the idea that experience is constructed, the problem of the limits of the human organism, the notion of schemas.

Q: What is the explanatory role of associations?

A: Associations have little explanatory value. Associations are descriptive, they do not provide explanations. The principles of associationism, such as "similarity," "contiguity," and so forth, are descriptive terms; they describe contingencies.

Q: People sometimes explain someone's behavior by saying it must have been associated in the past experience of the person behaving that way.

A: All you're saying is that there is a certain concatenation of events in the past that is inferred from present behavior. It's fascinating that very few people are doing any work on learning today [in 1975]. Cognitive psychologists so far are steady-state organism psychologists. We talk about semantic networks: How did they *get* there? That's left to the developmental psychologists. In that sense, there are now very few people who are interested in fundamental acquisition phenomena.

The interesting thing is that there are a very few cognitive psychologists who worry about the fact that they have no theory to explain the phenomena of conditioning. The data are there, but we've ignored them. When seems to be needed is a *good* cognitive theory that can encompass them.

Q: Is that because current cognitive psychology has no role for reinforcement and so on?

A: Yes. In fact, I think Skinner takes a reasonable position. He happens to be, on one issue, a "cognitive psychologist," and that is on the issue of the definition of stimulus and response.

Well, Skinner is *fundamentally* opposed to the S–R definition of stimulus and response. He's not an S–R psychologist. S–R psychology defines the stimulus physically, "out there." For Skinner, the stimulus is *whatever event* controls the behavior.

Q: Therefore, the organism becomes the measure of the stimulus.

A: Right. The response, for Skinner, is topographically neutral. It's not a particular response, as it is in the S–R theory of Hull. It is any event that reliably produces a certain consequence in the environment. That's the definition of an operant response such as a bar-press. But *how* the animal presses the bar, and what the topography of that bar-press is, is only of interest in the *second*-order theory, but *not* in the first instance as a definition. Stimulus and response are defined in terms of the organism's interaction with the environment. It's much more abstract than the physical idea of the stimulus and the response. It's really a cognitive theory.

Q: Is Skinner's definition of reinforcement similar then?

A: Exactly.

Q: Skinner is often viewed as the quintessential behaviorist.

A: He *is*, but the issue on which he is the quintessential behaviorist is the issue of theory, of useful fictions, not on the issue of associationism. Those two issues got all screwed up, because Watson was both an anti-fictioneer and an S–R psychologist, as was Hull.

Q: I am interested in the changes people experienced during the shift between the behaviorist and cognitive viewpoints — what they went through, how they adapted, or resisted, the new position.

A: I think that there are several fundamental changes between cognitive psychology and behaviorism. There has always been a cognitive psychology of the kind that we see now, going back at least 60 to 70 years, unencumbered by behaviorism! It just so happens that it wasn't very visible in the United States. It was present in England and in France, Germany, and Switzerland with Piaget. I think that American psychologists sometimes fail to understand that behaviorism was a *very* parochial event. Except for the Russians, who of course, developed a behaviorism of their own — my hunch is, for similar socioeconomic historical reasons.

Q: You would say that the Russians were behaviorists, then?

A: Yes, it's the tradition of Sechenov, Pavlov, and Bechterev. They were behaviorists, associationists, and antitheoretical. They said, "We're not going to make up any *psychological* fictions, we're going to use *physiological* fictions." Physiological fictions sound respectable. Let's leave the Russians aside for a minute. Pavlov and Watson were similar in influence, except that Pavlov was several orders of magnitude smarter than Watson.

Apart from the Russians, my impression is that the reaction of the Europeans during the '30s, '40s, and early '50s when we suffered through behaviorist orthodoxy, was "What is going on over there?" They paid very little attention to it. Europe had Claparède, Piaget, Bartlett, the Gestaltists, and Selz. All through that period people paid slight attention to that peculiar parochial movement in the United States. That is one of the reasons why I don't understand the hue and cry about the "paradigm-shift in psychology." If you look at it from a less parochial point of view — there was an aberration for a very short period in the United States.

In 1971 a British psychologist asked, "Did anybody ever take Hull seriously? I never understood what it was all about!" I couldn't explain to him what it was like. This was not somebody who was hindered by a language barrier, and he didn't know what was going on!

All the time there was a cognitive psychology, developing independently, but out of roots differing from the American roots.

We did inherit the Gestaltist movement during the Nazi period. The Gestalt psychologists, who were mostly Jewish or antifascist, came to the United States. Unfortunately, only a few people here paid any attention to them, because they came at the wrong time, in the '30s (Mandler & Mandler, 1968).

Q: What about psychoanalysis at this time?

A: I don't think experimental psychologists other than a few people around Hull ever saw psychoanalysis as a psychological theory.

Q: I've had the feeling that Hull's theory as a drive theory has a relationship to psychoanalysis.

A: Oh, yes, there's a common history, but that never came down to cognitive psychology. The European cognitive sources were different from our sources, but they were there, any time we were ready to come back home. When we returned to the mainstream, we picked up Piaget. Piaget is one of the major, consistent cognitive theories that we now have. No great explicitness, but more insights than anywhere else. He certainly did not come out of the background that we came out of. We developed cognitive psychology out of other influences.

One of them was *psychophysics*. People in psychophysics were blithely going along, inventing fictions, not dealing with S–R bonds. They were not behaviorists. If you look at what happened in the '50s, who came along with the new insights, you can see how many came out of psychoacoustics. Wendell Garner, George Miller, and McGill all came out of that environment. I remember a colloquium that George Miller gave in 1951. (I was a graduate student at Yale, and he was an assistant professor at the time.) The colloquium was on the mathematical model of learning. That was the first stochastic learning model, or one of the first ones.

Another influence was mathematical psychology. People like Bush and Mosteller couldn't have cared less about the issues that psychologists were so worried about. Bush was a physicist, and Mosteller, a mathematician. Bush's PhD was with Robert Oppenheimer at Princeton.

Q: People in psychophysics had the Weber–Fechner tradition going back to the 1840s, and they always had to deal with private experiences.

A: It never bothered them.

Q: Some of the behaviorists used to explain that by saying that psychophysicists were not really talking about a private event. They were talking about an objectively observable *response* such as "Yes, I hear it," "No, I don't," and so on. The verbal response was the datum for the theory.

A: Yes, but "This is bigger than that," and "That sounds like this," means comparisons, judgments, attention, and consciousness. They didn't need to talk about it, it was so obvious! And when psychophysicists moved into other fields, they were unencumbered by the behaviorist tradition of what you're allowed to do and what you're not allowed to do.

Q: That might have led to, for example, Shepard's work on imagery (e.g., Cooper & Shepard, 1973).

A: Shepard is an instance of yet another influence, and a very important one. Carl Hovland was Roger Shepard's teacher at Yale and also Murdock's teacher, my teacher, indirectly Gordon Bower's teacher. Bower was working with Neal Miller, but Hovland was around at that time. I'm not talking about the social psychologists—there's a whole generation of social psychologists whom Carl taught. Carl Hovland, Hull's student essentially, initially talked about cognitive approaches in terms of concept formation. He was a very, very liberating man.

By the way, he was one of the worst, and one of the most influential teachers imaginable. Carl believed *totally* in the Socratic method in his graduate seminar. We'd walk out of there utterly frustrated—because all he would do is raise a question, sit down, and let us talk and think about it. But within five years there wasn't anybody I know who became involved in cognitive psychology who didn't say "This is the man who influenced me most." By asking the right kind of question. But he was certainly willing to explore all sorts of possibilities, going far beyond Hull. An important contrast to Clark Hull, who was a humorless man, a dull man.

Q: Did Hull tend to believe his own ideas too much?

A: Oh, absolutely.

Q: Do you think that Skinner has really solved some problems?

A: Yes. I think Skinner is an important figure in American psychology.

Q: Even though many people would say today that the research community is moving away from his ideas?

A: That's because Skinner refused to be theoretical.

Q: But you believe that eventually cognitive psychologists will have to deal with Skinner's data.

A: Oh, yes.

Q: People talk about the feeling of anomaly toward the end of a paradigm. Behaviorism was perhaps not exactly a paradigm in Kuhn's sense, but did many people have a sense of discomfort — that there were anomalous results being unearthed?

A: There was a lot of argument, but I don't think there was anything in the way of being uncomfortable. You see, my senior research project as an undergraduate was on a Gestalt problem. When I started out, I was really a Gestalt psychologist. By the time I left Yale I was a Hullian, a polymorphous perverse Hullian.

Q: How was it that starting out from Gestalt psychology, you ended up with a behaviorist learning theory?

A: It was unavoidable, it was the seat of the Holy Grail!

Q: Yale must have been exceptional in that people did not make a strong distinction between experimental and clinical work.

A: This was in large part due to Carl Hovland. Yes, to me, the hero was Carl.

There's another influence, and that was the Simon and Newell direction, partly out of the cybernetic and the computational field, and partly out of European work. If you read the first Simon and Newell papers in the '50s, they paid their respects to a German psychologist named Selz. Otto Selz was a psychologist who influenced the Dutch psychologist De Groot, who did research on the cognitive abilities of chess players.

He had gotten to know Selz after he came to Holland to flee the Nazis. Selz was Jewish, an ex-officer in the German army, and he thought that he would be safe in Holland. When the Germans invaded Holland he was eventually killed. Selz talked about operators.

Q: Operators?

A: Functions that operate on concepts. That was 1911 to 1913. De Groot applied this work to chess problems, and Newell and Simon incorporated those ideas in their work on problem solving. So Newell and Simon used a European tradition, and came up with a cognitive psychology that, again, was *totally* uninfluenced by behaviorism. It developed not "in response to" but "independently of" behaviorism. Herb Simon, of course, has done everything — a very influential man.

And then, of course, there's Piaget. I don't know what people thought about Piaget at the time. They probably didn't understand him.

Q: Did Bruner study Piaget in the '50s?

A: Bruner wasn't doing developmental work until late. Bruner was doing selective perception in the late '40s and '50s, the "New Look" in perception. Bruner was close to Tolman, but a *maverick*, — smart and undisciplined.

I keep forgetting to stress that Gestalt psychologists, such as Köhler, Koffka, and Wertheimer, *were* in this country. Now, they were not at center stage, but they were around, and they had students. *Some* people talked with them. Swarthmore was *full* of interesting people. In 1940, Katona (another Gestaltist) published a book on *Organizing and Memorizing*.

Q: That sounds very much like something that might have been published in 1970.

A: Exactly. But the *experiments* are in there! Experiments on grouping are in there. It was possible to do that. And of course it took us a little while to follow up.

Q: What was Chomsky's role in all this?

A: It was all well along by the time Chomsky came along. My guess is that in 1958 most psychologists, if asked who Chomsky was, would say, "Who?" It wasn't really until Chomsky's review of Skinner's *Verbal Behavior* achieved prominence that psychologists started to pay serious attention to him (1958). George Miller, of course, adopted him as his patron saint. The Miller–Chomsky influence was very strong.

The major point I want to make is that all the influences were well put into motion before Chomsky came on the psychological scene. You have to look at the major experimental influences: There's no Chomsky in Bower or Shepard. Nowhere!

Q: Yes, but he unquestionably affected psycholinguistics.

A: That's understating it. His influence, in a sense, created psycholinguistics. But it wouldn't have happened as readily if there hadn't been a cognitive psychology that had prepared the field.

Q: Surely Transformational Grammar provided an initial theory for language processing?

A: Well, we buy our theories where we can find them, just as with signal detection.

Q: That's not a cognitive theory.

A: No, but it's *used* as a cognitive theory — ostensibly. That's the point I want to make: Chomsky's work was used in psycholinguistics the way signal detection theory was, which came out of engineering. Psychologists didn't invent signal detection theory; the engineers did, and we used it. That's sort of nice about scientists. They don't care what you do, and leave you alone to do your own work, but if they can *use* something, they'll say, "Aha! Yes, I can use that!" Cognitive psychologists were all ready to do language, but we didn't know how to do it. Chomsky showed us how to do it — *wrong* — but he showed us how to do it.

Q: One of the things that Chomsky's work seems to provide is a formal limit on the notion of associationism (Bever, Fodor, & Garrett, 1968).

A: Yes, but I don't think that anybody paid any attention to that outside of psycholinguistics. You know, human affairs and science are vague as well as overdetermined.

Q: Did Lashley have any influence on the shift?

A: I don't think that anybody really realized the importance of his 1951 paper until around 1960. I think that we understood Lashley's definition of the problem before we read Chomsky.

My guess is that somewhere between 1955 and 1965 all the significant influences reached critical mass. Not in one year, but in some five-year period, maybe between 1956 and 1961 or so. I think that one can show that by looking at the literature (see my *Cognitive Psychology*, 1985).

Q: Of course, the real question is why it happened particularly at that time, and why it didn't happen 15 years before or 50 years before.

A: Scientific events are a function of the particular society in which they happen. You can't divorce science from the rest of the world.

Q: What about the existence of machine analogies? For John Watson, the telephone switchboard gave him a machine model of the way in which mental connections could be made. Did the computer have a similar impact on contemporary psychologists?

A: Ah, the computer. I think the computer has been vastly overdone as an influence on theory. One can put practically *any* theory on a computer. The major role of the computer is that it is a great instrument for keeping people honest about theoretical predictions. But even *Hull* had a mechanical model — a machine to demonstrate correlation — and years ago it was agreed that one test of a theory is whether one can build a machine that will behave that way.

Q: But, surely, if the most complex machine that you can imagine is a switchboard, you would have trouble imagining a theory to account for human information processing?

A: Well, it was probably the other way around. More likely, the conditions that led to the development of the computer also ultimately gave rise to cognitive psychology.

Q: What about the influence of specific computer modeling of some human behavior, such as problem solving and so on?

A: That was significant in that people were forced to show that the theory really works. As a matter of fact, it would have been fascinating if we had had a computer in the Hullian days, and someone had tried to program the Hullian S–R theory on it. I think it would have turned out that the theory was much too inconsistent to make any predictions. But if somebody had tried to put Hullian theory on a computer, would that have made it a computer theory? No, obviously not.

Q: How do you see contemporary cognitive work?

A: I'm beginning to see the first signs of going back to the '40s or '50s, with *endless*, repetitive experiments.

Q: Why do you feel people tend to do that?

A: Oh, I would call that "normal science." There's an economic problem. There's a large number of people around who've got to keep busy. Many are not, or do not wish to be, theoreticians, so they say: Let's vary variable R at levels Y and Z! Let's see how that one works out. One consequence of success of the viewpoint is that it makes work. That's a negative view of the situation. Much of the experimentation is very useful, but I think there's a tendency toward overdoing things, and it was clearly overdone in the '40s and '50s.

Q: Do you think that is because the antitheoretical bias of the behaviorists is still around, so that doing experiments is safer and easier?

A: In part, but I also think it simply has to do with people having to keep busy.

Q: The whole question of the role of experiments is, I think, a very interesting one. The birth of scientific psychology is usually dated back to the first experiments in the 19th century. Experiments have been taken as the defining property of psychological science.

A: I don't see much of a problem, if one can find reliable data out there, to go without experimentally controlling the variables. After all, there is, if not the queen of the sciences, then at least one of the crown princes of the sciences, which has never done experiments at all — astronomy. Nobody says that astronomers are not scientific. Here's a bunch of people who are excellent scientists, who've never done an experiment in their lives! So, it *can't* be that the experiment is the defining characteristic of science.

There are now more and more people who are discovering that you can do very nice, controlled studies on real-life data. As one example, Mike Williams, working with Don Norman, is doing a thesis on long-term memory and retrieval, and he is looking at people's memory of their classmates in high school (Williams & Hollan, 1981). He got the yearbooks, he tracked down the people who went to that particular high school, and he's asked them simply, Do you remember who was in your high school class? Then he looks at how people retrieve that information, and the results look very much like the kind of results we get in arbitrary experiments. It's all of a piece.

Q: I still would like to ask about the problem psychologists had in the 19th century with unconscious processes. You have said that even James had trouble conceptualizing unconscious psychological processes.

A: Well, look at Freud at the same time. Freud worked theory into psychology by creating unconscious processes. If Freud had not used the terminology of conscious events to describe these unconscious processes, if he had not talked about unconscious *wishes* and unconscious *thoughts* and so on, there wouldn't have been any problem. What he meant to say was not unconscious *wishes* at all, but the processes (which are theoretical processes, clearly not conscious) that have the same *effect* as the conscious wish.

It all happened at the same time. People were starting to think about unconscious processes. Freud in the 1890s and the Würzburgers 10 years later started to say there are things that are causal, which aren't conscious and are not reducible to physiology.

Q: In what sense are they not physiological?

A: There is no claim that these are identifiable physiological mechanisms. When Freud talks about the dammed-up libido and the hydraulic model of drive and repression, he never claimed that if one looked hard enough one would find pipes flowing with libido in the head.

Q: So these were useful theoretical ideas.

A: Interesting and useful fictions. I am also concerned about the sense in which Chomsky's syntactic apparatus, which is unconscious, and Freud's unconscious apparatus are the same kind of thing.

I'm just as unconscious of the way I construct a sentence as I am unconscious of the reason why I make a slip or dislike somebody, or whatever. This gets into a discussion of consciousness. The difference seems to be that, in principle, Freudian mechanisms can become conscious. People can become aware of the "reasons" for their behavior. But it is probably true that one can *not* become conscious of the mechanisms that are responsible for syntactic constructions.

Linguists make up theories of what the grammar may be like. But that's very different from saying that I know that adjectives always precede nouns in English. Do I in any sense become aware of *the mechanism* that always makes me put adjectives before nouns? There is an interesting argument that one of my students recently made with respect to linguistic structures. Debbie Knapp maintained that the reason why we are not conscious of linguistic structures is because they are automatic structures.

Structures, like all others of which we were conscious when we first used them, but since our first use of them occurred at the time when we were developing language, there is no way of getting back to them. She has some very interesting evidence that the acquisition of new syntactic structures behaves like the acquisition of newly automatized behavior.

Q: I'm very much interested in the historical relationship between behaviorism and psychoanalysis and why the two viewpoints never got together.

A: But they did, for example at Yale in Dollard and Miller (1950).

Q: Yes, but that is at best a very farfetched set of correlates of psychoanalysis.

A: The major socially and clinically interested behaviorists were strongly influenced by psychoanalysis. Mowrer, Sears, Dollard, Miller, and so on and so forth. They tried to translate psychoanalytic concepts into behavioristic concepts. By that time the behaviorists had begun to overcome their dislike of fictions. Hull had built up his quasimathematical system, so it was all right to talk about internal processes. In part, people tried to translate psychoanalysis into behavioristic terms because psychoanalysis had become popular. A lot of them had gone into analysis. Many psychologists at Harvard and Yale were in contact with analysis in one way or another. They often went into personal analysis and then came out and said: "Isn't that fascinating. Let's make 'scientific' sense out of it."

Q: Present-day experimental psychologists seem to have very strong feelings against psychoanalysis.

A: I don't know if that's true. I think psychoanalysis is dying of its own success. The major psychoanalytic notions are around and everybody accepts them. It's not a big deal anymore. The superego notion, repression, analysis of anxiety as a signal, the whole drive-hydraulic notion, all of those things became part of the common understanding. They're often not recognized as psychoanalytic concepts anymore.

The notion that early development significantly affects later reactions to the world is, in part, what psychoanalysis is about. It is so generally accepted that nobody thinks about it as a pyschoanalytic concept anymore. Don't forget that before psychoanalysis it was not generally believed that the experiences of children when they're young determine their personality structure later on, but it is now. If we've got a paradigm, that's a paradigm. If somebody came along today with the notion that said that parent–child interactions are totally irrelevant to later development, people would look at him like he was some kind of a nut. All the arguments today are not about whether it's true or not, but where and when and to what degree.

Q: But certainly it's a paradigm without attribution to the people who originally developed it.

A: Oh, yes, but that's always the case. Do you think about evolution as necessarily Darwinian?

Q: But what about your background in clinical psychology?

A: That's the way I live, not the way I do research.

Q: So when you're talking about personality theory, it is essentially psychoanalytic theory?

A: It's the only one we've got at the present time. There are no useful personality theories except psychoanalytic theories. Oh, there are some hodge-podge notions of taking observed differences and trying to make a structure out of them. But the whole point of psychoanalytic theory is that every difference among people derives from some application of general principles, and that's the only way to go. *Atheoretical* individual differences are uninteresting.

Q: Do you have some conception of what psychology will be like in the future?

A: My most optimistic view is that we will have arrived, possibly by the end of the century, at a psychological paradigm. It will be something like this implementable fiction-rich thing called cognitive psychology, and that will be the way to think about human beings. Later, we will begin to clean house, which will look like a behaviorist reaction, but it will really be a housecleaning operation. It will be sort of a Hegelian spiral, getting back to the same place but at a higher level.

Q: Then you see behaviorism as representing a kind of housecleaning?

A: Clearly, anything that purports to clean up all those made-up processes sounds as if it's going back to behaviorism, but it won't. We'll never go back, but there will be a housecleaning, and that may, in fact, happen earlier than the paradigm shift.

I don't see how 20 years from now, running rats is going to be more than a parochial curiosity. When I say rats, I also mean pigeons, because the pigeon enterprise has become the nitpicking analysis of particular schedules of reinforcement.

Q: So you think it's become sterile?

A: Certainly. It's unfortunate, because it's a fun thing to do. What we really need is a good operant conditioner who one day wakes up and says, "Gee, we've got all those gorgeous clean data, what does it all mean?"

Q: But you don't think that's going to happen.

A: I don't know, maybe it will. That will be a real indication that the paradigm has taken over. Somebody comes up and writes a book that takes the operant data and puts them into the cognitive framework in terms of the organisms's knowledge, in terms of processing the information. The only thing I'm fairly sure of in reaction against people who've been yelling "paradigm shift," is that that's nonsense. We don't have a paradigm yet. We may be in the process of building one.[1]

1. *Postscript by George Mandler: 1985.* The preceding interview was conducted well over 10 years ago. Since that time I have learned much about the history of cognitive psychology and also about my own efforts in its construction. There are many statements in the interview that I would now amend and even retract, but I have let them stand as an example of how history looked in 1975 and as a reminder that our view of history changes with the present. In particular, I now believe that I understand better the influences that shaped the new beginnings in the late 1950s. I am also beginning to understand the rejection of psychological theory as it was exemplified earlier in this century and, I believe, as it is resurrected in different forms today. Finally, I have achieved a better appreciation of some of the people mentioned in the interview and some that should not have been left out. These newer insights are described in my recent book, *Cognitive Psychology: An Essay in Cognitive Science* (1985).

6

The Persuaders:
Nonbehavioristic Psychologists

Whoso would be a man must be a non-conformist. — RALPH WALDO EMERSON

Although behaviorism unquestionably dominated scientific psychology until well into the 1950s, there were numerous cross-currents even in the heyday of behaviorism. I have already pointed to social psychology as one field in which many of the major developments in the cognitive framework were foreshadowed (Chapter 4), and of course there were many other "protocognitive" trends in psychology. Many psychologists may have experienced considerable discomfort with behaviorism (*e.g.*, Roback, 1964). In fact, it was possible to come of age intellectually in psychology without ever really believing in behaviorism: The interviews in this chapter bear witness to that. Some psychologists such as Ernest R. Hilgard and Jerome S. Bruner flourished during the height of behaviorism without ever becoming behaviorists. And three of our interviewees — Ulric Neisser, Walter B. Weimer, and Michael Wapner — continue to disagree with the cognitive point of view, though they are clearly more cognitive than behavioristic. All these psychologists can be called "Persuaders" in that their fundamental stance *vis-à-vis* the larger community is an attempt to persuade the majority to change the dominant framework in some significant way.

All of the Persuaders are nonconformists, though in a sense all scientists have a nonconformist streak. If two scientists are doing work that is too similar, there is one scientist too many. There is a premium on being different in science, within limits. But the Persuaders have gone a step beyond the standard scientific independence of mind *by developing an entire point of view* that is different from the dominant one. The price such people pay is often a lack of communication with the larger community, and that has indeed been the case for all of the interviewees in this chapter. The price is admittedly high, but the reward can be very high as well when the community is persuaded to change and it accepts a successful Persuader as a guide for some time. Practically all the "great names" in the history of science can be viewed as successful Persuaders.

This chapter presents two apparently successful Persuaders and two relatively unsuccessful ones. At any one time there are probably *many* unsuccessful Persuaders in a scientific community. They may be said to represent the seeds of potential change; but most of these seeds fall on arid ground. The chances of success for any Persuader is small. Yet without the presence of such people, the scientific community would be left with no coherent program of development when its current course faltered.

Timing is a critical ingredient in the process of successful persuasion. In psychology as elsewhere, a receptive audience is one that has *almost* arrived at the same conclusion by itself. Thus, *Plans and the Structure of Behavior*, by George A. Miller, Eugene Galanter, and Karl Pribram, had a significant impact on the cognitive revolution, in part because it appeared in 1960, just as many psychologists were preparing to think more cognitively. Had it been published five years earlier, it would have been dismissed as too radical; five years later, it might have been neglected as too obvious.

By far, the most successful of these well-timed books was Ulric Neisser's *Cognitive Psychology* (1967), which presented the first integrated view of the snowballing empirical research. It named and crystallized a movement that was already pervasive, but until then was only vaguely perceived. As I pointed out in Chapter 4, the cognitive revolution did not define itself self-consciously until *after* it occurred "spontaneously" to many individual psychologists. Neisser wrote the right book at the right time.

The widespread impact of Neisser's book can be compared with another attempt to mold a revolution in psychology — the "New Look" in perception. The New Look came and went in the early 1950s, based on work by Jerome S. Bruner and Leo Postman (Bruner & Postman, 1947; Bruner, 1984; Erdelyi, 1974). That work advocated a view of perception in which biases and emotional factors would be taken into account as an inherent part of one's perception of reality. In many ways, the New Look was an attempt to make themes taken from psychodynamics, Gestalt psychology, and social psychology an integral part of the experimental psychology of perception. Though the attempt triggered a great deal of research, the New Look failed to persuade most experimental psychologists. (It probably has continued to influence some work in social psychology, however, such as work on person perception and attribution of personal causality.)

Another psychologist interviewed in this chapter, Ernest R. Hilgard, exemplifies some early attempts to move psychology in a new direction. Hilgard entered psychology as a product of the prebehavioristic Eastern establishment in experimental psychology, centered in Ivy League colleges such as Harvard, Yale, Columbia, and Cornell. These schools were the special province of an intellectual and social elite, and psychologists among them tended to be broadminded, widely educated, and cosmopolitan in outlook. Behaviorism acted on this tolerant world as a purge: It displaced the *in*clusive outlook with a much more *ex*clusive one. But psychologists such as Hilgard, who were trained in prebehavioristic psychology, continued to pursue a broader psychology.

Curiously, Hilgard's best-known work made him appear to be the essential behaviorist. *Conditioning and Learning* (1940), written with Donald G. Marquis, was for many years the core of the behavioral curriculum in graduate programs in psychology, together with its successor volume, *Hilgard and Marquis' Conditioning and Learning*, written by Kimble (1961). Learning was, of course, the primary focus of behavioristic research, and conditioning was the experimental paradigm that was thought to contain all the essential elements of learning. Until fairly recently, any graduate student had to know "Hilgard and Marquis" better than any other book.

But Hilgard never thought of himself as a behaviorist. In fact, when the book was completed, he and Marquis came to the conclusion that the behavioral program was fundamentally flawed: Conditioning could not, after all, provide a foundation for the whole psychology of learning. Hilgard expressed this in his next book, *Theories of Learning* (1948), but the message was apparently not understood by most experimental psychologists.

Psychologists are hardly unusual among scientists in turning a deaf ear to unconventional views. The two remaining interviewees in this chapter are more or less "scientific isolates," because they believe that current psychology fails to include some very important elements. Both men are extraordinarily intelligent and creative, and are concerned with very broad questions; each by temperament is more a theoretician than an experimentalist. In fact, neither Walter Weimer nor Michael Wapner have published experimental work, though both have been trained as experimentalists and completed experimental doctoral dissertations. (It is worth noting in this regard that contemporary psychology has virtually no professional niches for theoretical psychologists. Any theory not tied directly to a program of experiments is still commonly disregarded.)

It is well to recall at this point one of the themes of this book: the analogy of a scientific community to a biological species, exploiting and developing its ecological niche. When a biological species encounters a crisis occasioned by some change in its environment, its continued survival depends critically on individuals who differ from the mainstream, who have the genetic capability to exploit new niches. In just the same way, individuals who differ from the mainstream may begin to play a special role in times of crisis in a scientific community. Indeed, most of the great names in the history of science can be viewed in this way — as individuals who, 50 years earlier, would have been ignored as peculiar at best, but who seem to have had just the right solution at the right time for the scientific community when it came to a crossroads.

Thus neither Weimer nor Wapner are standard cognitive psychologists, though they are more cognitive than behavioristic. Both depart from the current cognitive perspective in significant ways. Weimer favors the viewpoint of "ecological psychology" (*e.g.*, Gibson, 1966, 1979), focusing on environmental determinants of perception and action rather than on inferred theoretical mechanisms. Wapner's viewpoint is more difficult to define. One thread is a theoretical metaphor that differs from the conventional "information-processing" metaphor; instead of talking about "representation," he prefers to talk about "adaptation" in the nervous system. Although these metaphors are often interchangeable, they tend to emphasize different aspects of human functioning.

Whether outsiders to the cognitive community can have any more influence than Hilgard and Bruner enjoyed in the case of behaviorism still remains to be seen. We would expect cognitive psychologists to have a more theoretical orientation than behaviorists, and this may lead to a greater openness to new ideas. Whether this will in fact happen will be interesting to see.

Ulric Neisser: Crystallizing the Cognitive Revolution

Ulric Neisser (b. 1928) is a prolific researcher who wrote the book that named and crystallized the new framework: *Cognitive Psychology* (Neisser, 1967). The book clearly shows influences from the field of Artificial Intelligence and Gestalt psychology. Neisser tells us that he was also much moved by the spirit of humanistic psychologists such as Abraham Maslow — in fact, he saw the cognitive approach as a more humanistic view of the human organism.

Ulric Neisser received a good part of his undergraduate and graduate training during the period of behavioristic dominance, but he never became a behaviorist. Many of his publications represent attempts to expand the framework of psychology, including some of his most recent work. Thus he has been critical of contemporary practices in cognitive psychology; in particular, his *Cognition and Reality* (1976) claimed, in effect, that modern studies of cognition have had very little to do with the reality of how human beings deal with reality. More recently, he has edited a charming collection of naturalistic studies of human memory called *Memory Observed* (1982), which attempts to show a better way of approaching the realities of memory.

Thus, like the other "Persuaders" interviewed in this chapter, Neisser continues to challenge the current framework, much as he challenged behaviorism.

Interview with Ulric Neisser

Q: How did you get started in psychology?

A: I got into psychology by a series of accidents. I was going to study physics at Harvard, but after a couple of years it didn't really sing to me. I took the introductory psychology course, which was taught by E. G. Boring, a rather old-fashioned little man; I had the feeling that I was the only one in a very large class who liked him. But I thought that the field was young, one could make a lot of progress, contribute some ideas. So I took more and more psychology courses.

I was particularly impressed with George Miller, a young professor at the time — about 1949 — and did an honors project with him. He was just moving into information theory when I took his course, called "The Psychology of Communication," around 1949. We used as a text the manuscript of his book *Language and Communication* (1951). It was all full of "bits" and "phonemes" and the like. Chomsky had not yet been heard from; none of the new linguistics existed yet.

I read a lot, and became particularly interested in Gestalt psychology. It had an idealistic quality that appealed to me. To the Gestalt psychologists human nature was something wonderful, worth exploring, worth knowing about. They were constantly doing battle with the behaviorists, who seemed to see human nature as a mere collection of conditioned responses or blind associations. From the Gestalt viewpoint, the mind is something beautiful, well-structured, in harmony with the universe.

After my bachelor's at Harvard, I went to Swarthmore for a master's degree. There I met Wolfgang Köhler, the leading Gestalt psychologist, and his collaborator Hans Wallach. I also met Henry Gleitman and Jack Nachmias at Swarthmore, and the three of us became very close. In Gleitman's seminar we went through all the behavioristic learning theorists: Hull and Tolman, Spence and Guthrie. Out of those sessions came a paper authored by the three of us on the S–R reinforcement theory of extinction (Gleitman, Nachmias, & Neisser, 1954). We had a wonderful time discovering that Hull's theory of extinction was logically contradictory in several different ways, and also unsupported by any evidence. I didn't continue to work on those problems later, but they seemed important then.

Behaviorism was the basic framework for almost all of psychology at the time: It was what you had to learn. That was the age when it was supposed that no psychological phenomenon was real unless you could demonstrate it in a rat. To establish whether there was such a thing as thinking, for example, one attempted to show that rats thought. A very peculiar enterprise, it seemed to me.

After I left Swarthmore I went to MIT, where they were attempting to start a psychology department. I was one of four or five graduate students. There I did a study of perceptual set, using homonyms as stimuli. It became the first paper I published alone (1954). The point was to show that you could distinguish perception from response. That was the title: "An Experimental Distinction Between Perceptual Process and Verbal Response." In 1954, this seemed to be an achievement. The method was simple. I first let the subject read a list of words, then I presented some words very briefly, in a tachistoscope, to determine if they would be reported accurately. Words from the previous list, which the subject was expecting, were easy to recognize, but their *homonyms* ("phrase" instead of "frays," for example) were not. If the effect of perceptual set had been to facilitate just certain *responses* (mouth movements), the homonyms would have been easily reported, too. So the pure-response hypothesis was ruled out. Now it seems crazy that one would have to prove such a thing, but that is how deep in the Dark Ages we were.

I wasn't satisfied with the graduate program at MIT. Information measurement (in "bits") was more sterile than I had supposed. I was unhappy with what I was doing. So along about August 1954, I walked back into the Harvard Psychology Department, just down the road from MIT, went to the Chairman, and said, "Please take me back." I transferred to Harvard and got my degree there in a relatively short time.

In 1957, after some postdoctoral work at Harvard, I got a job at Brandeis, where the chairman was Abraham Maslow. He influenced me quite a bit. Maslow felt very strongly that psychology should be a force for good. He hadn't yet crystallized that idea into the rather one-sided "humanistic psychology" that it later became. At that time, Maslow was very proud of his experimental psychology background—he liked to have hard-nosed people around him. Nevertheless, he kept saying things like, "Why doesn't psychology study *positive* aspects of human nature, such as courage, or love, or self-actualization?" I thought that he really had a point.

Maslow was trying to establish a "third force" in psychology. The other two "forces" were behaviorism and psychoanalysis. The third force would be humanistic, he thought, and would draw on existentialist traditions from Europe. It now appears that cognitive psychology became the third force instead. Maslow didn't foresee that; no one could have foreseen it. The word "cognitive psychology" was not in the lexicon at the time, at least not with the modern meaning.

Another person I met in those years was Oliver Selfridge, who is one of the smartest people anywhere. He's not a psychologist, and has no doctorate. His undergraduate work was in mathematics, and he was a pioneer in what has now become Artificial Intelligence. Oliver and I got in touch somehow and found that we were interested in the same things. I knew about perception, and he worked on pattern recognition— a kind of interaction of information theory and perception. I spent a lot of time with him at the Lincoln Laboratory at MIT, and learned a great deal (see Selfridge & Neisser, 1960).

Q: What was your view of behaviorism at that time?

A: I thought it was crazy. It was so constrained, uptight, full of prohibitions. There was nothing you could do. Everything in psychology had to be translated into that funny theoretical vocabulary. Ostensibly they were trying to prevent too much speculation, you know; to be tight and firm with operationally defined concepts. But actually they explained everything with hypothetical constructs such as the "r_g"—the fractional anticipatory goal response. It seemed to me that describing mental processes in terms of internal stimuli and responses only made it much more difficult to think straight. Most of the research was dull. They were bogged down in it. There were controversies about "latent learning" and "place learning," but they had run out of steam by the early '50s.

It seems to me now, in retrospect, that this sort of dominance by a narrow theoretical vocabulary and a few simple methods is a typical development in psychology, and maybe in social science generally. Once you get a couple of schools established and some methods developed, there is always a lot to think about. Why didn't this experiment work? What about this or that effect? Such questions tend to be answered in terms of the prevailing theory rather than in terms of fundamental assumptions about human nature. The behaviorists were just getting further and further away from the important questions. I had an unthinking negative reaction to them long before I figured out why.

Nevertheless, it could be fun to play their game. Gleitman and Nachmias and I had a great time working through Hullian theory. I was at an age when I liked to play chess and solve puzzles. There was an affinity between game playing and playing S–R psychology. You pushed the r_g's around according to certain rules, to see whether you could accomplish a certain theoretical demonstration or not.

A very similar feeling underlies my rejection of some of contemporary cognitive psychology. Modeling information processes is now becoming a game similar to the one the S–R psychologists played. Many people today explicitly call it a "game." I am surprised by the number of formal papers that set out to do science in that way. When people talk about "models," it always reminds me of what kids do in hobby shops. The authors often insist that they're not interested in the truth, but only in whether the "model" can be made to fit. It seems to me that psychology ought to be serious business; it's about human nature. Maybe I'm making a political objection. We're really worth our salt as teachers or researchers only if we're doing something that's worthwhile — trying to unravel some significant mystery in a serious way.

Incidentally, this analogy with gaming applies much more to Hull's behaviorism than Skinner's. The trouble with Skinner is different: He just oversimplifies everything. My quarrel with Skinnerian behaviorism isn't based on his aversion to consciousness. Often I don't want to talk about consciousness, either. It's that behaviorists don't try to analyze naturally occurring psychological processes in their own terms; they don't want to *find out* anything. A response is anything you can condition; a stimulus is anything that has effects; they are linked arbitrarily by reward. That way of talking obscures everything that's unique about the stimulus and about the response. It makes human life seem banal and uninteresting, consisting only of arbitrary responses controlled by arbitrary rewards, like the worse kind of wage labor.

Q: Skinner would disagree with the idea that reinforcement must necessarily be materialistic; reinforcement for Skinner is not necessarily money or some material reward, but anything that increases the probability of the response which it follows.

A: Yes, including perhaps idealism and so on. But that only makes matters worse; there are just various kinds of things that you pay people with, various coins that are interchangeable.

I'm not now trying to make a formal antibehaviorist argument, but responding to your question, What is it about behaviorism that didn't appeal to me from the beginning? The answer is those two things: the "game" quality of Hullian theorizing, and the deliberate turning away from everything interesting that Skinner represents. When Skinner finally gets around to noticing the existence of war, or racial discrimination, or science, or art, he sees them just as additional examples of lever-pressing.

Q: Then it is true to say that even as a student during the heyday of behaviorism, you were never a behaviorist? Did you consider yourself a Gestalt psychologist?

A: Not quite. I was very interested in Gestalt psychology, but wouldn't have called myself a Gestalt psychologist then, either. I didn't know what I was. Perhaps *Cognitive Psychology* (1967) was an attempt to define myself. It's a very personal book. There was no field called "cognitive psychology" at the time.

Q: And your *Cognitive Psychology* clearly crystallized the new outlook for many people. It was remarkably well-timed and catalytic.

A: I got letters from people saying that they were glad that I had given it a name, because they were interested in all the topics I considered, but the area had not had a theoretical identity.

Q: You were able to speak with some authority for a group of experimental psychologists because you had published a number of interesting "cognitive" experiments very early. How did you get started doing that?

A: While still at Brandeis, somehow through talking with Oliver Selfridge I got the idea for the "visual search" studies for which I became known. The idea was that people who scanned down a list of letter strings, in search of a particular target, would have to spend a certain amount of time with each item, to make sure the target *wasn't* there. But they wouldn't actually respond until they had found the target, so their search rate was a pure measure of perceptual processes, independent of response time. I called it "decision time without reaction time" (Neisser, 1963a). It still seemed important to find a measure of mental activity that was not confounded with behavior. The work on visual search was one of the first modern examples of what has become *mental chronometry* (Posner, 1978). I also used it to look for evidence of *parallel processing*, of the ability to look for several things at once. It turned out that people can do that rather easily.

My students and I carried out a good many visual search experiments in the early '60s. By around 1964, which was a watershed year in my life for many reasons, I had a lot of things to say. I was convinced that *information* was a central concept, and that you could follow it inward through the organism. There were Gestalt processes at the beginning that were needed to partition the input, and constructive memory processes at the end with a sort of humanistic flavor. I decided to put it all together into a book. With sabbatical and Carnegie Corporation support, I spent two years in a quiet office at Martin Orne's hypnosis laboratory in Philadelphia writing *Cognitive Psychology*. It was published in 1967.

I was pleased with the book. I had taken what I believed and put it into a coherent package. The argument had a systematic scientific feel to it: starting with the input and analyzing information step by step, from iconic memory to the short-term store to the long-term store. Yet I felt it also had a definite humanistic quality. The processes were constructive and active. Information processing was not something that just happened to the perceiver, but something that he *did*. And as one got deeper and deeper into the system, motives and preconceptions and cognitive structures became more and more important. I thought it was a positive view of human nature.

The book had a definite impact. After it was published, people began to introduce me as the "father of cognitive psychology"; it was a little embarrassing. By now, though, there are many books on cognitive psychology, and the field has moved a long way beyond what I knew in the 1960s.

Q: I remember that you defined the field as the study of "the vicissitudes of information" as it travels through the nervous system, much as Freud defined psychoanalysis as the study of "the drives and their vicissitudes." One of the curious aspects of experimental psychology is that it seems almost untouched by the ideas of Freud, in spite of his enormous influence in so many other areas.

A: Well, I tried to bring that connection in a little bit. I had been self-educated in psychoanalysis and such things, never having had much formal coursework in it. It just seemed to me that Freud had a lot of good points. My attitude has always been that many different approaches to psychology have a piece of truth. Freud was probably right to claim that there are unconscious processes as well as conscious ones, and that there are primary and secondary thinking processes. Information theory was also right, in a way, and so was Gestalt psychology. Well, how could that be? In a sense, my 1967 book was an attempt to show how all those approaches could be reconciled.

Later in my life, I met James J. Gibson (*e.g.*, Gibson, 1966). After a while, I realized *he* was right, too. Then the problem was, How could he be right, along with the rest of us, when he was starting with such different assumptions about perception? So my later book (1976) was an attempt to show how that might work as well.

So, to get back to the book *Cognitive Psychology*, it appealed to clinical people and humanistic people, but also experimental and perceptual psychologists. Even some of the Artificial Intelligence people liked it. For example, the idea that speech understanding involves "analysis by synthesis," which I strongly supported in that book, came out of AI.

Q: One of the paradoxical things is that for experimental psychology, the computer has been a largely humanizing influence. That may seem surprising to many people who see the computer as an antihumanistic, mechanical sort of thing.

A: Yes, and of course it was important for me, although even in the 1960s I was already becoming disenchanted with Artificial Intelligence. The computer was, as you say, a very humanizing device, because it legitimized talk about information processes, about pattern recognition, information retrieval, and even executive routines. If they could be put into computers, there wasn't anything metaphysical about them. Without the computer, the resistance of the behaviorists to the new cognitive mode would have been much stronger. They would have dug in their heels and said, "You can't talk about such processes, it's mentalistic." But how could a process be mentalistic if a machine was doing it?

I said in *Cognitive Psychology* that the study of cognition was much like trying to find out the program of an operating computer. (I wouldn't put it that way today.) Such a question seemed answerable, sensible. And it was not the same as asking about the *hardware* of the computer, so the study of cognition was separate from neurophysiology. Incidentally, it was really Donald Broadbent who first formulated the question about the flow of information through the organism. Broadbent and Treisman and the other British psychologists were a great influence on me. I used Broadbent's (1958) book *Perception and Communication* in a seminar at Brandeis in the early '60s. The students hated it, but I thought it was neat.

I've always been in the position of liking what other people don't like, so I was a little surprised when cognitive psychology caught on so well. Of course I had fantasies of success, but I generally think of myself as a marginal, critical theorist. I was caught by surprise, because I'm usually on the outs. And you'll see that I very quickly reestablished my position on the outs. I can't handle the mainstream very well.

Q: In fact, I don't know of any critical reviews of your 1967 book at all. One from a behavioristic point of view by Kurt Salzinger, perhaps (1973).

A: Yes, and even Salzinger wasn't very critical. I was disturbed by that. When he said that behaviorists could accommodate Neisser's concepts very easily, I thought, "I must be doing something wrong." And I was, as it turned out.

The person who was most sustainedly critical of the book was the philosopher Hubert Dreyfus (1972). I was irritated with him at the time. He included me in the Artificial Intelligence community, which — in his view — was a pretty bad crowd. I thought he had misunderstood me, because I'd defined myself as more of an opponent of AI than as a friend. I *still* think he misunderstood me in part, but I have more sympathy now for his argument than I once did.

The first couple of years after I finished *Cognitive Psychology*, I hardly had an idea in my head. I had poured it all out. Of course I continued to do experiments and published a little bit, but not much was happening in my mind. I now realize that it takes a while to recover.

I came to Cornell just after the book was published. It was then that I came into contact with J. J. Gibson, whose ecological approach to perception seemed very strange to me at first. Gibson (1966, 1979) denied *everything* about information processing — even that it occurred. His ideas took a while to sink in. When I first met him, I thought he was merely clever. Then some more time went by, and I thought, "Gosh, he's stubborn; why does he keep saying 'The information is in the light'? He just likes to argue." It took about 3 years before I began waking up in the middle of the night, realizing that he was right. The information *is* in the light. Of course it's in the light; where else would it be? That realization ultimately led to my second book, *Cognition and Reality* (1976), which is partially an attempt to reconcile Gibson's insights with my own ideas.

There were other factors besides Gibson's influence. I didn't like what was happening to cognitive psychology. It had become very popular, and everybody was doing it. Hundreds of models appeared, and experiments were done to decide which of seven models was the best. The experiments invariably showed that none of the seven existing models was appropriate, but that the eighth model, proposed by the author, fit perfectly. I found that I no longer enjoyed reading most of what was being published. I didn't quite know why yet, but a good rule of thumb in science is: If it bores you, there's something the matter.

Political factors also seemed somehow relevant. There was a war on, and a lot of people were asking searching questions. What are you doing? Why are you doing it? They reminded me of commitments that I had made decades before. Psychology should be about human nature, and it should contribute in some way to making the world better. It seemed to me that cognitive psychology was running full tilt into a little academic corner where nobody would care about it. There were occasional attempts to apply it (to the problem of reading, for example) but they did not seem to work very well.

But the message I brought in *Cognition and Reality* was not as popular as the one I had brought in 1967. At that time I had wanted what everyone wanted. I hadn't exerted great "leadership" or anything: I was just lucky to write my book at a time when people wanted to do those things anyhow. I gave them a framework. But now, I'm saying that what people want to do may not be worth doing; maybe they should be doing something else. That's not such a popular message. Cognitive psychologists seem very self-satisfied, very sure that they know a lot, that great progress is being made. My opinion is different. It's true that clever experiments are being done — some of them are fabulous — but we have not learned very much about human nature that we didn't know already. We need a more ecological approach, more oriented to understanding cognition as it occurs and less to testing clever theories in complex experiments.

Q: How would you summarize the situation today compared with the way things were in the '40s and '50s?

A: Let's see, what has cognitive psychology found out so far in its brief existence? We know a lot about the first few seconds of memory. Some of the early interpretations of the iconic memory work, such as Sperling's (1960) experiment, have turned out to be wrong. Things are more complicated than we thought at first. But we are making some progress in analyzing the first few seconds of memory: There is working memory, recoding, articulatory loops, and so on. What else has cognitive psychology discovered? Well, we have found out how recalcitrant the cognitive activities of everyday life are to experimental study. For example, the fact that we understand so little about reading after years of study is very impressive to me. Many people think we do understand it; there's an awful lot of theory about automatic processes, decoding, storing, and so on. It doesn't seem to me, though, that those models are particularly helpful. You can make any number of them, and none seems to help kids learn how to read. There is also a recent move by cognitive psychologists into the area of intelligence and individual differences, but it's too early to see how that will come out. I *do* think great advances are being made in the study of perception in infants — I that is part of cognitive psychology, too. There really are some new ideas and methods there, which are beginning to answer age-old questions about what's innate and what's learned.

The contrast with behaviorism is still striking. It's great to be free to talk about thinking and memory, seeing, knowing, and imagining, without having to look over your shoulder every minute, without having to explain that when you go back to your lab you won't do it any more. It's great not to have to use the vocabulary of implicit responses, not to have to pretend that all learning is due to reinforcement, or, alternately, to spend lifetimes proving that learning can occur without it. There were people who spent decades trying to prove that, as if they had never engaged in a conversation and remembered it afterward. It was a pitiful waste of talent and energy, imposed by behaviorism for 30 years or so. At least we're free of that, we don't have to do it anymore.

Now, what else have we gained? We have turned our attention to thinking, seeing, knowing, remembering, and now can we reasonably expect progress to be made? A little. Even Artificial Intelligence has led to some insights, though I have been critical of it.

Q: One of the arguments for AI goes that it is helpful to have a powerful theoretical language, and that certainly has come from AI.

A: It's not necessarily a great step forward to have a theoretical language. The question is what is being said. A step forward would be discovering things that we didn't already know. Finding a new language and using it can be such an exhilarating experinece that people don't bother to find out anything with it. I think it may be best to stick close to our intuitions about real situations. One of the important discoveries of cognitive psychology, for example, is Eleanor Rosch's finding that many everyday concepts are organized around prototypes (*e.g.*, Rosch & Lloyd, 1978). She came to the prototype idea by considering natural concepts—what do people mean by "dog," or "chair," or "table," or "furniture"? It turned out that those concepts don't have the sort of structure that had been described in the theoretical language of AI, or in the very similar language of earlier concept-formation theorists. Such discoveries will be made over and over again if we look at how things really are.

So we've freed ourselves from a certain set of unreasonable strictures. We're trying to think about interesting problems, but we've only gone a step. The step was toward the real world, but so far we have not gone very far. There is no cognitive psychology yet that helps us understand how I decide what to tell you today, or how you decide which cognitive psychologists you're going to interview.

As a psychologist you are always on a boundary between the commonsensical and the absurd. If you go far off, you either say things that are foolish and false, or things that everybody knows. But you *can* push the boundaries of common sense a little bit. If you do, your ideas will make a difference. That's what Freud did. Nobody in the 19th century would have said that Freud's insights were "common sense." Now we find many of them obvious, but that doesn't mean that he didn't accomplish anything. I suppose that we are trying to make some analogous contribution.

Ernest R. Hilgard:
Nonbehavioristic Trends in American Psychology

The career of Ernest R. Hilgard (b. 1904) began before behaviorism consolidated its influence, spanning the heyday of behavioristic influence, and reaching well into the cognitive era. As a graduate student at Yale, Hilgard helped to organize the 1929 International Congress of Psychology, which featured such historic figures as Pavlov and Piaget. After receiving his doctorate at Yale in 1930, he taught there for some years (overlapping Clark Hull's tenure), and then joined the faculty at Stanford, where he has remained since.

Hilgard is probably still best known for his textbook *Conditioning and Learning* (1940) (with Donald Marquis), which became so much of a standard that its successor, by Gregory Kimble, was called *Hilgard and Marquis' Conditioning and Learning* (1961). (Hilgard denies any direct connection with Kimble's book, however.)

Because the topic of "conditioning and learning" was the central concern of behavioristic research, and because Hilgard's book was a centerpiece of this literature, Hilgard could be thought to be a behaviorist. But he might better be considered a thoughtful (and very tolerant) eclectic, representing the period before the dominance of behaviorism, when many schools existed side by side (Heidbreder, 1933). In a sense, Ernest Hilgard is one of the last remaining representatives of the prebehavioristic "Eastern establishment" in psychology, which at one time included such figures as James, Tichener, and G. Stanley Hall.

By 1948, when his *Theories of Learning* appeared, Hilgard had already decided that the program of reducing all learning to conditioning was not going to reach its objectives, though he expressed great respect for the work of Skinner. His own interest now turned in other directions. Psychodynamics offered an interesting approach to psychological matters, but without any well-established empirical basis. Hilgard began to work with hypnosis in an attempt to test some psychodynamic assumptions, but became sidetracked from his original purpose by the fascination and difficulties of hypnotic phenomena themselves. Together with his wife, the psychotherapist Josephine Hilgard (1970), he has worked in recent decades to put hypnosis on a sounder scientific basis, culminating in his challenging book *Divided Consciousness* (1977), which concerns "split personalities" and other dissociative phenomena in hypnosis. He has explored the implications of this work for cognitive theory under the heading of "Neodissociation Theory of Multiple Cognitive Control Systems" (Hilgard, 1976). The facts Hilgard presents, and their theoretical implications, would seem to be of the greatest importance for the future of cognitive theory.

Professor Hilgard has received numerous honors, including the American Psychological Association Distinguished Scientific Contribution Award (1967), the American Psychological Foundation Gold Medal (1978), and the Howard Crosby Warren medal of the Society of Experimental Psychologists (1940). He is a member of the National Academy of Science and was president of the American Psychological Association in 1949.

Interview with Ernest R. Hilgard

Q: How did you happen to become a psychologist?

A: I was a chemical engineer originally — I graduated with a bachelor's degree in chemical engineering, though I never worked at it. I had been active in some YMCA activities at the University of Illinois, and the YMCA secretary asked me if I would stay on a year and run the student employment office, which was located in the YMCA. Somehow I didn't want to go on to graduate work at the time, and you can't do much with chemistry unless you have a PhD. Well, I had a good record and was offered a fellowship. But I think that experience with people's problems moved me over a little. As a matter of fact, at the suggestion of a famous clergyman, Harry Emerson Fosdick, I spent the first year after leaving Illinois at the Yale Divinity School, on a Kent Fellowship. That was a very good year for me, because it gave me an opportunity to work in areas that were rather foreign to me, like philosophy. I had very little liberal arts training in my undergraduate work. In fact, I was rather timid about it. I knew I could make good grades in anything precise or mathematical, but I didn't know that I could do anything like biblical criticism. But I did just as well there.

Q: Were you considering going into the clergy at one time?

A: No. The proposal was that people supported by the particular fellowship would go into teaching in fields related to values. I had to supplement my fellowship at Yale and continued to work in their employment office even during the year that I was at the Divinity School, and so it was very natural for me to move over into psychology, where I was more comfortable. It was kind of thesis–antithesis–synthesis I suppose. Psychology permitted me to use my mathematical and laboratory training along with the human interest side of it, and so, from a personal point of view, the shifts have not been as violent as they might sound.

This was prior to Hull's coming to Yale. The man with whom I worked was Raymond Dodge, a very fine person who was a psychologist's psychologist: that is, he wasn't well known outside the psychological profession. But he was very well known in psychology. He was president of the Psychological Association, and a member of the National Academy of Sciences. Today he's known in psychology primarily because he invented the mirror tachistoscope that is used for all tachistoscopic work. He was the first person to study eye movements in reading and some related problems. I worked with him on conditioned reflexes before Hull came. I had completed my dissertation on conditioning before Hull ever got there. So Hull and I were really colleagues, because by that time I was teaching at Yale.

I guess one of the best ways to define my career is to start with 1929, when the International Congress of Psychology met at Yale: That's over 50 years ago. I was already an instructor. Dodge was chairman of the program committee, and I was his "flunky": So I met everybody.

It was a most remarkable gathering. It was about the first substantial meeting after the First World War, after the recovery in Europe. Europe had been so torn up with inflation and all, but now they were comfortable enough and so all the famous names were there. Pavlov was there, Piaget as a young man, and his teacher, Claparède, Pieron from France, Carl Spearman from England. And from America: J. McKeen Cattell, who was president of the Congress; Karl Lashley, who was president of the American Psychological Association at the time; Wolfgang Köhler was there; and McDougall. So, it was a very exciting and broadening experience for me.

I met Kurt Lewin for the first time and became very fascinated by him and his work. In fact, my last year at Yale I applied for a postdoctoral fellowship to work with Lewin in Berlin. By that time Hitler was stirring things up, and Lewin left. He came to Stanford, and when I was appointed at Stanford, he asked me if I would accept the postdoctoral fellowship under him at Stanford instead of Berlin. But I wanted to get going on the academic ladder, so I turned him down, and I became an assistant professor here at Stanford in 1933. At Yale I did mostly work on reflexes and conditioned responses. I also worked with animals with brain extirpation; dogs and monkeys, with Donald Marquis. Dr. John

Fulton did much of the surgery. So I had the feeling of having a base in the conventional experimental and physiological psychology laboratory. But when I came to Stanford I never again worked with an animal. I was more interested in the human problem anyhow.

All along I've been interested in motivation and in the distinction between automatic and voluntary activity. I dealt with that a great deal in my doctoral dissertation on the relationship between the conditioned eyelid response and the voluntary eyelid response. When I came to Stanford I did work on conditioned eyelid discrimination, in which I actually used instructed "sets" to inhibit or facilitate the discrimination. I mention that because people wonder how in the world did you ever go into some crazy field like hypnosis from a substantial field like conditioning. Well, in essence, the same problem is involved. The subtitle of my last book, *Divided Consciousness: Multiple Controls in Human Thought and Action* (1977), is on control processes. The same interest is there, you see.

Q: By 1940, you and Donald Marquis had published the major textbook in conditioning and learning. That work and the second edition of it (Kimble, 1961) really defined the field of conditioning and learning for several decades. Because conditioning and learning were the central topics of behavioristic psychology, these books became the bibles to some extent.

Q: We didn't write the second edition. Kimble wrote the second edition; he just put us in the title, which was *Hilgard and Marquis' Conditioning and Learning*. It's not at all the same book. I mean he didn't even discuss with us the chapter outline of the book. It's completely Kimble's book. We were just tired of it by that time.

I think in essence we had rather hoped that in the process of writing the book we would be more convinced of the general utility of conditioning for psychology; instead, we both decided that it wasn't the basis for a general psychology.

Q: How interesting. When did you decide this? How did it come about?

A: We had already concluded this by the time our book was published, about 1940. I was already starting on my *Theories of Learning* (1948), which was really friendlier to something like Tolman's cognitive behaviorism. You see, none of the people with whom I studied were behaviorists. For instance, in our doctoral examinations at Yale in those days, you had to choose two authors, one living and one dead, and read all their works and take an examination on them. The dead author I chose was William James, and the living author was William McDougall, a great opponent of John Watson. These are both much more dynamically oriented, much more willing to deal with motivational problems, which is in essence my whole background. My teacher Raymond Dodge worked with objective methods, but he was never a behaviorist. Yerkes, with whom I worked quite closely — I spent a summer at Orange Park working with his chimpanzees — was a methodological behaviorist, but he never accepted behaviorism beyond that.

Q: I have a quote here from Boring's *History of Experimental Psychology* (1950) which is relevant to that period. He says, "After 1910 some psychologists were Wundtians, some radicals were functionalists, more psychologists were agnostics. Watson touched a match to the mass, there was an explosion and behaviorism was left. Watson founded behaviorism because everything was all ready for the founding. Otherwise he could not have done it" (p. 506). Your experience of that period seems to have been rather different.

A: Well, you see, Boring's interpretations are very personal. Boring's *History of Experimental Psychology* has almost become canonized. But now there's a revisionist history, and Boring is being torn limb from limb for his interpretation of Wundt by way of Titchener — because Titchener really hadn't interpreted Wundt correctly (Blumenthal, 1980). And think of the dominance of people like Woodworth and Thorndike, who never gave a hang for behaviorism. Now after a time, stimulus–response psychology was called behaviorism, but it was not really a behaviorist psychology. It was almost always a response to an entire situation, rather than to a simple stimulus.

Q: I'm not clear about that. What is the difference between stimulus–response psychology and behaviorism?

A: Well, for instance, John McGeoch (1942) was a functionalist who always used the terms stimulus–response when talking about memorizing nonsense syllables. Or Benton Underwood, who was a disciple of McGeoch and Arthur Melton. They were never behaviorists — they were stimulus–response psychologists.

Q: What is a behaviorist in the sense that you're talking about?

A: Remember now that there are of course many different definitions, but I'm talking about Watsonian behaviorism. Watsonian behaviorism described everything as built on reflexes. Of course, modern behaviorism in the form espoused by Skinner is an operant behaviorism, which isn't really a Watsonian behaviorism. Skinner isn't the slightest bit interested in the nervous system and reflexes in the classical sense.

All of this had to be restated in the perspective of the time. Tolman called himself a behaviorist, but he was much influenced by McDougall,

Perry, Holt, various people who were not themselves behaviorists. All Tolman meant was that he wouldn't deal with what he called "raw feelings"; so he liked to stick to the rat and make inferences to the intervening variables. That was the characteristic thing, and now that's become modern cognitive psychology. The stimulus–response people didn't like intervening variables very much, particularly the Skinnerian behaviorists, but the other stimulus–response people were perfectly comfortable with them. The concept of "meaning," for example—if you worked with the nonsense syllable, you were perfectly willing to classify things as having a degree of meaningfulness—even nonsense syllables. In a sense, meaning is defined operationally. Behaviorism blended into operationism (Bridgman, 1927) very easily, so people like John McGeoch and S. S. Stevens adopted operationism but did not have to call themselves behaviorists.

Q: When did operationism become known among psychologists?

A: There is a particular article by S. S. Stevens—"The Operational Definition of Psychological Concepts"—that is commonly used as the starting point. That must have been 1935 or so.

So it was in the air. Remember John Dewey had a pragmatic position, as in his *Experience and Nature* (1925). Those of us who were brought up on functionalism didn't see this as any change from what we had been thinking all along. I never had any sense of anything innovative about these things except for the extremism of Watson's behaviorism, which never attracted me.

Q: Why did you consider Watson extreme?

A: Well, for example his desire to convert all perceptual responses to conditioned responses, essentially denying imagery. I mean it seemed to me that imagery was just as communicable as anything else. If you have a person look at a bright light, and you turn it off and have the subject match his afterimage to a plate of colors, you can find out about his images quite objectively. Calling that "only verbal behavior" violates common sense. Watson wanted to be mechanistic, he wanted to be monistic, he wanted to be deterministic, and those of us who read philosophy were a little more sophisticated. We were quite satisfied to be probabilistic. We just knew that you can't predict human behavior that precisely. You probably never will, but you can predict it enough to get lawful relationships. So we were looking for lawfulness, not necessarily cause and effect.

Hull had really done more to make conditioning interesting by his hypothetico-deductive method. I was quite impressed by that: In fact, I still am rather impressed by it. Hull was just as ingenious as he could be about making these derivations of which the essence is that you derive propositions that don't look at all like the axioms from which you derived them.

Q: Did you feel that Hull produced a logically rigorous kind of a derivation?

A: I thought the outline of it was fine, though the substance of it was dreadful. I mean we always looked down our noses at Hull and his overemphasis on that little anticipatory response. Part of the problem was that Hull moved back and forth from men to rats. That was part of the lack of rigor in the thing. He'd take a generalization curve of Carl Hovland's on the galvanic skin response and make derivations from it about the length of an alley that a rat ran. The most searching criticism at the time was the review of Hull's book by Fred Skinner (1944). Skinner's a bright guy; he and I have great respect for each other. I don't like his system, either, but I think that's a temperamental matter — we just differ temperamentally. But he just sent me a copy of the second volume of his autobiography, in which he says that he pulled his punches a little in his review of Hull's book. He really thought that Hull's business was much worse than he said it was.

Q: Could you specify what you think is especially good in Hull's work?

A: The idea was to derive very general theoretical predictions. I think that's a beautiful logic, if we can apply that to psychology. Hull tried to do that, and when he made his first try at it, it was exciting. After that, the more precise it got, the more trivial it became. The whole thing fell apart when he tried to measure habit strength, which he really thought was his crowning achievement.

But the very first thing, which he called the Lepley hypothesis, to account for the shape of the serial position curve — that was just a very cute illustration. It was published first by Lepley (1932), who had worked with Hull. In any list of items that people learn, you find that the beginning and the end of the list are learned more easily than the middle. Well, Lepley proposed that in the middle of the list you have some remote associations, and those remote associations are going to produce delays, which, according to Pavlovian conditioning, are inhibitory. So he just counted up the number of remote associations and found that they would pile up in the middle of the list, and that would cause the greatest inhibition in the middle of the list, so you have a primacy and recency effect. You see, that's derived from an inhibition of delay in the conditioned response. So that was all of a piece. That was pretty.

Then Hull and his collaborators wrote this whole book on the mathematico-deductive theory of rote learning, which had symbolic logic and everything else in it. A terribly impressive book with a lot of authors (Hull *et al.*, 1940). But all the authors abandoned it after they studied it. For example, Hovland was completely fed up with it and never turned to that kind of thing again. Afterwards he went into social psychology. But — and this is true of a lot of Hull's followers — the only people who carried on were not his own students.

It's to Hull's credit that he really wanted to develop behaviorism into a serious general psychology, and he was concerned therefore to derive even the Gestalt principles. For example, he was interested in Lewinian field forces, and he tried to derive them by reductionism. Kurt Lewin had a very interesting movie of this baby trying to sit on a rock, and he just couldn't make it until he backed up to it. This baby had to look under his legs to get back and sit on the rock; when he turned around to see the rock, he couldn't sit on it 'cause he'd always be facing the wrong way. But if he looked between his legs and then backed up, he could sit on it. Lewin thought this could only be explained by Gestalt principles. Well, Hull finally got the baby to do that, theoretically. He was so happy when he finally got Kurt Lewin's baby to sit on the rock. And he had a theory of intellectual problem solving, which he called, "pure stimulus act," that is, an act designed to somehow produce stimuli in the brain. So Hull was not narrow.

Q: Hull's most famous proposal is the idea that goal-directed action can be explained by a chain of "fractional anticipatory goal responses" — little muscular and glandular responses that connect the final "goal response" to earlier behavior. Was he attempting to deal with the problem of teleology with that idea?

A: Well, this is really a kind of feedback notion, such as other people also proposed. Troland (1928) wrote a big book on the problem of motivation, in which he dealt with retroflex action. I once proposed what I called a "provisional try," so that you don't need teleology in trying out some future possibility. For example, in reaching for a pencil in the dark, the pencil doesn't become a stimulus until you reach it. Now did the pencil make you feel around? No, of course not. It's just typical operant behavior.

John Dewey (1896) had faced that already in his circular reflex idea. These ideas of feedback keep cropping up. If you were brought up in the kind of eclectic tradition I was, they all seemed so natural. That's why I don't seem to stand for anything, you see! I've never taken a very striking position, because I learn from other people.

Q: Do you think that the simpler your position is in psychology, the more widely it's going to be propagated?

A: Well, the more committed you are to it. It isn't necessarily simple. You can get people to be interested in theories that are quite convoluted, but they have to have some sense that "this is it." I suppose that it's almost like religious commitment. Think for instance of Skinner, of being just so committed to this thing that to his disciples he's just like a god. His early disciple was Fred Keller. They were graduate students together at Harvard, and Keller once said to me, "I'm so jealous of Skinner, I just hate him sometimes, and I would just love to find him wrong. But whenever I carefully study the last thing he's done, I find he's always right. It's so baffling." Much of Skinner's support when he was getting started and throughout his life has been from Fred Keller. You get that out of Skinner's autobiography. Fred is almost a St. Paul, except that Skinner didn't need a St. Paul to promulgate his theory. He was his own Paul, so I don't know; John the Baptist maybe is a better designation for Fred Keller.

You get the same influence in Milton Friedman's economics, for example. Friedman knows exactly where he stands, and so he is always calm, and people just question him and get so angry at him, but he always knows the answer. People always think they're suddenly going to get at Skinner on the deterministic issue by saying, Well, how can you write a book and plan it? He's met that so often that nobody's going to find an Achilles' heel. Or take Carl Rogers or Rollo May: These people really stand strongly for something, and they get quite a following. You know, they're names to conjure with.

Q: Do you think that psychologists who take a more extreme position are more likely to become well known than those who have a more inclusive viewpoint?

A: That's very clear: One remembers Watson and Titchener better than one remembers Woodworth. I think Woodworth was one of the most levelheaded psychologists that we've had. The sociology of science is a very fascinating thing: What makes these things come and go? Piaget, for example, I mean he knows where he stands. His genetic epistemology is not thought of very highly by professional philosophers, and many psychologists don't give a damn for it, but Piaget provided a substitute for Freud. If you needed a cognitive substitute for Freud, and you didn't have anybody, you'd use the word "cognitive" as loudly as Piaget did. Hence Piaget, once little known and rejected, was returned to favor when the time was right.

Q: As long as you mentioned Freud: It's rather clear that psychoanalysis created its own establishment outside of the academic establishment, at least in the United States. It's interesting to ask how much mutual influence there was.

A: With my interest in dynamic processes, it's not at all surprising that I was also interested in psychoanalysis. There's a curious way in which one must give Watson his due also. In his textbook *Psychology from the Standpoint of a Behaviorist* (1919), he had a chapter on personality, which is one of the first chapters on personality in a general textbook on psychology. And it was completely influenced by Freudianism. Watson, although influenced by Freud, translated him into behavioristic terms. The "unconscious" was translated as the "unverbalized." He talked about adolescent conflict and about the psychological triangle. In *Psychological Care of Infant and Child* (Watson & Raynor, 1928), Watson's recommendations for raising children were all designed to avoid the Oedipus complex, so he didn't follow the Freudian belief that the complex was inevitable.

Q: Was that the reason that parents were supposed to shake hands with their child rather than hugging the child?

A: Well, sure, because all the damage was going to be done if you develop these overattachments to your parents, you see. Hull was quite interested in psychoanalysis at Yale, and the Yale learning theorists incorporated psychoanalytic ideas.

Q: The traces are so subtle.

A: Well, they're partly subtle and they're partly sociological again. Healy and Bronner had been brought to the Institute of Human Relations at Yale to represent psychoanalysis. They had just written a big book on psychoanalysis (Healy, Bronner, & Bowers, 1929). It was clearly in the air. Some of the graduate students were being psychoanalyzed. Neal Miller went to Vienna to be psychoanalyzed, you know, and Dollard was a practicing psychoanalyst. All those fellows were deeply involved in it.

Q: One of the most common things today I think among psychologists is to treat psychoanalysis as a new form of witchcraft.

A: Yes, sure. Robert Sears (1943) wrote quite a nice survey of objective studies of psychoanalytic concepts in the early '40s and we rather hoped that we could take what were obviously some pretty important ideas in psychoanalysis, and see if we could domesticate them.

Q: Experimentally?

A: Yes. He tried to do with psychoanalysis what I've tried to do with hypnosis. I know that you get into bad company when you work with hypnosis — you get into bad company when you work with psychoanalysis, too. We had a little seminar before the Second World War, when Siegfried Bernfeld and Bernhard Berliner came to San Francisco. Bernfeld had been trained by Anna Freud, and Berliner received a PhD under Wundt. They both were established psychoanalysts, and they offered this seminar in our homes. We would all meet together. Tolman came and Kroeber, the anthropologist, and Jean MacFarlane. And then, during, and just after the Second World War it became very high all of a sudden. The psychiatry departments were all hiring psychoanalysts as their chairs. There was always "a couch shortage." All the people who wanted to be trained as psychiatrists immediately had to get an analyst when they arrived. Then this dropped, partly because of the bickering of the analysts, partly because of the ascendancy of two things: the drug therapies and the behavior therapies.

Q: Among contemporary cognitive psychologists there is also still a lot of hostility and rejection toward topics such as consciousness.

A: Yes. I think it's important to recognize that the development of cognitive psychology is not to be identified with the rise of interest in consciousness. Cognitive psychology is permissive with respect to intermediaries, with respect to hierarchies and control systems, and hence goes beyond the prevailing Skinnerian behaviorism. The models of short-term memory have moved *toward* consciousness by using ideas like Tolman's intervening variables. They're not the same *as* consciousness. The same thing is true with the introduction of mnemonic devices and imagery. There is a little fighting about whether it's really imagery or whether it's words, but that's the old behaviorism raising its ugly head. A nice illustration of this is Ulric Neisser, a cognitive psychologist who wrote a review of my *Divided Consciousness* (1977), in which he said that psychology is not yet ready for consciousness (Neisser, 1979).

Neisser is very different from William Estes, for example. Estes was Skinner's prize PhD, who broke with Skinner; he was defiant early, and wrote his dissertation almost deliberately avoiding Skinner's terminology. And in the introduction to his six-volume *Handbook of Learning and Cognitive Processes*, (Estes, 1975 and later), he states that now that the restrictions of behaviorism have been relaxed, we're able to move on to a more general theory. Since we've reintroduced introspection, you can ask a subject what he's doing while he's trying to solve a problem. So Estes says we're bringing introspection back now. This is a little like arguments over instinct. We may not bring "instincts" back into psychology, but we can sure as heck bring "species-specific behavior" back.

Q: Exactly the same idea, just using a different word.

A: Yeah, and for my money, I never gave up instincts. There is a difference between the robin and the oriole in what kind of nest they build, and they show that, regardless of instruction by their parents. That's what we mean by instinct. The word itself doesn't necessarily *explain* something, but you have to classify things before you explain them. People throw away the class when they are trying to throw away the explanation.

Q: I am still very puzzled about why this was felt to be such a successful maneuver: to get rid of words such as "instinct" and all the other commonsense words?

A: Well, it's because words get so familiar that they seem to explain things better than they really do. Just to say "inferiority complex" explains too much. Or "free-floating anxiety," and so on.

Q: An occasional semantic housecleaning might be useful.

A: Well, that's part of it. I think one has to be careful that in that process you don't just turn over the mattress and get the same mattress anyhow, with a different label up. This does go on. For example, when "anticipatory responses," "expectancies," and the like were out of vogue, we used the word "set." "Set" sounds causal; it's a push rather than a pull, you see, and that avoids the connotations of "purpose," which always sounds like teleology. Whereas "set" sounds like "ready, get set, go." It's something you do in preparation. But the fact that you wanted to run like hell — that you don't have to mention.

My own tendency toward Freud was encouraged in many ways. We had a very small department at Stanford, and that's a good thing. When someone went on leave, another one of us would simply teach his courses. So, I just taught everything at one time or another. I certainly taught sensation and perception, action theory, personality, interviewing, and abnormal psychology. Later I taught Calvin Stone's course on psychoanalysis.

Then during the Second World War, which came just after we'd finished the conditioning and learning book, I went to Washington and was invited there to work for Rensis Likert, who was working on consumer surveys and public opinion surveys. That's where I learned Rogerian forms of interviewing techniques, and IBM methods of analyzing masses of data. As a matter of a fact, I'd had some interest in social reform, so I was one of the early people in the Society for Psychological Studies of Social Issues. I worked with Theodore Newcomb, and with David Krech in Washington. I had the broadest acquaintance with different people. During the war you just did your job; they didn't worry about what your background was. I moved from the Likert thing to become an economic statistician for a while.

A few years later I became a graduate dean here at Stanford, and that was a time when the Ford Foundation was rather heavily supporting the behavioral and social sciences. During my deanship and while working with the Ford Foundation, I was on the National Advisory Mental Health Council of the National Institute for Mental Health. The Ford

Foundation had invited me to head a committee to see about giving some money to mental health, and three of us did the groundwork. I was chairman, and Merton Gill and David Shakow were the others; both of them were deeply psychoanalytic. We came out with a report proposing essentially that investigators try to see if they could make some scientific sense out of psychoanalysis. Now this was as late as 1953. Both of them had been interested in hypnosis, and so we got some money in our proposal, and the Ford Foundation put aside $15 million on the basis of our proposal (which at the time was a lot of money). They put aside some for hypnosis. Nobody came in for it, so I submitted a proposal for it. I thought of hypnosis as a very useful way to get some analogues of psychoanalytic concepts, for example, of repression and amnesia, recovery of childhood memories, and dream phenomena; you could produce dreams using hypnosis. I really proposed to initiate a kind of a laboratory of psychodynamics. As a matter of fact, in my presidential address for the Psychological Association in 1949, I had proposed a laboratory in psychodynamics. I used the word "hypnosis" just once in that article, but I was thinking along those lines. Increasingly my interest in learning was moving toward an interest in motivational factors in learning, and in motivation generally.

Q: And so you've been working with hypnosis actually for more than 25 years. Clearly you feel that it has paid off. Do you feel it has paid off in terms of the original idea?

A: No, it didn't. We got diverted from the original idea. There was so much that was unknown about hypnosis itself, and it takes so long to find out anything. We spent a long time developing better hypnotic susceptibility scales, and when we had those scales we couldn't predict what the correlates were. My wife, Josephine Hilgard, with all her psychoanalytic training, did an elaborate interview study showing that hypnotic susceptibility correlates mainly with the ability some people have for imaginative involvement (J. R. Hilgard, 1970). We thought maybe it would turn out to be parental dependency, but it didn't work out that way.

Then the whole application of hypnosis to therapy was so shoddy that we thought we could get a hold of that by going to some clear problem, such as pain. Se we did our laboratory studies on pain. My wife has just completed three years of study on pain and anxiety in children with leukemia, carrying hypnosis into the hospital to show that we're not just in the ivory tower.

Q: Was it possible to relieve the pain of those children with hypnosis?

A: Particularly pain due to the very severe treatment — bone marrow aspirations and the like. So it's been quite satisfying, what we've done. But we thought we'd work on pain a couple of years, and ended up working a dozen years on it. We've had several incidental studies of the psychoanalytic thing, but we've really never developed a full program in that.

Q: Do you think there would be an audience for that type of thing within experimental psychology, if you had made claims about psychoanalytic ideas?

A: Oh yes, there still is. It turned out actually that hypnosis was more closely related to Morton Prince's ideas and Janet's ideas than it was to Freud's. Although when you try to get down to basics, you realize that the nervous system doesn't care whose theory it is. I think there'll be a resurgence of interest in Freudian ideas. A lot of it is in our culture still: rationalization, defense mechanisms, and interpretation of many things: reaction formation, psychosomatic medicine. It hasn't gone. One thing I think is pretty clear is that the long-term psychoanalytic therapy was a very clumsy technique. Freud was really more interested in theory than he was in therapy, and a lot of the analysts have felt that they were doing research in the depths of the human mind, and that therapy was really quite incidental. Freud was not a very good therapist. Franz Alexander tells of being at a dinner with him when he was concerned over the departure of some of his disciples. Freud's aunt said, "The trouble with you, Siggie, is that you just don't understand people" (Jones, 1953).

I've closed up my hypnosis laboratory now, and I'm turning to the history of psychology. I started as an instructor in 1929. Over 50 years I've known most of the people who have developed psychology in that period, and my professors studied with William James and G. Stanley Hall. Though I didn't know James and Hall, I have kind of a warm feeling toward the things that have happened. Everybody thinks I'm a behaviorist because I wrote a book on conditioning, you know.

Q: But in a real sense you've never considered yourself a behaviorist?

A: No, and if anyone looks at that book, that's where we really introduced the notion of expectancy and anticipatory responses and things. We favored Tolman. Tolman was quite surprised to find himself in a book on conditioning. Classical conditioning just wasn't viable in covering the complexity of human behavior and experience. Whether Skinner's is viable or not I don't know. But in the Yale days we had professors who were behaviorists, functionalists, and visitors who told us about McDougall, the great opponent of Watson, and about Gestalt psychology.

But by 1933, when I left, most of these people were gone, and Hull was dominant, so that the flavor was more behavioristic than it had been in my time.

Q: Now, among other criteria for behaviorism, one can talk about the rejection of mental terms such as ideas, purpose, expectation, will, or consciousness. Was there agreement among people who did not consider themselves behaviorists that those were not good things?

A: No, on the contrary. Edward Robinson, who was a very influential teacher then, said, "Now let's not get us caught in this 'you mustn't say' psychology." I've quoted that occasionally as his objection to "You mustn't say this and you mustn't say that." "Don't get tongue tied. If you want to talk about afterimages, just talk about them. If you want to talk about your dreams, talk about them. We've got no taboos around here."

A: As for the stimulus–response business, it seemed the right approach for quite a long time. The limits were not really explicit until you got to Miller, Galanter, and Pribram (1960). They made it explicit that stimulus–response really wasn't the right unit.

Q: Is that right? And you feel it wasn't made explicit until then?

A: I think that's about as explicit a place as any. Information theory was terribly important in substituting the bit for the reflex. The analogy with the thermostat instead of with a prod. That's quite a difference in analogy.

If you think of behaviorism as a reaction against Titchener's introspectionism, Watson's effort was not to restrict psychology. That isn't the thing. Watson's purpose was to *expand* psychology, so you could really include animal behavior and talk freely about insane people and children. Because you couldn't do that very well in Titchenerian introspectionism. You couldn't interview animals. You could only talk about psychologists trained to introspect, and so you got silly things, such as Margaret Washburn's theorizing, in an otherwise important book on the animal mind, on introspection in the amoeba. She decided that the amoeba probably didn't have images. Titchener thought that maybe the ant had originally been conscious, and now this complex social behavior in the ant had become automatic, because in our own experience you often have a decline of consciousness as behavior becomes more automatic. It always had to be referred back to the question whether or not the ant was ever conscious. And Watson said, "The heck with having to always worry about that." So historically, behaviorism was meant to be a liberating movement. Unfortunately, it often ended up by restricting the domain of psychology rather than enlarging it.

Walter Weimer:
The Rhetoric of Scientific Revolutions

Walter Weimer (b. 1942) is a rather successful nonconformist in the psychological ecosystem. For some 50 years the *sine qua non* of scientific standing has been the publication of some apparently significant set of experiments. Weimer has published none, but he has nonetheless exercised real influence through his participation in the "ecological psychology" movement (Weimer & Palermo, 1974; see also the interviews with Neisser and Jenkins in this volume), by his writings on the philosophy of science (Weimer, 1977b, 1979; Weimer & Palermo, 1973), and several interesting theoretical papers (*e.g.*, Weimer, 1977a).

Weimer received training in both philosophy and psychology. In good part because of his philosophical background, he entered his graduate training at the University of Minnesota with considerable skepticism about behaviorism, thinking, in his words, that it was the sort of thing "only a fool or a philosopher could believe." Nevertheless, he learned the behavioral point of view thoroughly, to "push it as far as it would go" — and discover the limits of the framework. While at the university, Weimer participated in the summer seminars organized by Jenkins to expose Minnesota students and PhDs to the new point of view (see the interview with Jenkins); there, he became persuaded of Chomsky's views on the inadequacy of behavioristic theory. But Weimer has not followed other cognitive theorists in the direction of the computational metaphor. Rather, he agrees with the ecological psychology group — that cognition is not likely to be modeled by computer simulation.

Interview with Walter Weimer

Q: How would you characterize your work?

A: It's been a cause for amusement to some people. Psychologists regard me as a damned philosopher who comes in and meddles around. I also teach philosophy and I carry a philosopher's academic credentials, but philosophers regard me as a damned psychologist who occasionally muddles things up trying to do philosophy. So I'm a classic case of an interdisciplinarian. I am as much interested in philosophy of science and methodology as I am in cognitive psychology, aspects of linguistics, economics, speech, and communication. I'm simply interested in whatever it is that the human head does whenever it does whatever it is that the head does. So, for instance, I look at the history of science as data for a cognitive psychologist to learn something from.

I received a BA in psychology and philosophy at Pittsburgh in 1964 and went to graduate school at Minnesota because it was the only place in the country that had both first-rate psychology and first-rate philosophy departments. To many philosophers at the time it was already clear that behaviorism was a position that only a fool or a philosopher could believe in. But in psychology at Pittsburgh, I had gotten a traditional S–R rat-running background. So I was getting conflicting messages between disciplines. That conflict came to a head at Minnesota. The Human Learning Center at Minnesota offered a summer program in 1966 that was to include courses from three people: David Premack, Jerry Fodor, and Walter Reitman. So I talked to Jim Jenkins (the HLC director), and I gave him my 20-minute spiel about "Look, this is what I'm interested in, this is what I want to do." I wanted to take the Fodor and the Premack courses — Premack for the learning theory content, because he was obviously violently opposed to Chomsky and everything that even looked "revolutionary," and Fodor for the Chomsky point of view.

Q: Fodor was obviously already very close to Chomsky at this time.

A: Fodor has been close to Chomsky from day one: roughly, from 1960. Jerry Fodor and Jerry Katz and all the classic names (such as Paul Postal and Bob Lees) became the first generation of Chomskyite linguists. Chomsky was at MIT for about 5 years before he had any following, except for the graduate students. His first established convert was Bob Lees, who went around to linguistics conventions and got the ball rolling. Then Jerry Fodor (whom I tend to call a *fodorus pontificatus*, which is a very interesting, very rare bird) went around and made the arguments to psychologists. Now this is somewhat hilarious: It is really a case of the blind leading the blind, because Jerry is a philosopher. Jerry knew literally nothing about traditional psychology. But simply by listening to Chomsky and by listening to the behaviorists around, he taught himself enough psychology that he could interact with psychologists. So, by the summer of '66, we had a summer school session with Fodor, Premack, and Reitman, designed by Jenkins to be polarized in three directions. Premack represented one direction — trying to resuscitate behaviorism and be "sophisticated" by saying we can address all those higher mental processes, too. Premack was playing catch-up ball, but without knowing he was playing catch-up against Dallas in the last minutes of the Super Bowl. Another direction was Fodor, who just stole the show. He was already so involved in the linguistic argument that he was doing normal-science transformational work, that hot-off-the-mimeo-presses, "This is the latest grammar from MIT." He was already doing normal science in the new linguistics, and saying to us "All right, this is what you must do in psychology to catch up."

The relative rates of progress (between linguistics and S–R psychology) brings up an interesting tangential point. There's the old saw about Jenkins having asked Chomsky and the linguists, "How come you can get so far ahead of us?" and Chomsky allegedly replying, "It's no problem at all, we can do ten thousand experiments a week. You guys are lucky if you can do one experiment a month. All a linguist has to do if he wants to find out what's going on is to talk to an informant who speaks the language you're interested in." Whoopee. No wonder they're ahead of us. We were green with envy.

Walter Reitman's course was a discussion of his then new textbook, *Cognition and Thought* (Reitman, 1965), which was meant to address mathematical modeling and computer or AI research. I sat in on enough sessions to see that it was not relevant to psychology, and even though not overtly behavioristic, was not opposed to behaviorism; nor was it obviously compatible with Chomsky's work. That course appealed to the methodologists and experimental design people, but never seemed to engage the conceptual arguments of Premack and Fodor. Reitman's approach simply wasn't *cognitive* enough, and the only computer theorist that made an impact was Neisser, with *Cognitive Psychology*, published in 1967. But Reitman's course influenced only the technicians, not the theorists in psychology.

As you can imagine, that summer was really quite chaotic. It was mainly Fodor shouting at people, saying, "You don't know what you're talking about," and then preaching that "This is the way it's got to be." It was very indecisive at the time. A lot of us were really turned off by Fodor (as the subspecies *pontificatus*) because of his loud mouth and histrionics, and a lot of us were equally turned off by Premack, because he never addressed an issue that Fodor brought up and always had this "Well, we're obviously superior scientists, and they're mentalistic jerks" attitude, so that we were all pretty much ready to forget the whole confrontation. But somehow I got initiated enough to go back on my own and look at Chomsky's *Syntactic Structures* (1957) and *Aspects* (1965), which had just been published. At that point it started to finally make sense, because I had retained from Fodor enough context to interpret Chomsky in *Aspects*.

The next year Jenkins offered a year-long seminar in the psychology of language. Jenkins is a superb lecturer, incredibly organized, and he has the ability to take somebody else's unintelligible comments and spit them out in the form of coherent sentences, saying, "Isn't that what you meant to say, and wouldn't you really rather go from here to there, and to there, and then to there?" Jenkins was the "great man" of the Human Learning Center; he supported all that interdisciplinary cross-purpose chaos. Seeing that, I gravitated more and more into the Learning Center. I was technically a Milton Trapold advisee, and my thesis advisor was the philosopher–methodologist–clinician Paul Meehl, but the biggest single influence on me was neither Meehl nor Trapold, but Jim Jenkins. Toward the middle of the language seminar, I sort of took over Trapold's evening rat-running seminar, and immediately polarized everybody in the experimental program into those who were for radical change and those who were never going to change. And that is an interesting sort of thing: There are several characteristic responses to crisis.

A good case in point was one faculty member in that seminar, who said after about three weeks, "I know, I see what you're saying, you're putting things clearly enough now so that I can understand the arguments. And you're right. But from my background I can't do research in this field. What the hell am I going to do?" If you're a member of the "old school," and you are intellectually persuaded that there's a more coherent way to do psychology, but you can't think that way, because you've been trained as an experimentalist, and you can't now generate experiments in the new mold, you go crazy. And that's literally what this person did, effectively leaving the field of psychology to become a dean, and having no real contact with the psychology department anymore.

Another representative case would be Wally Russell, the other half of the Jenkins and Russell work-association studies in the '50s. Wally was teaching history (and doing a superb job) at Minnesota by the time I was there. And yet Wally led Jenkins down off the behavioristic tree (to use Bertrand Russell's metaphor about how G. E. Moore led him away from idealism). And he was smart enough to say, Well, I don't know where to go in research now; and so he left — he went into history, and later, after leaving Minnesota, into departmental administration.

What I've seen in the established, older-generation people who come to a crisis is that they've really got two possible responses. They can try desperately to learn the new language well enough to dream in it, in which case they can then do research in it; or, they can go into another field. As I said, Wally Russell eventually left Minnesota and went back to Iowa, into administration. Trapold didn't leave, but he got out of doing rat-running psychology and into administration, with minimal contact with his old field. Kenneth MacCorquodale wouldn't take the bait, never really admitted the challenge, and consequently never grew. His course notes when I was there were based on '40s lecture notes from Skinner, and he never updated them. He never had the courage to engage in the intellectual battle. He never reached a crisis point. One incident is indicative of his response. He came to my first presentation in the evening rat-running seminar, and afterward told me that I had done an excellent job and that he had found it very informative, but added that he was sorry, but he would be unable to attend the next week because he had to be out of town when the seminar met. The next week at 7:25 p.m. I went to his office and borrowed a reprint from him. The seminar started 5 minutes later.

Q: Why was Jenkins able to go through a transition relatively successfully, when other people couldn't?

A: I think the answer to that is fairly clear. Jenkins is a very applied researcher who is an eclectic "robber of interesting items" from anywhere in psychology. Jenkins was never indoctrinated into a particular *theoretical* position, but rather trained as a "rigorous" researcher in individual differences. He was encouraged to search out everything that looked interesting, no matter where he found it. So Jenkins "got converted" in the sense that he adopted his *first* coherent theoretical position as a result of the Chomsky–Fodor influence. He was not previously a rabid Skinnerian or a devoted Hullian or anything like that. He was familiar with all those positions, of course, and he was capable of reading the literature and interacting with the practitioners. But he was never a convert himself. He was young enough to be a "neo" behaviorist, or a "neo-neo" one, and realized the inadequacy and enormous change that already had occurred. His commitment was to generating informative research in psychology, and his behaviorism was of secondary importance.

Jim is roughly 20 years older than I am, but he's a lot like I was in terms of attitude. I never really bought S–R psychology, except perhaps for a term as an undergraduate. I was smart enough to know that there was something wrong with it, because too much was either stretched to fit or left out. Initially, at least, I sure as hell did not know what to do in its place. But I think Jenkins and I came out of the same, more encompassing framework. We knew the S–R approach was wrong, even though there were interesting tidbits in it that any position is going to have to encompass. But we initially had no coherent alternative. So we were sitting there marking time. Jenkins had abandoned the position as a result of "rigorous" experimentation culminating about 1960, which showed that the S–R mediation model of language, the four-stage paradigm, could not be experimentally corroborated. Thus, the explanatory power of the account dropped to zero for him, and he latched on to Chomsky as the first explanatorily adequate framework to take its place. I was marking time because of more philosophical doubts, and got caught up in conversion about five years later than Jenkins, and in substantial part because of his influence.

Now, come back to the Minnesota group circa '65 to '69. The Learning Center was composed of crazy guys like Terry Halwes, who was doing speech perception and converting the masses; outside non-HLC renegades like me who came in to deliver seminar presentations and terrify people; and a group of really first-rate graduate students: among them John Bransford and Jeff Franks, who were office mates. They were very quiet in classes. Bransford once said later that I used to terrify him in the seminar presentations because I would say something and it would always be reasonable, and he was afraid that if he'd say something then I'd say, No, that's nonsense. And he'd find out the hard way, right there. I don't know whether that's false modesty or not. But Bransford and Franks were quiet, whereas Halwes and Weimer were noisy, obviously *pontificatus* variants.

What happened was that Bransford and Franks, instead of preaching to others, got to thinking in conjunction with Jenkins about ways to do research — research that would show that the head is an active organizer of information, instead of a passive, associationistic, stamp-in-the-linkages-between-incoming-stimuli entity. So they sat down and said, How can we design a situation to show that? And, Let's play in the central ballpark of memory, because what we want to do is show that people can remember more than they think they do, and that they know more and remember more than the S–R approaches will allow for. Bransford and Franks came up with the idea that one could take compound "sentences" (or sets of ideas) and break them down into three or four short ideas. The same set of ideas can be expressed in a single long sentence, which integrates the ideas expressed in the short ones. In essence, subjects are presented with some of the short sentences, and afterwards they are asked to choose from a list of sentences those to which they had been exposed. The Bradsford–Franks phenomenon basically is that a subject will recognize one of the integrated long sentences as familiar, even though it was never presented, and be more confident of having heard it before than of having heard the shorter sentences, which he actually *did* hear. The more integrated sentences are falsely recognized as familiar — as having been heard before. The point is that the head does not integrate information in anything like the particular form in which it was initially presented. Syntactic and surface form are irrelevant in our ecological niche: Our knowledge and memory operate on semantic and pragmatic dimensions that exhibit creativity or productivity.

Q: The Bransford–Franks experiment is impressive not only because it is so elegant and effective, but also because the task is so natural.

A: That's it. Good psychology is not different from good business, no different from anything else in human life. Take somebody like

Johnson, who invented the Band-aid and becomes a billionaire, simply because he sold you a product that once you had it you just couldn't live without it. The Band-aid was so natural you just had to have it. The Bransford–Franks research paradigm is the same way. Once you hear it presented or once you see it done, it is so natural you cannot believe that people haven't known about it for a thousand years.

Q: What kind of challenge did this present to the S–R viewpoint?

A: The whole point of the study was to show that in the real world, the head utilizes information in a way that cannot be accounted for in a stimulus–response–reinforcement paradigm. The integrated sentences are totally novel. They did not occur at all during the acquisition phase. They demonstrate that the head is productive or creative. As Harvard psycholinguist Roger Brown used to say in his lectures, the mind has the ability to make infinite use of finite means in novel but appropriate fashion. The linguists had been arguing for a decade, since before 1960, for that point. This throws the burden of proof on the stimulus–response psychologist to come up with bigger and more coherent units of analysis, but that tends to create an intolerable conflict. The S–R theorist claimed as his scientific birthright (Premack's sneer at the mentalists) the fact that he is a physicalist, that his stimuli are physically specifiable, that his responses are overt, observable, and measurable. The only way the S–R theorist can account for this sort of phenomenon is to say that the subject learned a complete thought. To this, the response of the linguist is, OK, Professor Postman (who in fact tried that tack), how do you define a "thought" operationally? Their answer: Well, it's whatever the subject learned. And that's the end of it. The downfall of the stimulus–response approach in this case is simply that in order to account for the data, the account must be *ad hoc* and paraphrastic of the data to be explained, rather than being genuinely explanatory. The theoretical terms must become accordion words to such an extent that everything in the universe becomes a matter of stimuli, responses, and reinforcement. And if everything in the universe is a matter of the co-occurrence of stimuli, responses, and reinforcements, then you have a pleonastic system that explains nothing.

Q: Pleonastic?

A: A "pleonasm" is a logically vacuous word. To account for the exceptions, the oddball data that the Chomskyites and the psycholinguists kept poking at the S–R people every day, the S–R account became vacuous. It could account for everything and therefore could account for nothing. It could *post hoc* everything, and as a result it could predict and explain nothing. The revolution "hit" when it became obvious that the "oddball exceptions" were actually representative of reality, and the S–R study cases were in fact unrepresentative, laboratory artifacts, rather than ecologically relevant.

Q: Do you think that Bransford and Franks's work is perhaps the most fundamental experimental challenge to S–R psychology?

A: There is no question that it is. It's been demonstrated at nearly every major university in the country at this point. What was interesting is the extent to which people picked up on it. They didn't believe it at first; then they were run as subjects in it, saw what happened, and said, My God, how could I ever have been so stupid as to not believe this? In that sense, the Bransford–Franks paradigm is the single most persuasive empirical datum that experimental psychologists have generated on their own.

Q: An intelligent person who's never taken a psychology course in his life might not be surprised about this phenomenon.

A: That's it, that's precisely it. We are back to the point where it's clear that a position as "sophisticated" as behaviorism was is so absurd that only a fool or a philosopher could seriously propound it. A college sophomore will tell you that the S–R approaches are counterintuitive, and that they make the subject work with one hand tied behind his or her back. Jerry Fodor's constant argument that summer was that it should not surprise one that whatever a subject can do with one hand tied behind his back (in S–R fashion) he can also do with his hands free. It's the same sort of thing. It doesn't surprise the college sophomore. The college sophomore would require a detailed explanation of how we could, as a field, have been so stupid as to have forgotten basics like that.

Q: It's not unusual, in mathematics, for example, to believe that something is true and yet not be able to prove it.

A: Sure. Gödel and recent metamathematical research have indicated that that outcome can be expected.

Q: And being able to prove something, even though it seems to be obvious, is not at all trivial or useless in science. The question is, however, where do you go next?

A: A very good question, and a very good question with regard to the Bransford–Franks work. In various forms, that paradigm was milked to death for 10 years, and it's still being milked. It's still reasonably productive. But it's hard to find informative alternatives to the Bransford–Franks research. And this is part of the reason that there is real personal malaise among the older, more established experimentalists. For a while the Bransford–Franks stuff could give the Charlie Cofers and the Jim Jenkinses a new lease on life. They could do derivative studies in the new basic paradigm. Modifications on the paradigm would still grind out good publishable research, and they didn't have to come up with new creative, innovative frameworks or research paradigms.

Q: But the opposition is certainly no longer what it used to be.

A: The opposition has changed quite considerably. The opposition is now, if you will, a residual old-fashioned cognitive psychology that is basically S–R psychology translated into information-processing and computer terms. This is represented in the work of, for example, George Mandler, Gordon Bower, Herbert Simon, and numerous other younger researchers. Now these are individuals who are very sophisticated, and always regarded themselves as *avant garde* stimulus–response psychologists and who, even when they embraced Chomsky and psycholinguistics, never really moved very far at all. They adopted a new terminology, but they're still thinking the way they thought 20 (or more) years ago. Instead of talking in stimulus–response–reinforcement terms, they're talking in terms of information processing and computer simulation, but conceptually it's behaviorism, pure and simple.

Q: There are some computer simulators, such as Herb Simon, who could not reasonably be said to be behaviorists. What is the distinction between the two different groups that you perceive?

A: Let me make a distinction between three representative classes of theorists. On the one hand, we have the old-guard psychologists who think they are being very *avant garde*—the Mandlers, the Atkinsons, the Bowers. In the middle, we have somebody who's never been a psychologist, such as Herb Simon, who really has no reputation in psychology, despite the Nobel Prize, despite his fame, and so forth. He is not often regarded as a psychologist. He's in industrial and organizational behavior, whatever that is. And on the other hand, let's take somebody such as Mike Arbib or Seymour Papert or Marvin Minsky or one of the other Artificial Intelligence people who occasionally do psychology as a sideline. I would put Simon and others in a middle category. Simon doesn't really have too much to say to cognitive psychology.

Everybody in psychology knows he's great, but nobody's ever read him. I never have taken him seriously, and I can tell you why. When you have a man who sits there and looks you straight in the eye and says the brain is basically a very simple organ and we know all about it already, I no longer take him seriously. And Simon tells you that constantly in his books and lectures. He will tell you that in ways that just don't add up, because half of what he's saying is incredibly sophisticated, and the other half of it is unbelievably naïve. The Carnegie–Mellon group builds unbelievably powerful and sophisticated computer programs. But Simon is not a human psychologist; he is a machine psychologist. Artificial Intelligence is exactly that: artificial. He is doing, if you will, machine work. And what he has to say to real cognitive psychologists, I don't know. I don't think very much. On the other hand, if I had to go to somebody and say, "Find a way to bootstrap a computer to do something," I would sure as hell go to a Herb Simon.

Q: Don't you think that building a simulation that actually performs, say, speech perception, would give you some insight?

A: Yes and no. It's crystal clear that technology in the computer realm is going to get to the point where in a finite number of years, say 400 or 500, we will be able to duplicate everything that human beings can do with machines. We will be able to do all the translation stuff, we'll have solved, in a real sense, the voice-typewriter problem, etc. But the real issue is, will we have done it by constructing unbelievable machinery that doesn't bear any relation to the way the human head does it, or will we have done it by mimicking the human head? And the answer is, we will not have done it by mimicking the human head unless we just happen to be unbelievably lucky.

There is a real difference between building a machine that works the way the head does versus building a machine that simply outputs what it is that the head can output. Now if I had to bet on who would do the latter task, I would pick Herb Simon, no question about it. For that, he's great. But I think he's only kidding himself when he tells us that we already know how the head works. That is not cognitive science, but abject cognitive scientism.

Q: I think his claim is that to understand people you've got to look at the constraints that the environment imposes, and the goals that people need to achieve.

A: In so far as he says that, I obviously agree. That's completely correct. It's when he couples something like that (which I find eminently reasonable) on one page with the claim, on the next page, that we already know how the brain works that I reject Simon as a serious psychologist. I don't want it to look like I have a personal feud with him, I don't. He can run rings around me in terms of mathematical sophistication and everything else, but he does not do cognitive psychology. He does something distantly related to it, but he doesn't do it.

Q: You said that in 1964 you saw no real alternative to stimulus–response psychology, but you knew there was something wrong with it. What about George Miller's work at that time? He was beginning to take off on Chomsky's work.

A: The only work of Miller's that I knew at that time was "The Magical Number Seven" (1956), which pointed out that people can keep only about seven separate items of any kind in mind (immediate memory) at any one time. Probably the majority of psychologists at that time knew Miller primarily for that one article. George Miller was highly respected (also for the book *Language and Communication* in 1951), but he was always a little suspect among the experimentalists. He was regarded as basically a good guy, but sort of way-out, like Leon Festinger, the originator of cognitive dissonance theory.

That caliber of the individual was regarded as being sufficiently "beyond the pale" that although you knew of one or two of his studies, you never really bothered to look up his *vita* and read everything he did. So we didn't really know Miller. Miller, despite the fact that he is a first-rate psychologist, didn't really have much of a reputation outside of Harvard except in the last 10 or so years. He's a famous psychologist, and he's a good psychologist. He's a psychologist's psychologist. He is known to all the pros in the field, but his research, aside from the magic number 7, did not make it into basic psychology textbooks, and was not discussed readily in introductory courses.

Q: At some point Miller bacame proselytizer for Chomsky within psychology. When was that?

A: From 1960 on up in publications, and earlier in personal contact. If you go back to 1960 there's the infamous Miller, Galanter, and Pribram book, *Plans and the Structure of Behavior*. A funny book. A lot of us bought it, looked at it, and said, What's this? We couldn't make head or tail of it. So we threw it on the shelf and never came back to it until *after* the revolution. Then we went back and looked at it as part of our homework. We also picked up the math handbook chapters he did with Chomsky.

Q: I wonder, by the way, if that was a characteristic phenomenon for many people. You go through this change by yourself, and afterwards you suddenly realize that somebody wrote about it before, only you didn't know how to understand it before you'd changed.

A: Precisely. You've got to realize that those three authors are odd-balls in psychology. George Miller was beyond the pale in verbal learning, because he did interesting things and because he was a sophisticated mathematician. Here's a guy who can talk and think rings around you in the verbal learning–human experimental area. Old Geno Galanter, with his black leather jacket and his motorcycle and his mathematical psychology, effectively disappeared and was never heard of after that. And then, crazy Karl Pribram, the *prima donna* of physiological psychology, tells you he's the greatest thing since his mentors, Köhler and Lashley. And yet in the last decade, he's become exactly that: His ideas have finally caught on. He really was saying things in the '50s that are just now beginning to catch on, and his neurophysiological speculations are decades beyond other physiological work.

Q: You were saying that outsiders seemed to be more creative than the insiders: You consider yourself to be an outsider, like Fodor, Chomsky, Pribram, Miller, even Jenkins.

A: Yes. Weimer's first rule is that good psychology is never done by psychologists, and a corollary is that good cognitive psychology is not done by cognitive types, but by those outside that special field.

Q: Now, do outsiders play this influential role only when a field goes through a revolutionary period?

A: No, it's true any time, but it is noticed, because it is painfully obvious, during a revolution. If you look at the age curves on creativity, you'll find something very relevant. These studies indicate that there is a bimodal distribution, so that at age 20 or 30 (depending on the field studied), you've got a peak of creativity, then it drops down, and then at 50 or 60 or 70 there's another peak. Why that second peak? The answer is usually that there is a period (near retirement age) when somebody leaves his original field and looks at another field and says, "Well, you dumb bastards, this is the way you do that!" And he then applies to the new field what he already knows from a lifetime in the first field. And so there's that second peak of creativity of an older outsider who comes in and says, "This is the way that has to be, so how come you haven't been doing it that way?" Consider Michael Polanyi, a superb physical chemist, who became a philosopher, emphasized the tacit dimension, then became a second-rate psychologist, doing good work there (as in *Personal Knowledge* (1958) and *The Tacit Dimension* (1966)). The examples are legion. Lots of people make revolutionary applications within a new field, even though they are not particularly revolutionary in their original field of endeavor.

I separate the set of "scientists" into people who are basically normal-science researchers, come what may, and people like myself, who get bored with a field and leave it as soon as normal science sets in. Psycholinguistics, for instance, is for me, a dead issue. I have to teach the course next fall, but I haven't looked at it in five years, and I'm kind of scared. Why? Because it's become normal-science puzzle solving, and that sort of material no longer challenges me. That's not the way I look at the world. Like Jenkins, like the other outsiders, I am a synoptic overviewer who operates primarily at the metatheoretical level and who would prefer to say, "Look—you morons are playing in the wrong ballpark, get the hell over here," and then let them worry about the details. Normal-science detail is not my strong point.

I tend to regard Kuhn's *The Structure of Scientific Revolutions* (1962) as a very useful personality test. It seems to separate not only psychologists, but just about every other scientific community that I have any experience with, into people who are basically normal-science puzzle solvers, come what may, and revolutionary metatheoretical conceptualizers who occasionally stoop to get their hands dirty in the laboratory, but who are really much happier thinking than doing.

Q: You would claim that one could be a good scientist and never get into the laboratory.

A: There's obviously a continuum. I, for instance, am known only as a theoretician, and have never published a single experimental study I've done. I've done about 15 or 20, and so it doesn't mean that I'm afraid of the laboratory. It's not that I don't do that sort of thing or that I don't like it or consider it a waste of time — it's that I prefer to allocate *my time* in a different way. There's a lot of other people who also think that, but because of pressures from their grant and job commitments wind up publishing a lot more "experiments" than they really want to. Let's face it — it's a helluva lot easier to publish a silly little experimental article than it is to publish a theoretical article in psychology. The privilege of a theoretical article is usually reserved for the established pros.

Q: At least until recently we haven't really had an accepted theoretical language.

A: True. We have not had the journal that would take a theoretical article, and we have not had the theoretical framework in terms of which to cast the article to begin with.

Q: Certainly *Psychological Review* would claim that it accepts theoretical articles.

A: Yes, but I don't regard that journal as publishing theory at all. In fact, I regard the *Review* as one of the least informative theoretical sources in psychology. What the editors and referees for the last several years have regarded as a theoretical article is a normal-science puzzle-solving *series* of five or six studies that are fairly closely related, with three or four pages of discussion at the end. Their conception of a theoretical article, in other words, is normal-science puzzle-solving, not theory in the sense of integrative explanation or metatheoretical questioning of where we ought to go. It's interesting, for comparison, that the "hard" physicists don't have any problem with that sort of "speculation." If you look at *Physical Review* or similar sources, they will publish the normal-science theoretical integrative stuff side by side with the farthest-out speculation.

Q: You wrote in several of your articles (Weimer, 1973, 1979) that *facts* in science are "deep-structurally ambiguous." What do you mean by that?

A: What constitutes a fact is only what your theory says a fact must be. This is why "what the facts are" for the Skinnerian behaviorists are not the same facts as Chomsky's and Fodor's. That's why, to a large extent, paradigm debates are literally at cross-purposes — the participants are not talking about the same things at all. The best case I know of in physics, for instance, is that of Brownian motion. If you dump finely ground particles into liquid solutions, you'll get this funny rapid agitation of molecules. Here's a phenomenon that, empirically speaking, was discovered in the early 1800s by Thomas Brown, and in a literal sense no one knew what it was until 1905, when Einstein published, and it then became crystal clear what that funny stuff in that bottle is. But, with Einstein's publication 80 years later, the phenomenon itself literally changed.

Q: For Brown it was an observation.

A: It was an observation. You have a phenomenon. If you pour, say, finely ground clay into water, all of a sudden it will be uniformly cloudy, and you'll be able to see funny little things hopping around.

Q: And to Einstein, you're saying, this was a different phenomenon.

A: Precisely, because for Einstein it is not just that; it's an instance of interaction at a subatomic-particle level, which can be explained only in terms of quantum effects.

Q: And the observation is perceived to be different with the new framework?

A: Precisely. In a real sense Brownian motion wasn't a fact until Einstein. It was not a *theoretically motivated* observation, and facts are theory-motivated observations.

A typical case in linguistics is Chomsky's rediscovery of something that's always been there — *deep-structure* ambiguity. Before Chomsky, there was really only word ambiguity and surface-structure ambiguity. But deep-structure ambiguity is different: No surface bracketing of constituents will resolve it. The sentence, "Praising professors can be platitudinous," cannot be parsed into its separate meanings. The Necker cube in perception is, after the fact, an obvious example in psychology, but it was not known *as such* prior to the revolution in linguistics.

Q: Was the phenomenon of deep-structure ambiguity observed before by linguists? It must have been observed.

A: Sure. Humboldt seems to have noticed it in the 1800s, so as a casual observation it's been around for a while. But until there was a theory that made the observation relevant, it just didn't exist. People looked right through it. It wasn't there. You could hit them in the face with it and it wasn't there. All science is like that. What is or is not a fact is theoretically determined. What theories do, if you will, is to provide an alternative surface interpretation of a reality that is, in essence, deep-structurally ambiguous, because we can read reality in as many ways as we can make theories. And almost all those theories are at least pretty good. That's what's frightening to the methodologist and research-er alike.

Q: Then it might be very difficult to make decisions about what is true and what isn't.

A: Precisely. We make decisions about what's true, and we make them all the time. But we do not make them on any of the accepted methodological criteria that you can find in the textbooks for the masses.

Q: What's wrong with the usual ideas on the way scientists decide to accept a theory?

A: Funny, I just published a book on that (Weimer, 1979). Here we are back again to the issue of scientism and the role of positivistic methodology.

Q: And by "scientism" you mean . . .

A: By "scientism" I mean the term as reintroduced by Friedrich Hayek, in 1952, in *The Counterrevolution of Science*, one of the two or three most important books published in that decade. "Scientism" is the attempt to utilize the readily available methods of one area in another area before you know whether or not they are applicable. Scientism, in other words, is the pretense of knowledge instead of the real thing. Now, psychology is without a doubt the most scientistic discipline I know of—with the possi-ble exception of sociology or economics. There is more lip service to hard-science methodology, "methodolatry" as I call it (Weimer, 1980), than anywhere else.

If you look at physics, which is the paragon exemplar of a science for the logical positivist and empiricist theorists, what physicists do bears no relationship to positivistic methodological prescription. They're not nearly as Procrustian as we are. They have a very loose, let-it-all-hang-out, let's-think-about-that-for-a-while, I-think-you're-full-of-crap-but-let's-discuss-it sort of attitude. We tend to say, No, you can't do that, that's not scientific; show me your data; don't think, just write down your data. That approach has never held sway in any science that I've never looked at. Psychology is the only area that is trying to live up to that Procrustian ideal.

Q: Do you think that's different in cognitive psychology?

A: No, I think it's only attenuated in so-called cognitive psychology. In fact, in that sense, I really don't think that the revolution we anticipated would result from Chomsky's impact has actually come to cognitive psychology. I think it's at least 15 or 20 years down the road, and I think it will take another series of Bransford–Franks type demonstration experiments and a quasi-well-worked-out theoretical overview to change that. Right now, cognitive psychology is information-processing terminology applied in conjunction with behavioristic methodology to simplistic situations.

Q: Some well-known psychologists feel that psychology still has no paradigm—that we are, in Kuhn's sense, preparadigmatic.

A: I agree, in that I haven't seen the revolution that I want. And yet I am still so far beyond the pale of most of my older colleagues that I have a hard time interacting with them. It's not because I don't want to; it's because what is an issue for me and what are appropriate things to explore just aren't problems for them. In a sense I tried to lay that out in the motor-theory stuff I did (1977a), saying, Look, here's an alternative conceptual framework in terms of which I prefer to see the bone being kicked around. The other approach I've tried is by looking at methodology (Weimer, 1977b, 1979, 1980) and saying, Look, science isn't what you guys think it is, so why the hell do you bother doing that?

Q: Is motor theory like "top-down" processing? That idea is becoming very widespread in cognitive psychology.

A: Precisely.

Q: To what extent is your claim different from that?

A: The traditional approach in S–R psychology was a linear chaining model. The first step up from a chaining model is a hierarchical structure, which is another way of saying top-down processing. There is nothing in top-down processing that cannot be adequately explicated by a hierarchical model, if you spell it out. I claim that even the hierarchical model, even though it's an enormous increase in sophistication over chaining, is totally inadequate, and, at best, all that it can account for is a limited subsystem of a particular system, such as an aspect of the visual system. It cannot possibly account for the organization of the head as a whole.

Robert Shaw talks in terms of "coalitions" and "coalitional structures" (Shaw & McIntyre, 1974). He borrowed the terms from crazy old Heinz von Foerster at Illinois, one of the hoary old forefathers of automata theory, who was so beyond the pale in his field that they never claimed him.

Von Foerster's (1962) point is that there are coalitional structures that have as components a lot of hierarchical processing mechanisms. But the only way to understand the structured complexity of the whole is in terms that are, shall we say, devastating to the idea of the explanatory sufficiency of a hierarchy. If you take a hierarchical model and go to one of the higher branching points and disrupt it, according to the model, performance should be debilitated. Well, you know goddamned well that this does not happen to either a human being or an experimental animal in the physiology laboratory—if higher-level information is lost, the human being or animal still gets along quite well. We know that in rough terms, the Lashley (1929) equipotentiality notion is right! The decrement in performance of an experimental subject roughly correlates with how big a hole you make in its brain, not where the hole is located. Coalitions have the property that if you wipe out a node, the system has alternative ways of getting out the same responses. We are integrated in ways that are beyond the capabilities of a hierarchical structure. We still haven't learned Chomsky's message about explanatory power, in other words. Standard cognitive psychology is as far behind Chomsky as associationistic psychology was.

The motor-theory approach is the beginning of an attempt at looking at the structured complexity of an integrated nervous system. I have only one head, and it's both sensory and motor. It both acts and perceives, and my perception is actually action. This approach is at least potentially testable, and it seems to me infinitely more fruitful than the traditional sensory snippet stuff, as I have stigmatized the information-processing or sensory models in the motor theory article.

Michael A. Wapner:
The Vital, Invisible Role of Scientific Isolates

An unavoidable bias of this book is that it selects individuals who are widely recognized in the psychology community. They are generally highly intelligent and creative people. And yet there are unknown numbers of perhaps equally intelligent and creative individuals who are not recognized by the scientific community at large. Some members of the community are simply "desynchronized"—too far ahead or behind the rest of the group to share a genuine common language. But even more broadly, there are individuals who follow a valid direction all their own, which is, however, so different from the beaten path that it may *never* be recognized by the wider community. Such "scientific isolates" (see Esper, 1966) are often very interested, deeply committed individuals who have the strength to stand alone and bear the consequences of being out of step with their peers.

What is the function of scientific isolates in the development of science? One view might be that they play no role whatsoever—that they are a side show on the stage of history. But there is another way of viewing isolates which suggests that scientific development requires diversity as much as biological evolution does. In the evolution of a biological species, diversity is important; it creates flexibility for the future evolution of the species in the face of sudden, unpredictable changes in the environment. If in the evolution of genus *homo* there were no genetic variability with respect to brain size, our species would never have grown into *homo sapiens* — man with knowledge.

One can make the case that many of the "great" men and women in the history of science were isolates and nonconformists who happened to exist at a time when the community was ready for their contributions. It may be true that such men and women exist at all times, but that they simply are not recognized unless the community has encountered a crisis in the received approach. Einstein, for example, was clearly a noncon-formist — his career was going its own way, obscurely, when he wrote the early papers that ensured his fame. For some time, he walked together with the physical community. But when physicists turned to quantum mechanics, he balked for philosophical reasons, refusing to believe that "God played dice with the universe," and the majority of his colleagues deserted his path. Certainly Galileo, Copernicus, Kepler, Mendel, Darwin, Dalton, Pasteur, Priestley, Mendeleev, Pavlov, Freud, and other revolutionary personalities in the history of science might easily have been overlooked. The fact that they are so well known is not just of their own doing, but also a matter of being in the right place at the right time saying the right thing. How many Galileos and Darwins have not enjoyed the limelight of history?

If this point of view is correct, scientific isolates represent the gene pool from which the community, for better or worse, selects only a few exemplars to follow. They are the heirs-apparent waiting in the wings of history. Although only a few will ever be accorded great recognition, their invisible presence is necessary to present the scientific community with choices when it is confronted with some unresolvable fundamental problem along the lines described by Kuhn.

It may be inevitable that such individuals multiply toward the end of a shared community framework. They may be far quicker to spot the weaknesses of the conventional wisdom than others who place more value on their membership in the group. But, precisely because they are ahead of the norm in this respect, they risk their ability to be understood by others.

Michael A. Wapner (b. 1935) seems to be very much in this position. Having received his PhD from UCLA in 1965, when it was still a stronghold of behaviorism, he experienced a deep and continuing sense of dissonance toward psychology, including his own specialty, psychophysiology.

Wapner's ideas seem comparable in depth and interest to the other participants in this collection of interviews. Perhaps the most important of his ideas has emerged from Wapner's rejection of a "filter theory" of attention — the attempt to account for our apparently limited attention, for the fact that much information goes by us "unawares" (*e.g.*, Norman, 1976). "In fact," Wapner says, "the idea of a system rejecting [information] while being insensitive [to it] is a contradiction." And he argues that if a system *is* sensitive to information for the purpose of rejecting it, what is gained by rejecting it? As much processing capacity is needed to reject is as would be required to accept it, and thus rejection does not help to lighten the load on the system.

Wapner proposes, rather, that incoming information which is "unattended" becomes part of *the context* with respect to which the focal information is processed. It becomes part of the "ground." This viewpoint takes off from a weak spot in current cognitive theory and seems to lead in a potentially fruitful direction.

Cognitivists are engaged in the curious business of thinking about thinking. Very naturally, then, one's conclusions begin to affect the very process of investigation, and *vice versa*. Thus Michael Wapner's views on the nature of context begin to double back to influence his ideas concerning the nature of experiments, of theory, of science and knowledge.

In all, I believe this is an exciting interview, and one well worth rereading.

Interview with Michael A. Wapner

Q: How did you get started in psychology?

A: When I was an undergraduate, it was the time of the "New Look" in psychology (Bruner & Postman, 1947) and the idea that what one wanted or needed or expected influenced *what* one perceived. It was an extremely potent idea to me. It was part of the idea of the influence of language on perception, and of the Marxist idea of the influence of economics on perception. The whole idea of a relativism, a cognitive relativism, a perceptual relativism, an idea that somehow there was a *problem* about experience — it just got me.

When I got my bachelor's degree, I dropped out of psychology. I was going to go into psychiatry, partly because I was interested in doing therapy, but also because I was very disillusioned and really confused. Psychology didn't have the substance I was looking for. I *loved* the image of being a psychologist. That is an idea of a way of being that has always had such power in my life, but there wasn't anything tangible in psychology, except a lot of questions.

Q: What is a "psychologist" in your way of looking at it?

A: A psychologist is somebody whose central concern is the nature of life as it is lived. The idea that knowledge has a central place in lived human experience, as opposed to an academic, effete, scholastic kind of thing. It's really been an incredible image to me, really very important. When I finished my bachelor's degree, somehow psychology didn't do it. And so I got out. In fact, I was out of school for 3 years. I sold jewelry.

What I discovered was that I was not going to be able to exist at all outside of an academic setting. I just could not. I was not going to make it in business. People got bored hearing me talk about things that had nothing to do with business, and I got bored hearing them not talk about that stuff. So I went back to school. Anyway, I got taken by physiological psychology in graduate school, and particularly the Reticular Formation (Moruzzi & Magoun, 1949). The Reticular Formation was the soul, pure and simple, clearly and obviously. [*Note:* The Reticular Formation is a structure in the core of the brain stem and midbrain that seems intimately involved with the control of consciousness and attention.] Interestingly, the thing that I found significant about the Reticular Formation was different from what most people were seeing in it.

Many people at that time saw the Reticular Formation as an arousal mechanism, as a mechanism of "general drive," with no informational value at all. They talked about the primary sensory pathways as a kind of communication channel to the cortex, and about the Reticular Formation as mediating waking and sleeping and general arousal, but having *no* informational function. The Reticular Formation woke up the brain, and the sensory channels gave it information. But to me, what was really so significant about the Reticular Formation was its relation to perception in the absence of specificity. I knew goddamned well that all neural mechanisms of perception were not going to end up having the kind of specificity that people were looking for in the sensory systems.

Q: How do you see the way people are looking for specificity in sensory systems?

A: Well, it was clear that they were looking for a switchboard, and if it wasn't a naïve switchboard with a point-to-point correspondence, then it was a more sophisticated switchboard with a more complex neural code. It might be different for all the different senses, but its main function was still reliably to represent the world in the brain.

Of course the Reticular Formation couldn't perform that function because it is an area of incredible *convergence*, and also great *functional variability*. A verticular neuron responds in one way to an input if it's primed one way, but completely differently if it's primed a slightly different way; so that the responsiveness is highly contingent, as opposed to the supposedly higher reliability of the specific sensory areas. If you have a recording electrode in the brain of a cat, your *whole* response pattern is very changeable. Depending on how you look at it, that is, sure, there's a pattern. You throw away your transient changes in the neural activity — everybody throws away transients. If you hold all other things constant, after you get your system stabilized, then of course you have pretty good reliability, if you don't look too closely. But, if you pound the table, or if you tilt the apparatus that is holding the animal's head, or if your respirator is changed so that the amount of oxygen getting to the animal is changed, you get considerable variability — not to mention the variability you get when ordinary environmental stimulation is not controlled.

Of course these are all seen as experimental deficiencies, deficiencies of the preparation. But it seemed clear to me that they were more central. I think it was Warren McCulloch at MIT who talked about how you needed a perceptual system that was relatively insensitive to extraneous changes. But the system is *not* insensitive to extraneous changes. The system has *got* to change with background changes. You do not find a system that maintains some sort of mapping independent of large changes in input. Let me put it another way: The independence from extraneous changes is an *accomplishment of integration*, not of insulation.

Q: That's very interesting. Let me backtrack a little bit. What you're saying is that if you have something in the outside world, and the organism has to deal with it in a fairly invariant way, then that is a *result of* the neural process in the organism, and not some sort of ability of the nervous system to reject irrelevancy at a low level.

A: Yes. In fact, the idea of a system "rejecting while being insensitive" is a contradiction. And in fact, it's the central contradiction in the concept of "attention as a filtering mechanism" (*e.g.*, Broadbent, 1958, 1971). Filtering is based on the idea that the system must save information-processing capacity for other things, so somehow the system doesn't deal with everything, although it still has to process the stuff before it knows what to reject. That's a paradox, and a contradiction. I think it's the result of a central misunderstanding of how the thing works. The question of what the system does when it rejects, and what the system does when it is responsive, I've seen as a problem for a long time. In fact, that's why I've been very interested in neural habituation. For a long time it's been clear to me that habituation cannot be inhibition, because if the system is going to filter by inhibiting, then it's going to need every bit as much information to inhibit with precision, as it would to deal with the information in the first place! If I were to give you a pencil and say, "Cross out only these letters," you would need as much information about which letters to cross out as you would about which letters to leave in. It's no good for inhibition or habituation to be crossing out things.

Q: It does not save you any work.

A: That's right. So that habituation has to be another thing. What is it that happens when a change can occur in the environment that ordinarily the organism would be sensitive to, but which now has no stimulus-value for the organism? That's what happens in habituation, right? It's something that under other circumstances would have brought about a response, but now for some reason does not. And so we say the organism is habituated to the stimulus — but the idea that somehow the input's being filtered out or rejected is not viable. The other alternative is that the input is somehow *being included*, and that now, what's happening is that it's *constituting part of the ground*, part of the very code with respect to which whatever is being processed is being processed.

Q: You mean that it is presupposed? It becomes part of the context?

A: Yes, that's right. And that's a particularly powerful thing, because, you see, now that allows the organism not only to "attend" to something, but simultaneously to monitor what it's not attending to. Because an unexpected change in what's habituated brings about an alteration in what is being attended to, like a figure changes when you manipulate the ground. What happens is that when you alter ground gradually enough, a person may not know that you're altering ground, and he experiences it as a change in figure.

We know that the perception of color, brightness, and various things like that are relational. But you don't *experience* them as being relational; you experience them as absolute, because essentially one of the relata is taken as a constant, and the figure is experienced with respect to that.

Q: So you have the illusion that the object is changing, when in reality the context is changing?

A: We have to redefine what we mean by a perceptual object. An object is not simply an entity that is discreet and separate from ground regardless of context or frame of reference. The objects of experience are the results of particular stategies of differentiating ambient stimulation. So that an object is a very high-level abstraction. An object is a relational event, a relational thing. To experience "a change in ground" as a change in the object is not an illusion. Essentially, it is just calling on the inherent ambiguity in the entire system.

I'm expressing it in one way; you have structured it in another way, so you call my mode of expressing "an illusion." These are points of view that have really come up against the whole problem of the relationship between how a system is characterized and what are taken as absolute standards of measurement. Then the question arises: Well, if this relativity of perception is true, then what do you mean by a valid perception? How can there be any reliability, if every time I get hungry, somehow my world changes as a function of that? Or, if you speak a different language, you're seeing a different world? If you take it to its extreme, it's absurd. I think the reason a relativistic view has taken so long in gaining influence in psychology is that people have looked at the absurdity of what they saw as the logical extension of this relativity and have rejected it.

That's why I think the New Look in psychology was rejected, because the way people saw it, it had absurd implications. One of my concerns, then, was to see how, on the other hand, this kind of relativism could be incorporated in a way of thinking about perception that didn't make a mockery of *validity* and *solidity*. I'm not a solipsist — I don't want to argue that somehow everyone perceives a different world; that doesn't make any sense to me. So one of my real concerns was how to reconcile the relativistic and realistic aspects of perception. I think that is where cognitive psychology must go. If you take a kind of naïve realistic view, any contribution to perception that is made by expectation, by motivation, by need, has got to be an *interference* with valid perception. If perception is optimal when it is just a straight correspondence between the representation and the world, then any contribution by "need" has to influence it negatively, make it less accurate.

My feeling, however, is that *in the absence* of a contribution by what we'll call for now "need" or expectation, the stimulation is unstructured, and that it is a primary function of the cognitive process to introduce order. I could just as easily say *discover* order.

Q: To introduce bias.

A: That's right. There is an ambiguity in events, if you like, and it is the cognitive processes that essentially resolve the ambiguity and integrate it, so that out comes a coherent formulation. My feeling is that perception is the result of that process, and that vision, for instance, is to be understood as the achievement of integration of all of the influences inpinging on the organism.

Q: Not just visual input, not just light?

A: Yes, not at all just light. There's good reason to believe that there are all sorts of influences on vision. We know this, for instance: that there are kinesthetic influences on vision. We know that a person who's moving with respect to something perceived has to integrate the rate of his movement in order to perceive it with constancy.

Q: He has to compensate for the fact that he's moving.

A: That's right. And when he starts moving in a system for which he cannot compensate, his visual experience is distorted, as in seasickness. In seasickness, the movement of the ground, or the system within which the person finds himself, is so erratic that he cannot compensate. Until he compensates, his visual experience is disorganized, and he gets sick. A sailor "gets his sea legs" essentially when he integrates, *as context*, the movement of the ship and the water and the like, and when he functions with that as a stable, predictable ground. When the sailor goes on shore after an extended period of time at sea, he experiences much the same kind of pitching and instability on land, clearly an indication that he incorporated, as a stable criterion, the movement of the ship.

Q: To go back to what you were saying previously, it's not that the movement of the ship is being *inhibited*, but rather that it has become part of your way of analyzing the world.

A: Yes, exactly.

Q: And now, when he goes back on land —

A: He's got to reorganize. When he makes the transition more and more often, the reorganization itself becomes the higher-order process, so that eventually he can make it as often as necessary without being disturbed.

Q: But when he feels unstable as he first steps on land, he is actively processing "land" as if it were "sea," in a sense, and making predictions that are not true for the land experience. And you think this is a general process?

A: I think it's absolutely general. I think not only is it general in this sense, but it's clear that *conscious experience encompasses essentially the domain of mismatch*. That is, what constitutes the conscious experience are just those smaller changes that a person has to make in order to compensate for the misanticipations. And in those cases in which he anticipates perfectly, there is no conscious experience. I think the business of stabilized retinal images is just one example. If the retinal image is perfectly stable, the experience of it disappears.

By the way, I think this is really significant, with respect to another area that I think is much misunderstood: that is sensory deprivation. If a person has habituated to the whole ambience, if you then remove that ambience, essentially you're *stimulating* him. It's not deprivation, it's stimulation, because you're doing what you do whenever you stimulate a person. That is, you alter some aspect of the ambience that he's habituated to and require a reorganization. Only in sensory deprivation you don't give him the wherewithal for reorganization — he has nothing to organize *with*.

I think that's how you can understand memory in general. Memory is the reorganization of the coding schemes, in an attempt to find one that will make sense. Looking into the past is essentially reconciling the past with the present.

Q: In other words, memory is not primarily a question of storage.

A: It depends on what you mean by storage. Memory is not a storage device if by that you mean something within which records are placed so that they can be retrieved and somehow viewed again. All retrieval is *change* in the memory, and I think the evidence is good that to remember is to change what is remembered.

Q: But obviously there is some retention of something that happened originally. It's not as if it is completely a creation of the moment.

A: It's not that it's a creation of the moment, but when you say "retention", this is again the problem of identity.

Q: Can you say that in some other way?

A: The person who finds that his mode of organizing is not valid, because it keeps leading him into unfulfilled expectations and disappointments and surprises, has got to reevaluate and reorganize the basis of his expectations.

Q: So if you're a child and not much aware of things in your world, so that you expect things that are not true about the world, you're forced into doing something about it.

A: Yes, a child or anybody else. Piaget really talks about it beautifully. Piaget talks about the need of a child to find a way of viewing, so that when he takes another step and changes his relationship to the object that he's viewing, he doesn't come to see a different object. Piaget calls it objectification. For Piaget, objectification is the way in which the child achieves stability across changes in perspective.

Q: He has to find something in common among all those different perspectives.

A: That's the sense in which to remember is to change. To remember is not merely to change in terms of the moment, because then there would be no stability. But rather, to remember is to find the sense in which "now" *can be reconciled with* "before." So that one finds a different perspective, a reconciliation. To remember is a reinterpretation of the past. It's not to invalidate the memory, it's rather to integrate it with respect to the present. What is remembered is remembered primarily within the context of the present, so that you can predict the form of a memory by knowing what the person is doing when he's remembering (*e.g.*, Bransford, 1979).

It has to be that way. If memory did not operate with respect to the present, it would be totally dysfunctional. You'd be continually bombarded with memories that are totally irrelevant to what you're doing now. They have to be functional with respect to now. Not only that, but to the extent to which memory is problem-oriented, it has to not only be a representation of the past, but has to be a representation of the past *with respect to* the problem that you're confronting now.

When you rethink the past, or when you remember, essentially: *One*, it indicates a *problem* in the present. I think that's a general principle. You remember when you're in trouble, you remember when you're stymied, you remember when you're frustrated. *Two*, you remember with respect to the situation that you're in now, so that memory has this thing in common with perception, that it is also a function of context, it's a *perspective*. *Three*, not only is it a function of the context, but the very record is altered. The alteration is not somehow a wiping away of the previous thing and now it changes, but it's altered in the sense that the "now" and the "then" is reorganized.

To remember is a commitment. It is a commitment to make a change that has implications beyond the immediate memory. You are now confronted with things that have to be changed to be made consistent. I think this has very strong implications for repression and for clinical pathological processes. It becomes very Freudian, in the sense that you have to rework old assumptions in order to reorganize your adjustment to the present.

An analogy would be a broken leg that heals badly. You don't know that it's healing *badly*, it's just healing. And given the way it heals, you make accommodations in posture, and given the accommodations in posture, you may start finding that you have calluses on your feet and pains in your toes. When you get to the place where you have pains in your toes, your problem is an adjustment that you made way back, which seemed to be quite a good adjustment at the time you made it. It is only problematic now. What you have to do is rebreak the leg and get it to heal better.

Q: At some point, perhaps we should go back to some of your personal experiences of the changes in psychology.

A: I would be happy to. It's not a thing that comes very easily to me, first of all because I don't think I've really come to terms yet with my experiences in psychology so far. One of the things I think is both my strength and a terrible weakness, in a way, is that I have not been much influenced by anybody. As a student, I found it impossible to apprentice myself to anybody.

In a way, what I was talking about in terms of memory is a kind of a picture of me. In a sense, I take each step, and with each step I redefine where I've been, or I define where I've been for the first time, maybe.

In this respect, by the way, teaching has been an absolute godsend. In the class, I have the most patient audience I have ever had. I like to think that it's not just because they're a captive audience, but that a kind of rapport is generated, so they're extremely patient with me. In 10 or 15 weeks, I'm able to define a context within which I can start talking. Nobody else is patient enough to listen to me long enough to allow me to define what I'm saying. I have not been able to say it cogently and explicitly and quickly. I've tried to write, and I have, what is that phrase you use, it's really beautiful — "a combinatorial explosion." My writing is that. I write a few pages, and the next few pages after that will comment on the previous pages, and then the next few pages will comment on the preceding pages. I'm just searching for a stable point with respect to which I can go on without having to keep redefining what I just said. Talking and especially lecturing — I've been able to do that.

Q: Would you say that behaviorism was in fact an extension of logical positivism?

A: Yes. The program was formulated — well, I was going to say, long before the data was in. But of course it had to have been before the data was in, because when the data started to accumulate, behaviorism went down the drain. It is clear that it never had the data to substantiate its position, so that it was clearly a program. It was a moral position. It was an ethical and moral position about the nature of the way psychology was to be done. The nature of the kinds of things that could be said, and by extension, the nature of what there was in the world to be explained. You said it, it was an extension of positivism in that respect.

I think people like Spence essentially attacked the way other people did psychology. One of the things that comes to mind is the Spence attack on Kurt Lewin. Lewin was, I think, one of the most brilliant psychologists in the 20th century, without doubt, and clearly one of the forerunners of cognitive psychology. The Spencian attack on him was that Lewin had an R–R approach rather than an S–R approach, therefore he could not make the kinds of predictions that one could with an S–R approach, because he did not have a well-defined independent variable. He could only predict one dependent variable based on another dependent variable (that's an R–R approach). Spence paid no attention to the incredible breadth and depth of the phenomena that Lewin was able to deal with, or at least was able to *talk about* and to make an approach to dealing with. I don't know Spence, and maybe I'm doing him an injustice, but from the way it looked to me, he really rejected it out of hand for quite doctrinaire reasons. He was going to prescribe what psychology could be and would be.

Q: Who changed, for example?

A: I think of James Deese as one person who, in his book *Psychology as Science and Art* (1972), really expresses extreme reservations about the viability of the whole position that was taken by his old brand of psychology. I think an incredible thing was the Koch article (1959). Here's Sigmund Koch, who's commissioned to do a survey of psychology at midcentury, doing seven volumes of *Psychology: The Study of a Science* (1959), and essentially he writes this chapter talking about psychology as having trivialized the whole human experience, being essentially bankrupt — psychology not only having nothing to offer, but having so obscured the issues that it's been more a hindrance than a contribution. Really incredible. By the way, I don't think Koch is a cognitive psychologist. I think Koch just essentially rejected what he felt to be wrong.

Q: Do you view behaviorism in an entirely negative light?

A: No. In fact, I think it was part of a process; it was almost good that psychology went through it. The feelings that I have about it, maybe, are strong, but they do reflect a personal experience as well. At the time when I was first thinking about those things — in '57, '58, '59 — it was a disturbingly common experience to try to tell somebody about what I was thinking about, and having them say to me, "Well, *that's mentalistic*." I was brought up short, and made to feel that I would not be able to express what I was thinking, because somehow I could not couch it within the forms that were provided by this way of thinking.

Q: What does "mentalism" mean from a behavioristic viewpoint, as a criticism?

A: One thing it meant was that the person who was listening to you did not have much faith in your ability to translate what you were talking about into operational terms — to do an experiment. Actually, in discussing experiments I may have introduced — not an irrelevancy, but not quite the right point. The very idea that two people in psychology cannot have a long discussion without immediately thinking about how it's going to be translated into an experiment is itself an incredible constraint on thought. The idea that it is somehow anathema to just talk, without, for the moment, worrying about whether you can perform the experiment! And it isn't just a matter of talking to other people, because that mode of thought gets internalized so that it becomes the way you think even when you're alone. You find that there's an incredible constriction in the breadth of thought that psychologists are willing to entertain because some idea doesn't allow itself to be translated into an experiment immediately.

Q: Why is it so difficult to translate our thoughts into experiments?

A: I think that psychology, for one, has totally misinterpreted the significance of the experiment in science. It is a caricature of empiricism carried to a bizarre absurdity. The idea that the only meaningful conclusions that you can come to are somehow the *results of* experiments, and that the only meaningful statements that you can make are somehow those that can be translated *into* experiments—it's ludicrous.

Q: Let me play devil's advocate: What's so hard about putting things into experiments? Why couldn't you put notions such as "reward" into an experiment—what is the difficulty there?

A: Turn the question around and say, What is the advantage of *thought* over *action*? That is, why is it that we have some advantage by being able to think about something without having to do it before thinking about it? Because to do an experiment, you have to deal with things that are largely irrelevant to the main thrust of your thought, so that it may take years to get the apparatus functioning to finally operationalize something that you thought years back.

Now, of course, conversely, operationalizing in that respect is really a very good check to the extremes of thought that allow you to slip over and ignore what in fact cannot occur. That's what's great about computers. You're forced to make explicit things that you never thought were relevant, and you realize then that it can't be done, for reasons that you didn't think were connected with your problems.

I'm not throwing experiments out, but on the other hand, take any fairly complex proposition, and think about how many aspects of that proposition are in principle testable. If you wanted to question *every aspect* that you could think of, any single complicated proposition would have more testable aspects than you could test in a lifetime. That is, how many things must in fact be true for the proposition to be true as a whole? Any noun–predicate combination has so many assumptions—that *this* is in fact the case, and that *that* is an instance of the more general class of things, and that *these* are to be found together, and so forth. But it's not necessary to do all that.

Q: You're saying that explicit empirical verification of every proposition is not required.

A: Yes. The absolute distinction between thought and observation
is invalid. The idea that there are some ideas that are somehow the result
of activities occurring only in the head, and therefore, are not a reflection of what's going on in the world, and that there are other ideas that
are somehow a direct representation of something in the world, that are
"empirical" — that distinction is baloney. The fact of the matter is, as we
know from cognitive psychology, that the very act of experiencing is in
some sense a prediction. Perception always involves an expectation, a
proposition put to the world, such that it is in some sense confirmed or
not confirmed. The very act of thought has an ongoing empirical dimension; it is always being tested.

On the other hand, the most empirical of empirical statements has
a *rational* dimension, in the sense that there are no purely empirical observations that are independent of assumptions that are not totally present
in the world.

What that does, then, is to reintroduce, in a different way, the role
of thought. Thought can encompass things that ultimately, in principle,
are not encompassable in experiments. So that thought is no longer merely that process by which you put together the data of a whole bunch of
different experiments. Thought becomes some process that takes you
places where experiments can never take you, and generates a kind of
data that must *complement* the data of experiments. That's why I think
the demand that everything that you want to talk about be operationalizable is essentially an unrealistic one. If you demand it too stringent-
ly, it ultimately is stultifying to your science.

The analogy that I use in class is of a wagon train heading West,
and it's approaching some mountains. The people in the wagon train
are fearful of Indians and snow and all sorts of terrible things. They send
scouts out to explore the mountains and to see whether it's favorable to
cross there, or whether they ought to go around to some other place. The
scouts go up into the mountains and look at the ground and the surround-
ings. All of a sudden they get so interested in the rocks and mountains
that they become geologists. They stick around studying the ground.
That's all very interesting and very nice. No one can fault them for being interested in geology. Meanwhile, the wagon train has to fend for
itself without the kind of information and intelligence that it needs.

In some sense, psychology has done that kind of thing. Psychology
is essential because it has to deal with aspects of human experience that
are problematic and which we are worried about — aspects that we cer-

tainly would like to know a little bit about, so that we could deal with them, or at least know how to think about them. To the extent to which that's important, then all the programs of psychology and its methodology are important.

To the extent to which *methodology becomes criterial*, and the extent to which the particular internal issues become important, the stream of human experience is abandoned. But that's not the whole story, because that is not to imply that the geologists who are in the mountains are not also humans. What has happened is that now *their* circumstance becomes the context of human experience. That is, they *become* their own wagon train. One of the things that happens, then, is that to the extent to which the meaning of experience is a function of the ongoing context, the people in the original wagon train will have a different context from the people up in the mountains. What you have here is the origin of separate cultures. To the extent to which they all cling to and pursue to increasing depth their respective interests and languages, you have a fragmentation. So that what is discovered in one context is communicable to the other only with great difficulty, if at all. Even if the scouts did come back and tried to tell the wagon train what they had found, it would be like somebody coming back after five or six generations, having evolved a whole new language. Now, having something important to say, they find that they just don't know how to communicate it bvecause their whole way of thinking about things has changed. It's not even clear whether they're still talking about the same problem anymore.

One of the things that's important about teaching psychology is that students come in with interests, with concerns — they come to psychology because presumably it's got to do with their experiences — and rather than psychology having answers or ways of thinking about their experiences, students of psychology are asked in effect to *give up* their way of structuring their experience, and to restructure their experience in a way that psychology can deal with. So it's not so much that we have answers to the students' questions, but that we demand that they *reformulate* their questions in a way consistent with our methodology.

This may well be true of all disciplines; it may well be a characteristic of structure. I think that this involves an extremely fundamental principle in the genesis of universes. When I say "the genesis of universes," I mean physical universes as much as mental, although actually I mean that there isn't a distinction to be made. It's a way in which *differentiation* takes place, insofar as a substructure evolves from within a parent structure, such that the substructure becomes too complex for the parent structure to accommodate. And when the parent structure can no longer accommodate it, there's a separation and fragmentation, and they become separate structures. When they become separate, simultaneously they generate a space that may accommodate the two of them. That's what I mean by the generation of universes. I mean this is not only true with respect to the birth of an organism, for instance, but I think that this happens in the growth of plants, in budding and the like. I also think that it is a fundamental principle in the genesis of physical systems.

Q: The behaviorists were very sympathetic to Bridgman's operationalism (1927) precisely because they felt that it was the unstated *presuppositions* that people had about psychology which could lead us astray, and we would start asking the wrong questions. They focused on experiments, very much because they suspected the assumptions of common sense.

A: That's a very good point. It's really interesting that you bring up Bridgman. I think Bridgman is really focal to this whole thing. His initial idea was that one could overcome the problem of the revolutionary experience that Einsteinian physics generated for physicists by operationalizing the theoretical constructs of physics, and he suggested that one should equate a *concept* with an *operation*. When one speaks of "distance" or "time" or "space," one has to specify the concrete way in which one means it. It's an expression of a hope that is not realizable, but it is not necessary for it to be realizable.

Let me put it another way. Korszybski (the founder of the General Semantics movement) proposed something really quite analogous. Korszybski suggested that when we speak of John, the person, that really we're speaking quite ambiguously. We could mean John today, John yesterday, John at 20, John at 30, John as a child, John in New York, John in San Francisco. And what we really ought to do is *date* and *localize* our reference, so that when we say John, we have a subscript, and it's "John, as referred to on January 23rd in San Francisco," and the like. That is quite like Bridgman, because he's saying you have to specify what it is you mean when you say something. But, of course, the problem in both cases is that there's a failure to grasp the significance of a concept. John becomes a concept because it is some abstraction that can be found either in San Francisco or New York. A concept is a potent device precisely because it *doesn't* demand that you do that, and precisely because it accomplishes things that can never be accomplishable in those terms.

Two points. One point is this: to demand that you label your concepts is to fail to recognize that "January 23rd" is equally a concept, and that "New York" is equally a concept, and that you have not overcome the problem by adding labels, because the labels are also concepts! If I were then to ask the question, "What do you mean by San Franscisco? Do you mean San Francisco on January 23rd, do you mean San Francisco as limited by the city limits, or do you mean greater San Francisco?" And so forth. Then you find that what you have thought to be delimiting is only a delimiting process insofar as you don't look at your operation, because the operation also turns out to be abstract! Precisely the same thing with Bridgman. Bridgman can demand operational definition as long as nobody asks him for an operational definition of the operational definition, because he can't provide it.

Q: For example, as in "What is a ruler?"

A: Precisely. A central issue is that rulers function only as insofar as you don't demand that they be operationalized along *all* possible dimensions. That is, there are aspects of experience that must not be questioned in order that other aspects of experience be questionable.

Q: You can't specify context exhaustively?

A: That's right. Also it means, that what constitutes *context* and what constitutes *content* is not fixed.

It goes back to experiments. Experiments are only meaningful to the extent to which the experimenter and the people for whom the experiment is being done share a common frame of reference, such that there are things that are unquestioned. That's what is untenable about behaviorism, and I think that's what is salutary and important about the cognitive revolution: namely, that it's a rediscovery of the fact that there are always implicit dimensions, and that there are conditions under which you can in fact demand too much. It's meaningless to talk about something without presuppositions. In fact, I think it gets to the fundamental relationship between presuppositions (or context) and data such as empirical statements coming out of experiments. The behaviorist bias comes out of the positivism of the Newtonian era — the idea that one had to rid oneself of the idiosyncracies of particular perspectives, particular frames of reference. To the extent to which a statement could be made that was not a function of a particular frame of reference, it was objective, and if it was not objective, it was invalid. Now, in a sense, the behaviorist–positivist point of view was an attempt to totally rid oneself of this kind of contextual or implicit information. But it's not possible to rid oneself of context: more importantly, *without context, there are no data*.

Titchener and Wundt did not recognize the extent to which their views of conscious contents was very much a function of their particular technique, their particular mode of introspection. Under the attack, for instance, of people who believed in "imageless thought," they got embroiled in very provincial kinds of controversy, trying to defend and reiterate the legitimacy of their methodology. And so it became sterile in that respect. It didn't go on, they were defensive.

The behaviorists can be seen, then, as people who threw up their hands and said, Look, *forget it*! It's just not profitable to continue that controversy. They said, Before I let you ask those kinds of questions, I want you to show me what it is you mean in some tangible way that allows me to deal with it. So in that respect I think the behaviorist movement was really good.

Also, it brought in the whole issue of the significance of evolution in psychology. Essentially, what behaviorism said was, We need a technique and a psychology that does not so totally separate human experience and activity from the animal domain. That is, the whole business of consciousness as *the* issue in psychology, without any clear relationship to behavior, was an anti-evolutionary point of view, an antibiological point of view. I don't know about the story about Watson being more comfortable with animals than with people—but I think nonetheless that behaviorism was good in that respect. For instance, it did create a bridge between psychology in America and what Pavlov was doing.

Q: What is consciousness from your point of view?

A: Consciousness, I think, is going to be *the process within which changes of context occur*. I think consciousness is going to be that process within which structures evolve. To the extent to which to perceive is to reorganize forms of perception, consciousness is a manifestation of the ongoing change in the relationship between what is taken to be the object of perception and what is taken to be the process of perception.

The analogy that I use is between consciousness and energy. Say you look at "heat" in terms of a bunch of molecules in a bottle, and you ask, Where in that bottle is the energy? It is not *in* any of the objects, but it is that which is generated by the reorganization and rearrangement of the objects. Now I go one step further, and I say even that is superficial, because from a relativistic point of view, it is not strictly the relationship among the objects that is to be thought of as energy, but in fact one has to realize that it is in the very *definition* of the object that energy is involved. The differentiation between an object and a relationship is not a final differentiation. There are some points of view with respect to which what you have called an object will end up from another point of view to be part of a relationship. So that the very identity of objects and relationships is subject to change. That's a thing that modern psychology has not yet come to.

I see experiments as a *transaction*, as really what people like Ittleson and the Transactionalists have been saying (Allport, 1955). It's an act of communication. The experimenter has a way of structuring *his* experience. You then measure something about the ability of the experimenter to *manipulate* to bring the subject around.

Traditionally, the experiment has been structured so that the experimenter's way of structuring the world is not subject to question. *That* constitutes the world. To the extent to which the subject deviates from that, you say that he's inadequate, that it's a limitation, he has failed to learn, he doesn't perceive appropriately or accurately or something of that sort.

But it's clear that there are other situations in which you could allow the *experimenter's* way of structuring the world to vary as a function of interacting with the subject, and indeed that does happen, but typically it happens *across* experiments rather than *within* experiments. So when an experimenter finds that the subject is not responding well to the set of stimuli that he's got, in the next experiment he'll define the stimuli differently, which is to say that the subject's way of structuring the world has now communicated itself to the experimenter, and now the experimenter has *changed* his way of structuring. But it doesn't get reported that way.

For example, the "gambler's fallacy" is based on the assumption that the way we psychologists break up probabilities is somehow the "real" way, so that if a person sees nine heads come up in a row, it's a fallacy to bet on the tails just because it's improbable that ten heads in a row will ever come up. So we call that the "gambler's fallacy" without realizing that it's really an alternative way of structuring, and it's not until one brings up the whole problem of what you *mean* by "the domain of events" in probability theory that you realize that the gambler's fallacy hasn't been a stupid way to structure the world, it's been an alternative way that has some validity within some context. The gambler simply defines his domain over 10 trials, whereas the psychologist looking on defines it from trial to trial.

Q: You say that motivation is really just an aspect of the way in which we structure our experience of the world. But motivations certainly don't completely constrain experience — if that were so, our wishes would dictate our experiences.

A: It's not that motivations completely constrain our experience. They do not constrain. What you're misunderstanding, and what's critical, is that motivations do not constrain, in the sense that they impose form. Motivation is *the process by which we attempt* to achieve consistent form across all the domains of our experience, all of the contexts of our experience. So that if I come to conclusions in one area that lead me to structure my beliefs and my attitudes and my knowledge in a certain way, there may very well be experiences that will not fit. Either I was talking about, How would you know it if a person were not talking to you from your context? That is, how would you know when there is a violation of context? I think *emotion is fundamentally the experience of violation of context* and the reorganization to a new context. That is, an emotional experience is fundamentally a transition.

Q: But then emotion is closely related to your definition of consciousness.

A: Absolutely. What I'm saying is that perception is essentially an emotional event, in that what one is aware of is the process of experiencing violation of, and readjustment to, new situations. So that emotions tend to be those instances of violations of context that are sufficiently drawn out between the violation and the resolution, that we give them names. But it's clear, for instance, that the physiological symptoms of emotional experience are closely related to the orienting reflex (a physiological measure of conscious surprise). The orienting reflex is just the arousal response to a novel stimulus. You get heart-rate changes, changes in galvanic skin response, and brain-wave changes. What it indicates is discontinuity.

Research on emotion indicates that an emotional event must, on the one hand, be a violation. On the other hand, what you call the emotion that you had — whether it's a happy, sad, or disappointing thing — depends on the new context within which you have to resolve the violation. They've done studies, for instance, where they've given people adrenalin unbeknownst to the subjects, and then whether the resulting feeling is interpreted as fear or anger seems to depend on the concomitant context — whether it's reasonable to be afraid or to be angry in that situation (Schachter & Singer, 1962).

The experience of emotion is the same kind of transition that underlies perception, but extended over longer time periods.

Motivation I really see as a process of attempting to achieve some kind of integrity across contexts. "Meaning" is contextually constrained, but no person lives his entire life within a single context, nor can one person leave all the information that he's gained in one context *in* that context and go form a new life in another context. So the problem is that you're carrying things from one context to the next. You bring in expectations that are going to be violated precisely because it's not appropriate in the new context. Then you have to not only define it for the new context, but you're going to have to *redefine* it with respect to the old context. That's what we talked about as "memory," memory being that process of redefining the past in terms of the present. If you successfully do that, you find the ways in which the old and new contexts are similar. That is, you're uniting them, you're integrating them. So motivation is that process by which antagonistic contexts are integrated in order to preserve the integrity of the organism. I think that can be applied not only to motivations such as needs to know or to achieve in art, science, or the like, but it can be applied to hunger and thirst as well.

Q: I'm interested in what kinds of changes you have noticed in people during the change from behavioral to cognitive thinking—people who attempted to adjust to the shift.

A: I think there really is a very significant personal toll that it takes, not unrelated to the "paradigm-shift." It's not a shift to a new, well-defined area. That is, there's a whole, ill-defined transition period when it's not at all clear what's happening.

Q: It may be that now that we know what behaviorism is, we still don't really know what cognitive psychology is.

A: That's why we won't let the issue of behaviorism die. That's why we keep hoping there are real behaviorists, so we can flog them still, so we can define ourselves by them.

Q: Talking about flogging behaviorists, behaviorists define themselves by a set of pejoratives, which they apply to the introspectionists. Do cognitive psychologists do the same thing *vis-à-vis* behaviorism?

A: I think the most damning thing that can be said about behaviorism is that it trivialized experience and that therefore it really did contribute to alienation. One of the tenets of the cognitive or structuralist approach is that the very things that you can think about and deal with are a function of the ways you have of thinking about them. When you have a science, a context that has a set of categories, it determines the aspects of experience that you'll be able to deal with. The question becomes, "What happens to aspects of experience that you *cannot* fit into those grooves?" What happens is that those aspects of experience are rejected, externalized, denied; they are problematic and lead to problems in experience in the same way that unacceptable sexual thoughts led to repression or pathology in Freud's time.

The purpose of knowledge, as I see it, is to give form to experience. It is for that reason that knowledge must be active, vital, and progressive. Not all ways of thought will do justice to all experiences. The question then becomes: What happens when you are adapted to old modes of experiencing, and you start confronting new possibilities of experience that don't fit? You're put into a terrible conflict.

It's not that you *repress* hard-to-understand experiences, in the sense that you'll grab them and push them down. There will continue to be a problematic aspect, unstable and ill-defined, which is continually bringing about emotions that cannot be resolved, and continually demanding different attempts to structure it in order to contain it. You are not free to structure the new situation in any arbitrary way, because the new structures cannot violate what is already structured.

In the extreme you get the belief structure of a paranoid schizophrenic. You have a person who is desperately attempting to order and contain his experience, and who is forced into increasingly grand, complex, and intricate schemes for the sake of consistency. From this basis, it *cannot* be consistent, and so the person is *not* safe from the anxiety, is torn by anxiety, except to the extent to which he severely restricts the areas of his life experience. It's just pathological in that for the individual there is no resolvable way of thinking about it.

In the whole positivist and empiricist movement, you assume that there's a real-life set of experiences, and there's another set of experiences which have to do with fantasy. Fantasy is not real, but perception *is* real. Therefore, if there are big hunks of your life that you have to attribute to fantasy, somehow you have to separate fantasy from reality. If it's acceptable, OK. If you engage in fantasy (maybe if you daydream), to the extent to which you confuse reality with daydreams you're in trouble. But I think it's quite clear that the value of a fantasy life is precisely that it penetrates into your experience of reality, and *thereby* you get the benefit. And yet, what you're calling the reality keeps some constraint on fantasy, so you have this interchange. That's one of the things we were talking about before: the necessity to claim that there are empirical observations which are somehow uncontaminated by personal perspective. There's the need to deny the reflection of oneself in the context of one's knowledge. So that the knowledge of reality is separated from one's whole personal dynamics. But of course they're not indefinitely separable.

7

The Nucleators:
Contributors from Outside Psychology

In a scientific revolution, outsiders to the community can sometimes exercise great influence, because they often do not suffer from the conceptual barriers held by most members of the community. Sometimes they can bring helpful techniques or ideas from other disciplines, or show the relevance of whole new domains of evidence. This was very much the case with the cognitive revolution. When things had stabilized somewhat, the very landscape and boundaries of psychology had been altered. Suddenly linguistics, computer science, and even parts of philosophy were seen to be directly relevant to the pursuit of psychology. These fields had previously been held at arms' length, but now they were suddenly considered to be very relevant to the new psychology.

It is this *redefinition* of the boundaries of the community that concerns us in this chapter. In physics a "nucleator" is a particle that provides a center for other particles to gather about, much as a dust mote in the atmosphere will, under the right conditions, cause water vapor to condense and crystallize to create a snowflake. Because we do not have an existing word to convey this meaning, we borrow the term "nucleator" to refer to those outsiders who provided the focus for a new "psychological" subcommunity outside the old boundaries, which the new psychology saw as very central to its own concerns.

The four Nucleators interviewed in this chapter have contributed as much to our understanding of human beings as any "indigenous" member of the psychological community. Noam Chomsky singlehandedly created a cognitive revolution in linguistics, and thereby influenced the psychology of language in major ways. Herbert A. Simon has made historic contributions to economics (for which he received a Nobel Prize in 1976), to political science, and (in collaboration with Allen Newell and others) to computer science, and to psychology as well. Jerrold A. Fodor received his doctorate in the philosophy of science, but he also collabo-

rated on several classic experiments in psycholinguistics. He is currently a major philosopher of psychology, attempting to state the cognitive
view as precisely as possible from a philosophical perspective.

Our last interview looks to the future. Donald A. Norman came from
graduate work in electrical and computer engineering, and he has made
notable contributions to the study of memory, attention, and action. He
is one of the founders of the Cognitive Science Society, which attempts
to encourage an integrated approach to cognition, combining psychology,
Artificial Intelligence, linguistics, and philosophy. This new interdisciplinary field has sometimes been very fruitful in the past, and it may
continue to work well in the future. Norman is optimistic about a new
integration of psychological thinking under the aegis of cognitive science.

Noam Chomsky:
The Formal Inadequacy of Behavioristic Theory

Noam Chomsky's historic work in the study of language has no exact
parallel in experimental psychology. The field of linguistics, which was
behavioristic in orientation, went through its own "cognitive revolution"
as a direct result of Chomsky's work. Further, Chomsky (b. 1928) defined
a new goal for linguistics as a discipline, and demonstrated a methodology
for working toward that goal. In the process he also developed a set of
trenchant theoretical criticisms of general behaviorism, which had significant impact on the cognitive shift in scientific psychology.

The major events of Chomsky's career have a curiously accidental
quality. His early major work, *The Logical Structure of Linguistic Theory*,
although written in the 1950s, was not published until 1975. Instead,
a European publisher, who happened to learn of Chomsky's ideas, published a set of lecture notes under the title *Syntactic Structures* (1957). As
I mentioned earlier, this book essentially triggered the shift in linguistics
by its elegant refutation of several types of grammar that were, at the
time, thought to be viable. But, in part, the impact of this book was the
result of a fortuitous review by Robert Lees (1957) in the central journal *Language*. Lees became Chomsky's first influential disciple. Soon
thereafter, George A. Miller discovered Chomsky, and became his advocate among psychologists. And, finally, in 1958, Bernard Bloch, editor
of *Language*, asked Chomsky to write a review of B. F. Skinner's new book
Verbal Behavior (1957). Chomsky's review (1959) was highly critical, suggesting that behavioristic approaches *of any kind* were inadequate in principle to explain some of the very basic properties of language. In fact,
Chomsky's review of Skinner's *Verbal Behavior* has been far more influential than the book itself. His argument was ultimately extended beyond

language by Bever, Fodor, and Garrett (1968) to behavioristic theory in general.

Since that time, Chomsky has published other major works on phonology (Halle & Chomsky, 1968), on Transformational Generative Grammar (1965), on the history of linguistics, and a number of non-technical works on political issues such as the war in Vietnam. For our purposes, however, the early work is the most important, especially the criticisms of the formal inadequacy of behavioristic theory. Even though serious debate still exists about many of his specific theoretical proposals, there is little disagreement about Chomsky's general views, especially his formal arguments against behavioristic theory.

Chomsky's arguments are basically simple. First, language is not an entity that can be learned word-for-word. Chomsky and Miller (1958) estimated that a speaker of English can understand and produce more sentences than there are seconds in a lifetime, indicating that these sentences could not possibly be learned individually — they must be *generated* as symbol strings from a far simpler set of powerful rules, analogous to the rules of algebra. Indeed, Chomsky has defined the task of linguistics as the discovery of a "grammar," a set of rules that will generate all and only the correct sentences in a language.

The mathematical Theory of Automata permits one to specify the explanatory power of theories of various complexity, from a simple string of elements (a Markov Process) to a somewhat more complex hierarchical theory (equivalent to a tree-diagram), to a Transformational Grammar (effectively, a tree-diagram that is mapped into another tree-diagram). A Transformational Grammar is equivalent to a Turing Machine, which, as I say in Chapter 4, is capable in principle of computing *any* function, and therefore has maximum explanatory power.

Superficially, language looks like a string of symbols. But using Automata Theory, one can show that certain simple changes in a string of symbols must be explained by mathematical "machines" more powerful than Markov chains. Many behavioristic theories were effectively Markov chains. For example, Hull's account of goal-directed activity suggested that it could be explained by a *string* of internal stimuli and responses (r_g-s_g). If any behavioristic theory is effectively a subset of Markov chains, and if Markov chains are inadequate, it follows that behavioristic theories in general are not adequate to explain human processes.

A sentence appears superficially to be a chain of words. To account for the syntactic relationships in a single sentence, we need a tree-diagram (Figure 7-1). (This is just what many people have learned in grammar school as "diagramming a sentence.") But to explain the relationship between *two* related sentences, such as an active and a passive sentence,

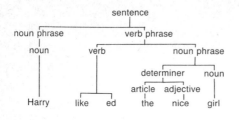

Figure 1. A tree diagram representing the constituents of a sentence and their relations to each other. Chomskyan theory suggests that only surface syntactic relationships can be represented by a single tree diagram, and that another, "deeper" tree is needed to represent other properties, such as the true subject and object of a sentence. From Postal (1964, p. 250).

we need a theory that will permit one tree to be related to another; and this is precisely what a Transformational Grammar is designed to do.

Chomsky also rediscovered a class of syntactic ambiguities in which the basic tree-diagram does *not* reveal the underlying ambiguity. Thus, there seemed to be syntactic information that required additional theoretical mechanisms. Specifically, there are "deep-structure" ambiguities in which the real subject or object of the sentence is ambiguous. For example,

    1. Visiting relatives can be boring.

— is it the act of going to visit relatives that is boring, or is it the relatives themselves? Or, consider another example,

    2. Flying planes can be dangerous.

— are the planes dangerous to onlookers, or is the act of flying the planes dangerous? To provide more evidence for the claim that simple tree-structures by themselves cannot describe all of the syntactic phenomena in a sentence, Chomsky also cites pairs of sentences such as the following, which have very *similar* surface structure, but very different underlying assignment of subject and object:

    3. John is easy to please.
          versus
    4. John is eager to please.

Notice that in the first case, "John" is the object of the verb, but in the next sentence, "John" is the subject of the verb. In all these cases, Chomsky argues, there must be another syntactic tree (called a "deep structure") that can represent the real difference between superficially similar sentences. The deep structure is, roughly speaking, related to the *meaning* of the sentence. A grammar that contains both a deep and surface structure needs to show the relationship between these two levels of representation: This is accomplished, in Chomsky's theory, by rules called transformations, and the resulting grammar is called a Transformational Generative Grammar.

Today there still exists considerable disagreement as to whether

Transformational Grammar tells us the actual set of rules people use in language, but there is now good agreement that any human grammar must have the formal power of a Transformational Grammar. All grammars used in Artificial Intelligence systems that are able to simulate human linguistic functions are formally equivalent to Transformational Grammars.

It is difficult to exaggerate the impact of Chomsky's work. In effect, he fundamentally restructured the approach to language in linguistics and in experimental psychology. For about a decade after Chomsky's first book, psychologists of language defined their enterprise in good part as a pursuit of the "psychological reality" of linguistic rules. In retrospect, this seems to be a questionable enterprise, given that linguistics itself deals with psychological evidence, though not experimental evidence. We need no experiment to tell us that sentences 1 and 2 presented earlier are ambiguous. Nevertheless, psycholinguistic work in pursuit of Chomskyan rules was valuable, because it gave psychologists experience with far more powerful theories than they had yet permitted themselves to use.

Interview with Noam Chomsky

Q: How did you get involved in linguistics?

A: I have an unusual history for a linguist. I had a very unconventional training, and I suppose that I would not be regarded as having professional qualifications. I did study linguistics as an undergraduate at Penn. I studied there with Zelig Harris, who was rather unconventional himself. After receiving a master's degree at Penn I went off to Harvard, where I was in the Society of Fellows. I didn't study any formal linguistics there. What course work I did was mostly in philosophy and logic, and I was working pretty much on my own. So I was very much outside of the field.

Not surprisingly, I was unemployable and I couldn't publish much. Virtually everything I published in the early years was either out of the country or in another discipline. The only major book I wrote at the time was not published until 1975. That was called *The Logical Structure of Linguistic Theory*. I submitted it for publication in 1966 and it was rejected. I did not pursue it very much because I thought the conclusion of the publishers was reasonable. It was so exotic that it didn't make much sense for it to be published at the time.

Q: It was circulated in manuscript form for many years, is that right?

A: Yes, George Miller had a copy. In fact, I think he had the only copy, which he rescued from a fire in Memorial Hall in 1955. He went plunging into the flames to pull it out, so I was told. Yes, it was circulated some, but it wasn't published for about 20 years.

Q: But did *Syntactic Structures* (1957) come out of that book?

A: Not really. *Syntactic Structures*, which came out in Europe, was more or less the class notes for undergraduate courses that I taught here at MIT. I may have changed it a little bit to make it more accessible to an audience of linguists, but fundamentally it was oriented toward MIT undergraduates. There were mathematicians here, and that's one of the reasons incidentally why there was a discussion of topics such as Finite-State Markov sources, which were a big thing here at that time. But they had not shown up much in linguistics.

Finite-State Markov sources and similar models were very highly regarded at the time. There was a lot of euphoria about such approaches to language. In part, it came from the prestige and achievements of information theory, which involved similar notions; in part, the statistical approaches to linguistics; and, in part, it had a kind of technological air to it. There was a lot of euphoria at that time in the area of linguistics in general, about the potentially great achievements that lay ahead along these lines. It was thought that they were already partly real. Then there was the potential of the technology that had come out of the war.

There was the sound spectrograph, information theory, and computers. The big technological revolution of the early '50s had created an atmosphere of considerable expectation in places like Cambridge, where a lot of people were interested in these matters. It was believed that concepts of information theory or Finite-State Markov sources, and so on were going to be unifying notions that would solve the problems of the behavioral sciences.

From things such as George Miller's book at the time (Miller, 1951) you'll get a sense that things were felt to be about to explode; many of the problems seemed basically solved, and others on the verge of solution. I thought that was completely wrong from every point of view, and I was particularly interested in seeing whether this crucial concept of Finite-State Markov sources could even in principle provide a way of dealing with the problems of language.

You could ask a question that for some reason investigators rarely asked: namely, can the proposed models *even in principle* account for the known facts? As soon as you ask that it becomes clear that Finite-State Markov sources can't possibly account for the known facts about language. So it falls apart.

But there was also a broader intent. In the back of my mind was the idea that Finite Automata seemed to subsume any conceivable notion of behaviorist psychology. Given that you could show that the grammar of a language could not be represented as a Finite Automaton, it also had to be true that anything approaching the structural character of language could never *in principle* be explained by any behavioristic theory.

For example, Hull, — obviously Skinner, but Hull's theory is richer than Skinner's — Hull's theory seemed to fall within the framework of Finite-State Automata. Anything you could by any stretch of the imagination call behaviorism seemed to me to fall in the domain of the theory of Finite Automata and Finite-State Markov sources and so on. As a matter of fact, they even included the ideas of people who were critical of behavioristic theories, such as Lashley (1951).

So my broader interest in studying these mathematical systems was that if you could show that they're impossible in principle, then you would show that any behavioristic theory is impossible in principle.

Now Patrick Suppes later gave a formal proof that stimulus-sampling theory (Suppes, 1969), which is arguably the most sophisticated variety of any quasibehaviorist learning theory around, could approach a particular subclass of Finite Automata in the limit. He interpreted that as a positive result for behaviorist theory. I would interpret it as an important negative result, because it's not just that they could only approach a subset of Finite Automata as a limit — *that's all* they could approach. They couldn't go beyond Finite Automata, and that means that this rich variety of behaviorist theory, which was well worked out, was demonstrably inadequate. Because we can show that *any* Finite Automaton is inadequate on grounds that such systems can't deal with very trivial properties of language. As I say, this is not Suppe's interpretation of his results.

Q: Your demonstration of the inadequacy of Finite Automata (*Syntactic Structures*, 1957) depends on the idea that people can handle strings that are infinitely recursive, strings that cannot be handled by any Finite Automaton. One of the things that psychologists clearly still have difficulties with is the degree to which you should take seriously the notion of infinite recursiveness . . .

A: Yes, I think some do have problems with that but it's a curious problem, based perhaps on a misunderstanding of what's at issue. The real point is that our performance can increase without limit as constraints on memory, attention, and time are reduced. Now of course those constraints can never be eliminated completely. Let's just for the moment forget language altogether. Suppose someone has learned the set "aa, bb, abba, aabbaa, baab, bbaabb . . . ," and in fact after a few examples has learned the whole notion of mirror-image. OK, that's easy to teach. I can teach it to somebody in three minutes or less.

And if people can do that, it follows that they can learn something that no possible behaviorist theory can explain, if the theory of Finite Automata subsumes such theories. The very fact that one can state that mirror-image rule and recognize any instance of it in principle shows that stimulus-sampling theory, and Hullian theory, and any other theory with the same limitations is inadequate.

Q: I'm surprised that you seem to be talking about your work as if it were an actual theory of mental structure and language comprehension. I've always thought that your theory was about the abstract structure of language, rather than about the mind.

A: Well, here again is a serious misunderstanding of my early work. If you look at *Syntactic Structures*, the main topic is "strong generative capacity." That is the question of what are the structures that *in fact* enter into language use and understanding.

Q: How has the myth come about that you do not mean it to apply to actual psychological structure?

A: Maybe because people don't read carefully. Well, in part the myth has come about because of the way *Syntactic Structures* is laid out. But if you take a careful look at the book, you'll find that that is what it's about.

Q: So it's inherently a theory of comprehension?

A: It is a theory of knowledge and of the structures that enter into comprehension. A similar misunderstanding exists about the relationship between syntax and semantics. Semantics, within linguistics, is the study of truth, meaning, and certain aspects of language use. I argued in *Syntactic Structures* that the claim that syntax reduces to semantics was not well founded. People thereupon concluded that I was somehow throwing meaning out of language or something. It is a pretty crazy inference. But I think that if you look at the last chapter of *Syntactic Structures*, it's absolutely clear and explicit. I wouldn't change a word if I could. Despite 25 years of misunderstanding, I can't see any way of saying it more clearly.

Q: Misunderstandings like this seem to be remarkably common in science.

A: Well, I don't call this science. I mean I think a lot of it is way out on the outer periphery of science, and I don't think misunderstandings of this nature *could* go on in science. But I think the point was fairly elementary. A large reason for the misunderstanding, it seems to me, is that in these fields people for some reason don't think clearly. I mean there's a block. There's too much ideology, there is too much mystical and quasireligious commitment to one position or another.

Typically, behaviorism — which in my view is basically a religious commitment — is based on the very profound dualist assumption that says that humans and animals in general simply cannot be understood with the canons of rationality that are standard in studying the physical world. Nobody can deal with the physical world on the basis of the criteria that behaviorism insists on, as a matter of principle. In fact, physics wouldn't have reached the level of the Babylonians if it had kept to these methodological canons. So in a very fundamental way behaviorism reflects a kind of dualism.

I think that a very funny thing happened about the 17th or 18th century. As metaphysical dualism was eliminated, a kind of epistemological dualism that was much more insidious took its place. Namely, this dualism said that the normal canons of rationality are simply inapplicable in the study of organisms. Take the criteria that are used to limit theory construction. Every variety of behaviorism imposes *a priori* constraints on legitimate theoretical notions. So radical behaviorism says that theoretical notions have to be totally defined in terms of what's observed. You can't postulate anything about inner structure. And other varieties of behaviorism say that you can have internal S's and R's, and you can have this or that, but any variety of behaviorism imposes some *a priori* constraint on theory.

Now what we should ask is the following: Suppose that one were to have insisted on studying the heavenly bodies in a similar way, imposing *a priori* constraints on legitimate theory construction. You wouldn't be able to have fruitful theory. This actually happened in the history of physics, when the Cartesians assumed that "action at a distance" was illegitimate. Things actually had to be in contact to influence each other. But of course in the common sense of the next generation, that obstacle was gone, and people recognized that there is no way to impose *a priori* constraints of this sort on your theories. Now imagine translating any variety of behaviorism into a physical domain. If you're studying some physical system and somebody comes along and says you're not allowed to talk about internal structure, you would laugh at him. But, nevertheless, such things are taken seriously in psychology.

Q: Of course behaviorists would say that they are so strict because they are suspicious of the tendencies people have to indulge in fantasies about psychology. They are suspicious of unconstrained theory.

A: I think that behaviorists represent those tendencies in a much more extreme fashion than anyone else, because in fact they have allowed various mystical and quasireligious views to enter into their theories about people. Behaviorists have raised all this to an absolute point of principle. They have made it a methodological requirement that you have to be absolutely irrational in dealing with organisms in general.

Q: Is it possible that in every science you have some people who are just concerned with data and suspicious of theory? In the history of physics, after all, you have people who were mostly data-oriented.

A: The issue is not concern with data. This does not distinguish behaviorists from anybody else, because everybody's concerned with data. Take a physicist who wants to figure out what is happening inside the sun. He's concerned with data too, but he doesn't limit himself to arrangement of data concerning the sun's exterior. He may accept an explanatory theory that he dreamed up about the invisible interior of the sun, which happens to work very well, explains lots of things, and is continuous with the rest of physics in some fashion.

Q: Didn't physicists like Percy Bridgman (1927) get involved with operationalism at one point, which was much like behaviorism?

A: Operationalism had a brief vogue, but physics was a well-enough established subject so that even though people talked operationalism it was pretty much irrelevant to what they actually did. No one, I think, abandoned physical theory on operationalist grounds. Psychology being in a much weaker position, was very much influenced by the fact that some people took operationalism very seriously and allowed it to constrain the kinds of work they did.

Q: Now Skinner would argue that you can restate any physical construct in functional terms. Instead of saying "electron," you could simply point to certain operations and the equations that connect those operations.

A: Well, I don't think that is worth discussing, frankly. Of course in some vague sense you can — but does anybody take that idea seriously in the natural sciences? Would anybody waste a moment's time trying to give a functional analysis in terms of arrangement of data for the concepts of, say, nuclear structure or biochemistry? The idea that you can give anything like a functional analysis in that sense is so farfetched that I don't think it is worth discussing. Which is exactly why nobody discusses it in the natural sciences.

But in the psychological sciences you can get away with that kind of thing because there are so few established results that you think, well, maybe it could work. As soon as there begin to be results, then of course you know that you're just constructing explanatory theories that are constrained by data. But apart from that, to insist that they be somehow reducible to observations, that's crazy.

You can see the influence of these quite pernicious ideas even in the terminology that's used. Take the phrase "behavioral sciences." It's a very curious phrase. I mean it's a bit like calling the natural sciences "meter-reading sciences." In fact a physicist's data often consists of things like meter readings, but nobody calls physics "meter-reading science." Similarly, the data of a psychologist is behavior, in a broad sense. But to call a field "behavioral science" is to say it's a science of behavior in the sense in which physics is a science of meter reading. Of course physics is not a science of meter reading; it's the study of matter and forces in the real world, and so on. Psychology is similarly not the science of behavior, but the study of the mind, mental organization, and mental structure, which uses behavior as its data.

Q: In your early work in the 1950s, how did your work catch on?

A: I had very little communication with linguists, but there were some, like Bernard Bloch (editor of *Language* for many years) who were sympathetic. That is why I'm at MIT, which was at the time a place with no vested interests in linguistics or the humanities and related social sciences. Bob Lees came here, feeling very antagonistic to my kind of work, but he became interested in it when he was here. When *Syntactic Structures* was published in Europe (1957), Lees wrote a long and influential review, which Bloch published right away (Lees, 1957). In fact it came out the same time the book came out, and that is what brought the ideas to the attention of linguists. Before that time, when I gave talks, it was usually to mathematicians and computer scientists.

Q: What about psychologists? Was George Miller your primary entrée into psychology?

A: Yes. He became interested in these things around '55, and he invited me out to an institute that he was running at Stanford. It was in the summer of 1957. We spent the summer together, did some work together, and stayed in contact for a number of years. Through him I got to know some of the mathematical psychologists, as well as others.

I think that George Miller brought back a lot of this kind of thinking to psychology. His book *Plans and the Structure of Behavior*, for example (Miller, Galanter, & Pribram, 1960).

Q: Miller agrees with Simon and Newell that, for him, the shift occurred in the middle '50s. I think that half-jokingly he places it as September 11, 1956.

A: The IRE Convention.

Q: Right. You were there; Newell and Simon, George Miller, David Green, and Swets were talking about signal detection, and so on. When did the shift take place for you?

A: Well, about 1953 I realized that the basis of linguistic behaviorism, which was the idea of a taxonomic discovery procedure, was wrong. That is, the claim was that the structure of language is exhausted by the classification of sounds into classes of sounds, sequences of these classes, classes of such sequences, and so on. I became convinced that there was no such thing as a taxonomic discovery procedure, and that human beings have to have prior knowledge about language in order to gain the mature knowledge they possess — knowledge of a system of generative rules. That conference in 1956 was interesting, and for me it was an opportunity to talk to other people about the work I was doing.

Q: Did you have a sense at the conference of convergence between your work and other people's?

A: Not really. I still don't. I mean Simon's type of work is undoubtedly interesting, but it doesn't seem to relate to what I've been interested in. There is some very serious work in Artificial Intelligence (AI). For example, the work on vision that comes out of David Marr's laboratory is first-rate and important (*e.g.*, Marr, 1982). There's a lot of computer technique, a lot of flexibility in using computers, that's valuable to have. But in terms of principles or theories coming out of AI, I don't think there is much to discuss, apart from work such as Marr's. Much of the work in AI seems to me misguided, in that it is too concrete. Also, it is trying to deal with how people solve certain problems that they solve very badly, instead of understanding how people solve problems that they solve very well, as Marr has pointed out. For example, one thing you do very well is to solve the problem of identifying an object in motion. But something you do very badly is proving a theorem in propositional calculus. The AI approaches are too concrete in that they are much too concerned with the actual algorithm — there may be many algorithms to realize a particular computational theory, and the study of algorithms requires a prior understanding of the structure of the problem being addressed. Again, this is a point that Marr has emphasized. To assume that your program *is* your theory is simply to abandon any hope for understanding what people are doing.

Q: One of the things that has been stated very clearly is the need for having many different levels of representation, and making available information from any of those levels to resolve problems at other levels. Top-down plus bottom-up processing, or "mixed initiative", and so on.

A: But you don't have to do any work to show that! It is pretty obvious without any inquiry that when you and I understand each other we're bringing in all sorts of information that has nothing to do with language. I don't think we have to show that.

Q: I suspect that for many cognitive psychologists and Artificial Intelligence people, and perhaps for some linguists as well, this may be a new idea.

A: I find that kind of astonishing, because it's such an obvious point.

I mean, if you want my frank opinion, I can only attribute what you found about that to the amazing irrationality of the study of humans. Because, after all, if you think for one minute, it's perfectly obvious that when you understand what somebody is saying, you are going to use all the information available to you: information about the person, about the topic, and everything—in fact, syntactic information may be very marginal. It's perfectly obvious. That's why you can often understand what somebody says if you hear a few scattered words, because you roughly know what it's about. Would that have to be demonstrated? Just go to a party and listen to someone under noisy conditions and it's demonstrated.

Q: Another thing that one might claim for AI work in language is that they have tried to deal with things such as question answering, ellipsis, and so on—often neglected topics in formal linguistics. At least in the sense that there are actual systems doing something like answering questions where there were none able to do so before, there has been progress.

A: Well, we perhaps have a real divergence with regard to what one might consider to be of interest. I think many of the topics that they are concerned with are perfectly interesting. The question is, do they have anything of interest *to say* about them? Are there any interesting principles? A flower collector is dealing with very interesting things; all of natural history is dealing with utterly fascinating things. I'm interested in flowers and sunsets and so forth. But if somebody asks, Does it have any intellectual interest? No, there is no intellectual interest, because there are no principles, no explanations, no theories, and so on.

Now as far as AI is concerned, let's just take what you said about question answering. Certainly that's an interesting topic, but at the level at which flower collecting is interesting. Is it interesting at the level at which, say, biochemistry is? Does it have any principles—one weak principle? Does it have one minor generalization? The answer as far as I can see is no.

Q: Has there been any opposition among linguists to your claim that linguistics is essentially a part of cognitive psychology? My feeling is that linguists are somewhat nervous about the autonomy of linguistics as a field.

Q: I'm really not the right person to ask about that, because I have very little contact with professional linguists. My own feeling is that you are probably right. But you know, as far as I'm concerned, all of these autonomy questions are of interest primarily to people who are concerned with how to organize departments in universities.

Q: You don't have a strong identification with linguistics as a field?

A: I don't even know what it is. I mean, what is linguistics? It's, in part, the study of one particular aspect of human cognition. How that should be conducted at some historical moment — it probably makes sense to have it conducted in relative isolation from some other topics. But perhaps not. Few articulate theoreticians in linguistics suggested that it should be an autonomous discipline unconcerned with other aspects of human psychology.

Q: You have said that there is no relationship between your political interests and your linguistic work, except in that there is some common notion of human nature involved in both. Could you clarify that?

A: There's a good deal of complete nonsense written about it. Some people claim, on the basis of gross distortion of what I have written, that I somehow claim to be able to deduce political theories from syntactic theories, and that alleged claim has been attacked. Well, it's difficult to imagine anything more insane than the idea that you might be able to deduce political theories from syntactic theories. Certainly it is not my view, or anything remotely like it.

But yes, I think you could say there's a certain feeling about human nature, about human capacity, that lies at the core of my political ideas and my linguistic ideas. Something having to do with innate structure, with creativity, with the fundamental need for creative work and activity. In some vague way these ideas show up in various guises. Contrary to some other people, I think that it is only on the assumption that people have a very rich, intrinsic, biologically determined mental structure, it is only on that assumption that we can develop any concept of human nature as flexible, inventive, creative. I think that the crucial factor in human creativity and freedom is that we have very heavy biological constraints.

Q: Environmentalism certainly is a theme in behaviorism, and it is typically part of the popular American view that you can turn people into anything if they only try hard enough.

A: Well, I think that is true, and I've commented on that. It seems to me that behaviorism, and empiricism in general, are in certain respects very manipulative ideologies. I think it's a fair question why these ideologies have achieved the appeal that they have. I don't believe it is possible to explain that appeal on either empirical or rational grounds. They are seen to be grossly false as soon as you begin to look at them. Therefore, the fact that they have had such an overwhelming power over the imagination is a question of interest, since they are so plainly false. Why should that be?

My own feeling is — I've suggested this and it hasn't made me popular, but I'll suggest it again — that the intelligentsia as an organized group have tended to be very closely associated with manipulation. They've tended very strongly to associate themselves with state power or with various coercive and manipulative ideologies, which is rather natural. That's how they hope to gain their prestige and influence and sometimes even power. Hence, I think they rather naturally tend toward manipulative ideologies, and an extreme form of environmentalism is just such an ideology. It's part of its appeal, I believe.

Jerrold A. Fodor: Psycholinguist and Philosopher of Science

Jerrold A. Fodor (b. 1935) received his PhD in philosophy in 1960 from Princeton University, working under the direction of the philosopher of science Hilary Putnam. During Fodor's graduate years, a strong movement was developing in philosophy against logical positivism, led by Putnam among others (*e.g.*, Putnam, 1975). Thus Fodor developed an intellectual ambience in which the philosophical foundations of behaviorism had little standing.

Fodor first came to the attention of experimental psychologists as a champion of Chomsky's views on language (see the interviews with Jenkins and Weimer, this volume). Even better known within psychology was Fodor's experimental work on "the psychological reality of syntax," as well as his attack on Osgood's notion that linguistic "meaning" was an implicit response or r_m (Osgood, 1953, 1966; Fodor, 1965; Fodor & Garrett, 1967). In collaboration with his colleagues, Fodor showed that clicks inserted into a tape-recorded sentence tended to be perceived as syntactic clause boundaries, even when they were physically located some distance away from the boundary. Gestalt psychologists knew of similar boundary phenomena in visual perception, but this demonstration of the perceptual effects of syntax did much to legitimize Chomsky's work with experimental psychologists. It is worth noting that Chomsky's own evidence was already psychological — for example, the existence of deep-structure ambiguities is a psychological fact. But it was not an *experimentally demonstrated fact*, and, hedged by methodological restrictions, many psychologists refused to believe mere "naturalistic demonstrations." Thus, from Fodor's point of view, these experiments did not reveal anything new — they provided a useful tool of persuasion, a rhetorical tool (see Weimer interview).

Since this work, Fodor has gone on to become prominent as a philosopher of psychology and a psychological theorist (Fodor, 1968, 1975, 1981). Taking the computational metaphor of mind as the core insight of cognitive psychology, he has elaborated on its philosophical implications under the label of "functionalism." (Needless to say, Fodor's functionalism is different from the psychological functionalism of Dewey, Angell, and even Skinner.) Further, in *The Language of Thought* (1975), he has argued in favor of a *lingua mentis*, a fundamental code in the nervous system that would symbolize and transform mental representations. Most recently, in *The Modularity of Mind* (1983), he has argued for a very strong view of specialization of function in the nervous system, a view that also implies a very strong nativism.

Among other honors, Professor Fodor has been a Fulbright scholar, a Guggenheim Fellow, and a Fellow of the Center for Advanced Study of the Behavioral Sciences at Stanford. He is now Professor of Philosophy and Psychology at the Massachusetts Institute of Technology.

Interview with Jerrold A. Fodor

Q: You have done such a great variety of things relevant to psychology — how would you describe your work?

A: I do a range of things, from experimental psycholinguistics to philosophical foundations of psychology. I think of it as "cognitive science" as much as anything. That seems to be the in-word at the moment. I was trained in philosophy. That's what my PhD is in, but I guess I've always been interested in philosophy of language and philosophy of mind. I got interested in psychological stuff in a sort of odd way. I mean purely serendipitously. I was appointed, when I was a visitor in the philosophy department at the University of Illinois, to a sort of a part-time position on a research project that Charlie Osgood was running in psycholinguistics. This was in the late 1950s! And I got to talking with a lot of graduate students down there who were doing empirical psychological work. In particular I got to talk with Merrill Garrett, with whom I've been working steadily ever since. And between us we stumbled into this click stuff, and did some of the original experimental work on it. We inserted auditory clicks into sentences and played them to subjects, and it turned out that subjects perceived the clicks to be at the syntactic breaks in the sentences, even though the actual clicks were not located there. This was taken to be an argument for the existence of syntactic structure in the perception of sentences. When I got back to MIT, I met Tom Bever, who was a graduate student at the time, and we did some more experimental work on clicks. And about a year after that, I got an opportunity to teach a psycholinguistics course in the psychology department. And it lead finally to a joint appointment in psychology and philosophy. The tie-up with the experimental stuff has all been fairly accidental. There was at that time in the Boston area a lot of interesting philosophy of mind and linguistic work going on at MIT, including Chomsky's work.

Q: Your background in philosophy raises some interesting questions. For example, there's a very clear relationship between the philosophy of logical positivism and behaviorism. They seem to arise at the same time historically, and also behaviorists frequently had recourse to the philosophy of science that came out of logical positivism to justify their ideas.

A: According to the epistomology that went with positivism and operationalism, you had to take a certain reductionist attitude toward serious science. If you were going to have a science for which epistemologic probity could be claimed, it had to be a science that was articulated entirely in terms of relations between data sentences. That is to say, between descriptions of observables. And that picture I think is central to the behaviorist movement. I think the application of that picture of science to psychology gives you something like Skinner's approach to mental events. In that approach theoretical entities can have only a heuristic value. They may be useful fictions, but they have to be eventually eliminated in a statement of the refined science. I think that this idea of science was taken as almost self-evidently true both in linguistics before Chomsky and in behavioristic psychology.

Q: Are there parallels in philosophy to the cognitive shift in psychology?

A: By the time that I got interested in this stuff in the mid-'60s, an antipositivist movement in philosophy of science was clearly in full swing. It hadn't yet begun to have much of an effect on the behavioral sciences, but it was very much evident in philosophy. One of the major figures was and is Hilary Putnam, who was my thesis advisor at Princeton. And Hilary at that time took the line that you have to have a philosophy of science that leads to a realistic interpretation of theoretical entities. You simply can't make sense of the history of science unless you do that. There are, crudely, two sorts of pictures that you can take. One is that when a scientist refers to electrons, that is just sort of a *façon de parler* — a manner of speaking — for talking about pointer readings on an instrument or something of that kind. If you adopt that picture for psychology, it says that when you talk about mental states and processes, that has to be construed as just the heuristic way of talking about behavioral inputs and outputs. And I take it that that is the picture which behaviorists inherited from the positivists and operationalists. The alternative is the realistic picture that when a scientist or a physicist says there are electrons, he means there are electrons in reality. There are little things out in the world that are charged in a certain way and move a certain way through orbits. And if you apply that picture to science, that is how Hilary Putnam at that time, and a lot of other philosophers more recently, are inclined to look at science.

Q: Then the real distinction seems to be a question of the ontology, that is, the reality of the theoretical constructs?

A: I think it's a question of how you interpret the truth conditions of scientific claims. In the first view, the one that underlies the behavioristic movement, if a scientist talks about mental processes, the truth conditions on those claims have to be specified in terms of stimulus–response relations. In the other kind of view, the truth conditions of the theoretical claims are to be understood in terms of the mental processes going on in the organism that mediate its behavior. That's the picture that was emerging in philosophy of mind in the 1960s, and it goes very naturally with the work in linguistics and in cognitive theory.

Q: Would you say, then, that the behaviorists in many ways extrapolated the view that came from philosophy of science to psychology?

A: Yes. It's a proper extrapolation from the way philosophers viewed the practices of other sciences. But that view is wrong. It is wrong about the other sciences, and it's not surprising that it turned out to be wrong about psychology.

Q: Do you think that psychologists such as the behaviorists were perhaps even victimized by the views of proper science that were prescribed by philosophy of science at the time?

A: I think philosophy did an enormous amount of damage in the behavioral sciences, and I think the damage is still being rectified. But I think it is also fair to say that if you look at the long tradition in philosophy, the operationalist and positivist period was really an aberration of philosophical tradition. I mean the great tradition in philosophy, back to Locke and Descartes and others, is a tradition of realism about mental constructs such as ideas. Philosophers convinced themselves for about 20 years or so that that tradition had to be abandoned, but the arguments were never very good. And they rested upon analogies from what was supposed to be going on in the other sciences. Unfortunately, modern linguistics, psychology, and sociology developed contemporaneously with this period in philosophy. So the philosophy these people learned was this kind of reductionist, behaviorist, fictionalist view of mental entities. It blew over rather fast in philosophy, but it lasted longer in these scientific communities. As I say, I think the damage is still being rectified.

On the other hand, it's clear that the behaviorists revolted against an introspectionist point of view, which was clearly sterile. And what's going on now in the attempt to develop an experimental cognitive science is an attempt to find techniques for measuring mental properties so that you don't have to rely on introspection to measure them. What happened in the behaviorist movement was really a systematic throwing out of the baby with the bath water. They thought that the way to avoid the introspectionist implications of the classical work in psychology was by avoiding the notion that the natural object of psychological theory is mental states and processes. That seems to have been a very natural mistake.

Q: Would you consider yourself a mentalist?

A: Well, if that means somebody who thinks that there are mental states and processes, and that they have causal relations to behavior and to affective states: sure. That does not mean that I am not a physicalist. I believe that it is possible to be a physicalist and still believe in mental constructs. What I find surprising is that despite 20 years of pointing out to people that this is a viable view, that you can in fact be a physicalist and still consider mental constructs to be real, that view seems to have made very little impact on people who were originally committed to the behaviorist line. It's made a lot of impact on the graduate students, however. I suppose that is not unprecedented in a Kuhnian sense. It's the sort of thing you might expect with a "paradigm shift."

Q: What is the role of consciousness for a mentalist in the sense that you mean that word?

A: I don't think that we have an account of consciousness as things now stand. We don't really know what it is for a mental state to be conscious. And I think it's no accident that the cognitive psychology we are developing is a cognitive psychology of beliefs rather than one of sensations and feelings.

Q: In other words, there can be mental states that are not conscious?

A: Presumably, some beliefs and desires are not conscious. How to understand the difference between mental states that can be conscious and mental states that must be unconscious is not clear.

Q: But still one can presumably make empirical claims about consciousness. Conscious experiences exist.

A: Well, I can't imagine why anybody would want to deny it. The problem isn't so much what the facts are, as how the facts are to be described, and how they ought to be explained. The kind of cognitive psychology that we're developing has not made very many moves in these areas.

Q: To get back to the situation you experienced in the 1950s, what was the situation like, especially around Cambridge?

A: You have to remember that in the early '60s, around MIT, there was a very small collection of people who were developing these things. You could find out all the linguistics that there was, at least within the transformational point of view, by walking down the hall and asking your friends. I remember relatively little discussion about the methodological issues we've been talking about, because everybody held roughly the same views — that the behaviorist theory was fundamentally dead, and that the problem was to reconstruct a kind of mentalism that would work, at least in some areas of psychology and presumably in linguistics, since that seemed to be where the action was. I got to MIT about 1960, and there was a small group of people then, mostly under Noam [Chomsky]. It was all very exciting, particularly by the middle and late '60s, because by then there was a vast amount of linguistics being done throughout the country. And the work was being done from a transformational point of view and with a sort of psychological malice aforethought. Much of this work was influenced by activity at MIT, especially by Chomsky seminars.

Q: Was there a lot of controversy between proponents of the transformational point of view and other people, either in linguistics or psychology?

A: I think there was some. But there was no blood in the streets, nothing remotely like that. On the other hand, it was certainly not true that the curtain was raised, and the scene changed overnight. There was a lot and there still is a lot of resistance to the transformational line. And, indeed, there isn't any single transformational line. There are a lot of ways of developing a Transformational Grammar, and there are a lot of people who accept the general picture that goes with Chomsky's stuff, and still don't accept the transformational story. So, I don't think there's any Kuhnian melodrama. Or if there was, I certainly wasn't involved in it. I don't remember any particular revolutionary fervor. There was a great deal of disagreement about how far these ideas could be pushed. And some of it was a disagreement about the assumptions underlying the methods. And that is as it should be. I mean, none of this is self-evidently true. But I would have thought, at least from an outsider's point of view, that the MIT linguistics people did pretty well pretty fast. I mean, even before I knew him, Chomsky was recognized as a force on the horizon.

I think it would have been amazing if the truth of these views had been acknowledged overnight. For one thing, they're not sufficiently well worked out, even now, so that a clear-cut question of truth and falsity could be asked. It took about 10 years, I guess, for the groundwork of assumptions to be made clear. And I don't think it was accomplished by any bloody clashes or anything. It was mostly a slow process of individual persuasion. By the time that Premack and I had our seminars at Minnesota debating those issues — this is about the late '60s — a lot of this stuff had been pretty well assimilated. Remember, there were things going on besides linguistics. There was the computer revolution, and the computer metaphor was making its effect felt. There had always been a tradition in psychology that was nonbehavioristic — say, in the theory of perception. And also, of course, the philosophical changes had made mentalists begin to look respectable again. So all this was beginning to have a cumulative effect. I think what linguistics did that was terrifically important, and still is, was to provide an example of what it was like to be successful in this area. There is no doubt — whatever you think about the way you do syntax — there is no doubt that an enormous amount has been learned over the past 20 or 30 years about the structure of natural language. It's all very well to do philosophical tub-thumping and claim that you ought to be able, in principle, to have a mentalistic psychology. But here was a group of people who looked like they were actually doing it. Things that people hadn't noticed before were suddenly being brought to the fore. Facts about how language worked were being brought to people's attention, and the data were very striking. I guess the same point can be made about the '60s movement in mentalism that you could make about the '40s movement in positivism and operationalism. What impressed people about the behavioristic point of view was that learning theory seemed to be making some progress. In fact, people were finding out about what happens to pigeons or rats under various schedules of reinforcement. Similarly, the cognitive shift has something to do with the fact that people were actually finding something out about mental functions. A little empirical progress goes a long way in methodological disputes.

Q: At what point would you say that a major change occurred? What range of years?

A: Well, I would pick the 1960s as paradigmatic, and I guess the change was mostly in attitude. More in the attitude of graduate students than of their teachers. There were a couple of relatively spectacular senior conversions. Jim Jenkins seemed to be moved by Chomsky's stuff, and seemed to seriously shift his view over a relatively short period. But I think the picture of conversion in general, the picture of an overnight shift, is really badly misleading. I mean, I remember talking to some of the first psychologists that I knew seriously, people from Haskins Laboratories, such as Al Liberman. People like that had been working for years and years on speech perception and were never remotely tempted by the behaviorist story. They immediately saw what was going on in syntax as continuous with the kind of questions they wanted to ask about speech perception. It was a very mixed picture. It was more like the gradual change of the center of gravity and a change in rhetoric rather than a religious conversion. It is also important to remember that although everyone agrees on the rejection of behaviorism and everyone is generally in a computational framework, there is still a lot of disagreement about the right research strategy. Witness the total discrepancy in research strategy between Chomsky and Schank, or between Chomsky and Minsky, for that matter. It's completely different. The bets about research priorities are entirely different. In any science the breakthroughs come with somebody finding the right question to work on, and despite all the noise and excitement, there have been relatively few breakthroughs of that kind in contemporary cognitive science. I personally think that it would be a serious mistake to underestimate the time scale. We're looking at the tip of the iceberg when it comes to understanding how mental structure is composed, even for those areas that we know how to talk about at all. I think it is going to be a long pull. What we are seeing now, I hope, is a quieting down of the methodological talk and the ideological activity and an increasing matter of addressing ourselves to actual problems of developing well-warranted empirical theories. And it's bloody hard. It's hard even in those areas in which it works best, like linguistics.

Q: One could make the argument that the cognitive shift was actually a metatheoretical shift.

A: Indeed.

Q: And that the shift was in principle methodological.

A: That's partly right. It's methodological, but it's sensitive to empirical results. On the other hand, I think that there is no guarantee that even making the right methodological moves pays off in solving all your problems overnight. That's certainly not going to happen. And I think it is utterly clear that the longer you look at the problems in cognition, the harder they get to be.

If you look at the experiments I did with Garrett and Bever on inserting clicks in speech to show that people perceive the clicks to be at the syntactic boundaries, that seems to be now a sort of amusing demonstration experiment. It was sort of fun to do, and everything is right on the surface, and the results are easy to interpret. I don't think that if somebody did that now, that anyone would be even remotely interested in it, and properly so. At that time the question was whether theories of perception were going to say things in terms of mental constructs, such as syntactic clauses. When that issue was very much in the forefront, those demonstration experiments had real sociological effects. Here's a piece of what looked to be hard science. This was a fully replicable, straightforward experimental paradigm, which still looked as though you needed to explain it in terms of the mental representation of the stimulus. And people found that very hard to believe. But people who had predominant commitments to, say, the Gestalt psychology of perception didn't find this surprising at all. They could show another half-dozen kind of effects of the same sort.

Q: But not with speech, probably.

A: But not with speech. In order to explain the click effect, you have to assume that syntactic structures must be used to explain the effect, even though the syntactic structures are not there on the surface of the stimulus. This is a truism now. But at the time it seemed strange and wonderful.

Q: In your experience, did people go through a kind of inner struggle between behaviorism and a cognitive point of view?

A: Well, I can only speak for my own case. Much before 1960 it was becoming very clear in the philosophical tradition that there was something badly wrong, not just with the Watson–Skinner view, but with much more sophisticated approaches to behaviorism, such as those of Ryle and Wittgenstein. I mean, people were getting very dubious about that stuff quite early on. In my case, Hilary Putnam was a major figure, because it seemed that a lot of articles that he was writing at that time against the behaviorism of people like Norman Malcolm were clearly right and devastating. So it didn't look as though it was an issue of behaviorism at all. That seemed to be fairly much decided. It looked as though it was an issue of whether or not there was a viable field in cognitive psychology.

Q: Was there a problem about physicalism? That is to say, was it difficult to explain how you could have a fundamentally physical universe and still be forced to talk about abstract things such as ideas and meanings?

A: Well, it depends very much on what you mean by "physicalism." The idea that psychology should reduce to neurology by some kind of laws is very likely to be wrong. I think what physicalism ought to suggest is that mental processes at some level will turn out to be physical processes. Suppose there were mental events in machines, or Martians, and suppose these machines or Martians were made out of silicon. Then, if their mental events are of the same type as ours, they could indeed feel pain, and as long as silicon is physical, this would be a physical event. But it would not be the same physical event that would make you and I feel pain. So there's an abstract level where we could communicate with the silicon Martian and transmit information back and forth, without it necessarily being true that my feeling of pain should be the same kind of *physical* event as a Martian's feeling of pain. That latter doctrine is what the unity-of-science view typically assumes. And I think it's wrong. I think there is every reason to think it's wrong.

Q: It seems to me that you're making a distinction analogous to the computer program versus computer hardware.

A: Yes, it's exactly a program-versus-hardware distinction. In fact, the functionalist movement in philosophy of mind that has developed along with all this psychological stuff has been based on exactly that distinction.

Q: Would you say that psychology is about information? Where information may be independent of a physiological or physical substrate?

A: Yes. That is the sort of picture that goes very naturally with the sort of cognitive psychology we've been talking about. As a research strategy, it may not work. For example, there are problems of certain kinds for the case of consciousness. But it looks like it works for a lot of mental states and functions and it's plausible, at least, for a lot of the area that cognitive psychology is actually being developed in. I mean the psychology of beliefs, intuitions, and so on. It looks to make a fairly good case there. And it's becoming sort of the official view of how you ought to refute Skinner. I mean, you can refute Skinner by saying, "Look, you can have a physicalism that is nonbehavioristic, and the way to do it is by having functionalist physicalism." That is, by saying that the information-processing tasks are independent of the physical mechanism that subserves it.

Q: Then this is partly a contribution of the computer?

A: Right. I think that's really the major contribution that the computer has made to the ideology of modern cognitive psychology. Not so much that we have computational models of this and that, but that thinking about the way that computers work gives us a picture of how there could be a science at the level of abstraction of computer programs. And that allows one to have one's functionalism and one's physicalism and one's nonbehaviorism all at the same time. That realization was very liberating. I mean, it's become part of the official ideology of the movement, and it enormously liberates the imagination. One seemed to have this dilemma before, which went: Either you're a behaviorist or you're some sort of central-state physicalist. So either you have no mental events at all, or you have physiological events that are only incidentally psychological. Thus, the functionalist computer metaphor seems to have shown a way between the horns of that dilemma.

Q: How do you see the future of this field? Certainly you seem to see it more as cognitive science, that is to say, as an inherently interdisciplinary field.

A: Yes. I have some sort of detailed expectations about how we're going to go. In terms of content, within the next 10 years I think we will be learning how to do things such as automatic parsing of language. And the work that is being done now by the theoreticians will connect in a new way with psycholinguistic experimentation. So one might actually see some substantive advances. As far as the structure of the discipline is concerned, I think it's very hard to tell. The actual detailed interactions among linguists and psychologists and computer scientists and so on have not really been very striking so far, and not really terribly productive, with a few exceptions. I think that we are going to see a rather different approach to graduate training in cognitive psychology. People are going to have to know more about the philosophical background of cognitive psychology, because a lot of what's going on in cognitive science has been basicallly the reinvention of philosophical positions that have been fairly well understood for several hundred years. So there's going to have to be a great deal more sophistication about the epistemology built into graduate training. And there will have to be a good deal of sophistication about computer science in order to do this stuff seriously. Aside from that, I find it very hard to predict what's going to happen. I'm sort of hoping that the propaganda will quiet down a bit, and that a period of reasonably normal science will set in. I don't think a case for the existence of this discipline has been made. I think the antibehaviorist case has been made all right, and I think the case for the possibility of finding out about the structure of natural language has been made, but the case for the existence of a cognitive science as a general approach to mental processes — it's just the best idea anybody has right now. But the way to make the case for it is not by showing that it's defensible in the face of behavioristic criticism. It's to actually make some progress. And I think the progress is going to be slow in coming and really very hard to make.

Herbert A. Simon: Pioneer in Cognitive Science

Even among an exceptionally creative group of contributors, Herbert A. Simon (b. 1916) stands out as something of a Renaissance man. After receiving his doctoral degree at the University of Chicago in 1943 in political science, he went on to do classical work in the economics of the firm, for which he received a Nobel Prize in 1978. During the 1950s, just as the computer was becoming a usable device, he became one of the pioneers in computer science, Artificial Intelligence, and computational modeling of psychological processes. This work was performed in collaboration with several other individuals, most consistently with his long-time friend and coworker Allen Newell, with whom he shared the prestigious Turing Prize of the Association for Computing Machinery in 1974. Their contributions ranged from the first high-level computer language (IPL-I); to the early development of the notion of recursion, which has been of fundamental importance in Artificial Intelligence; to some of the earliest simulations of human short-term memory; to major studies of chess playing and problem solving in human subjects. The range and depth of this work is breathtaking, some of it indeed so revolutionary that psychologists concerned with some of these issues are just now beginning to understand it in detail.

Among Simon's most important writings are *Administrative Behavior* (1947) and *The Sciences of the Artificial* (1969/1981). He has published numerous papers in collaboration with others, showing that logic theorems can be proved by a computer (Newell & Simon, 1956); on a General Problem Solver, simulating human central processes (Newell, Shaw, & Simon, 1960); on chess-playing programs (Newell, Shaw, & Simon, 1958b); a report on a 15-year research program on human problem solving, called, naturally, *Human Problem Solving* (Newell & Simon, 1972); and a review of protocol analysis as a general method for gaining insight into human thinking (Ericsson & Simon, 1980).

In addition to the Nobel Prize in Economics (1978) and the Turing Prize in Computer Science (shared with Allen Newell), Herbert A. Simon has received the Distinguished Scientific Contribution award of the American Psychological Association, as well as numerous honorary doctorates. He is currently Professor of Psychology and Computer Science at Carnegie–Mellon University in Pittsburgh.

Interview with Herbert A. Simon

Q: Do you consider yourself primarily a psychologist, a computer scientist, or an economist?

A: I consider myself primarily a behavioral scientist who's been working basically in psychology for the last 20 years or so, with excursions into other areas. But the continuing thread through all of my work is the interest in human decision making, which led me to my general interest in human cognition.

My PhD is in Political Science, but the political science department at Chicago was very forgiving, so that I had a good slug of economics at the same time. I studied some logic and some mathematical biophysics as well. When I got my bachelor's degree, I got a job studying the problem of evaluating municipal governments, with a lot of attention to decision making in general, and budget making in particular.

Q: Even in that early work there seems to be a consistent thread that can be found later on.

A: I like to think so. Very early on, it seemed to me that one of the most fascinating problems was that, because of the complexities that organizations deal with, the human beings in the organizations had only very partial views of the total situation. So they were always making up pictures of what the situation was from the standpoint of their particular locations in the organization. And then the question was, How does that affect organizational decision making? Further, how do you design organizations that take into account those human cognitive limitations?

Those cognitive limitations have been a central theme in almost all of the theorizing that I've done since then. Limitations such as those of short-term memory are fundamental. They are in fact very important limitations on human rationality, particularly if the rationality has to be exercised in a face-to-face real-time context.

Short-term memory limitations are much less important in more extended decision processes, where things are recorded on paper. But even here you get limitations, because the typical size of the problem space is just enormous compared with the ability people have for searching it. So any exploration of a problem space is highly selective. Only a tiny fraction of the things that could be looked at do get looked at. The discrepancy between the capabilities of the human mind and the complexity of the world is a very deeply built-in limitation, and one that we alleviate only slightly when we have aids like computers.

In human decision making what we're talking about is a serial system, a one-at-a-time system, that's groping around in the long-term memory and in the world through its senses. And it really does see only a tiny bit, because it can't search all of the information in any reasonable time. At any given moment it sees only the infinitesimal fraction of the whole. That's the short-term memory problem.

Now we usually cope with that when we gain experience: The limits of short-term memory are measured by the number of familiar items or "chunks" that you can hold at any one time. As you gain experience with things, whole collections of chunks become single chunks.

In this way you have in short-term memory a kind of recursive structure. Take Lincoln's Gettysburg Address—if I've misspent my childhood by memorizing it, that one label "Gettysburg Address" can evoke a whole string of things from long-term memory. I can bring each one in gradually. So, in a sense, that one label constitutes one chunk of short-term memory and points to a whole lot of other chunks of information. That's a principal reason why a person who is experienced in a particular field can, by noticing some features of a situation, immediately access a lot of information about what's relevant to that situation.

Q: And there is a contrast between the limited capacity of short-term memory and the enormous size of long-term memory, so that there *is* a lot of information in memory; it's just hard to get at one time.

A: Right. Well, when we—that is, Allen Newell, Cliff Shaw, and I—started out in '55 or thereabouts to try and simulate some human problem-solving processes on the computer, it was clear that we had to have a programming language that didn't require us to know in advance how much of various different kinds of information there was going to be, and how they were all going to be uniquely related to each other. It's not like a simple algebra problem where you know ahead of time exactly how much information you need. In a problem-solving search you've got to build a big search tree and you don't know where it is going to branch, or how big it's going to grow.

Furthermore, you want to be able to store structures that you can reorder and restructure. If you have two items adjoining, you want to be able to stick a third one between them that you didn't know of before. So, we tried to think about a programming language that would have that kind of flexibility—which standard algebraic programming languages didn't have. Remember, this was quite early on—there wasn't even a FORTRAN then. There essentially were no higher-level languages.

We wanted to have a higher-level language that would have this kind of flexibility, and we asked, Well, where can we get ideas for that? Well, one place you could get the ideas was psychology. People have been talking about human associative memory since Aristotle. So we tried to see how the human mind had solved that problem, and some of the ideas of *list processing*—its basic associative character—are in fact drawn in a very obvious way from what we know about human psychology.

Q: How would you characterize "list processing"?

A: Well, a symbol list is simply an ordered set of items. In developing IPL-V (which was the main programming language we developed), we found we needed lists, and then the items on a list had to have the capabilities of being lists also. That's what we called list *structures* — arbitrary lists whose members could be lists, whose members could also be lists, and so on.

And then we discovered that we needed something else that was anticipated by psychologists — we needed *directed associations*. We called them "description lists," or "property lists." If you want to know that a "dog" is a member of a class called "animals," you need a directed association that is asymmetrical. "Animal" is superordinate to "dog," but not *vice versa*. So there was an obvious need for directed associations. Those were the basic ideas that were embedded in the IPL languages.

Q: Those languages are recursive in the sense that any item on the list can itself be a list.

A: Yes. They're recursive in a lot of ways: For example, programs were also recursive in that the definition of a particular subroutine could contain that subroutine in it. It was one of the first languages that had recursive capability in subroutines.

Q: You have pointed out that recursiveness is such a powerful property that it eliminates certain theoretical controversies that psychologists have had for many decades (Newell & Simon, 1972). For example, the controversy between associationistic and Gestalt viewpoints in psychology — associationists deal with connections between units, and Gestaltists deal with holistic properties of human experience. But with a recursive representation you can talk about units and about holistic organization using the same representation.

A: We said something like that in our 1958 article (Newell, Shaw, & Simon, 1958a), the first paper we wrote to try to introduce psychologists to this point of view. If you will enrich the S–R association concept a little bit, you get a lot more power: You need not just simple S–R associations, but the notion of labeled or directed associations. Then, you have to have the notion of *program* as well as *data*: things that *act* as well as things that *know*. You need the notion of a branch, the ability to *choose* alternatives on the basis of what you know. Those notions were really lacking in the formalisms of behaviorism.

But the Gestaltists and other European groups had paid a lot of attention to these ideas, particularly the Würtzburg group. They didn't have a good formal language for those ideas, but they knew that such things were important in complex mental performance. It takes a little bit of hindsight, but you can go back now and read Selz (1913; Frijda & de Groot, 1981), who was one of the Würtzburg group, and rediscover the same ideas. Selz was very influential in the research on chess. De

Groot (*e.g.*, 1965) met Selz in Holland when he was a refugee from the Nazis. Later Selz was carried off and gassed during the Nazi occupation of Holland. But you can go back now and read Selz, and translate him into our modern information-processing formulas very directly.

Q: Much of Artificial Intelligence research is done in the computer language LISP, which is based on the concepts you just outlined. In LISP you can clearly represent symbolic processes that are very complex and yet very holistic.

A: Yes. Well, that's due to the fact (a) that you can name any list and then deal with the name, and (b) that you can name any function or subroutine and deal with it by the name—in this way, *anything* can become a chunk.

Q: It's a remarkably elegant system. With a very small number of simple properties it seems to accomplish a great deal. For example, you and Allen Newell have discussed the definition of "symbol" (Newell & Simon, 1972)—how would you define that?

A: Well it's ordinarily a string of bits in a single machine address. It designates, it points to something, which is its meaning, essentially. The something it points to may be other information in computer memory, that is, other structures of symbols, or it might point to a routine. If you execute that routine it may, for example, perform a test on something in the outside world, so the symbol that designates "blue" in my memory allows me to get access to a test that allows me to say that a piece of paper over there is blue.

Q: So there's a procedure that you can go to to find out whether something that might be blue is actually blue, and this is in part the meaning of the symbol "blue."

A: Right.

Q: Your position *vis-à-vis* other people in computer science and psychology is very interesting. Within computer science you are seen as pursuing an "experimental" approach rather than a formal one, which must be upsetting to many mathematically-oriented computer scientists. In psychology, your position is exactly the opposite—certainly for many years, you have been far more formal and theoretical than the great majority of experimental psychologists.

A: Computer science was from the beginning heavily populated with people who had training in mathematics. I suppose a majority of early computer scientists were either mathematicians or engineers. The mathematicians didn't feel very comfortable with a field that didn't have theorems, so they found something called automata theory and later on complexity theory. To many mathematicians, *those* are computer science.

One reason Allen Newell and I put the stress on an *experimental approach*, as we did in our Turing lecture (1976), was to point out that the mathematical view is a very partial view of things. Now another, to us more interesting, view of things is to say: "Here is the computer. Here's this great invention, here's a new kind of organism in the world. There weren't any of them before. They are very big, complex things, capable of behaving in complex ways. Let's have a science of them in the same way we have a science of *Homo sapiens*". The two sciences are related, but you study how computers behave.

Q: And you try out something experimentally and see what happens?

A: Right, right. Again, if one takes bounded rationality seriously, and I guess I ought to, human beings aren't very smart. Human beings can't even write a 10-line program and predict what it's going to do when you put it on the computer. Why—without actually running the computer, programming it, and studying it—why should we be able to understand what this program is all about, just because some human being invented it and put it together? It's like saying there's nothing to economics, it's just people behaving, so "obviously" people understand it! Well, there's something wrong with the "obviously" there. There's something wrong with the idea that "obviously" we understand computers because we built them.

Q: There's something paradoxical in what you're saying. When I perceive the world, for example, I must be doing something very, very complex, and in that sense I must be smart, although these smart mechanisms are certainly not conscious. If I were doing it consciously, I would undoubtedly get lost in all the information. So in what sense would you say that people are smart or not smart?

A: Well, of course "smart" and "not smart" are very relative terms. The only way we usually measure this is by comparing people with other people. Some are smarter than others. But if we make a rough division between those parts of the human nervous system that are the interfaces with the world, and those parts that are central, then I think it is pretty clear that it is the peripheral parts that are smart. The eye and the ear are very complex mechanisms. They've had a long time to adapt through evolutionary processes. The central nervous system, in particular the parts that are in the cerebrum, are fairly new structures, and compared with something like the eye, they seem to me to be incredibly simple. Maybe not simple in their neurophysiological structure, but simple in the range of capabilities they seem to have. So when human beings have to do anything with the central parts of the nervous system, just close their eyes and ears and do it all inside, there isn't very much they can do. Lie in bed tomorrow morning when you wake up and multiply two four-digit numbers together in your head—1776 by 1492, you can remember those two numbers—do it lying in bed with your eyes shut. It isn't easy. That sort of marks the limit as to what people can do with this nervous system.

Q: So people are good at perceiving and acting out but not good at thinking.

A: And pretty good at remembering, once they can by a slow and painful process get the stuff inside. A lot of the things we do that we think are smart are *recognition* sorts of things. For example, if you look at the abilities of chess masters, the one thing they do well is to *recognize* a very large number of situations they encounter in playing chess.

Q: Some people are shocked by your claim that the human nervous system really is simple. How would you deal with that kind of objection?

A: By pointing out that they're wrong! Again, "simple" is a slippery term, and I think in *The Sciences of the Artificial* (Simon, 1969/1981) I used it partially for dramatic effect. "Simple" relative to some of the mythical conceptions that people have of the wonderful things going on in the human head. Now, there are some complexities in the human system. I mentioned the eye as a fairly complex pattern recognizer. At least the things it does seem quite difficult to do. Second, of course, by the time long-term memory gets loaded up with a lot of things that can be accessed by recognition, the system looks complex. But it's only complex in the sense that an encyclopedia is complex. Is the *Encyclopedia Britannica* complex? It looks to me like just strings of ink on paper! That's what it looks like to me. Now, it has something called an index, which allows you to go zing! and find particular things in that big five-foot bookshelf. And that's what makes it look pretty impressive. That's what makes the human mind look complex.

Q: And so the critical question becomes, how do you index information in your model of the human mind?

A: This was one of the things we were trying to get at through the chess perception research.

Q: Some of the most dramatic findings in that research involve the memory for chess positions in chess masters and beginners. Chess masters are very good at remembering positions that make sense, but no better than beginners at remembering arbitrary chess situations (Chase & Simon, 1973).

A: Right. So this seems to us a pretty clear demonstration that what's held in short-term memory is, again, just a small number of chunks, but the chessmaster's chunk is a pretty rich thing. It has a lot of information.

Q: I believe that you estimated that a chess master needs to have about 50,000 chunks in long-term memory. The question is, of course, How do you find the right chunk for the situation you see on the chess board?

A: And that's the recognition process. You look at a chess board, and there's an open file there, and you say, Gee, maybe you ought to put a rook on it. Or the pawns in front of a king's position have been jumped forward, and you say, Gee, there's a loose king's position — a kingside pawn attack should lead to a working combination.

Q: And a grand master does look at only a small number of possibilities.

A: That's what all the evidence indicates. He looks at the *right* ones. That's what George Baylor and I did with the Master chess program. It rediscovered a lot of the real brilliancies that you can find in all the chess books.

Q: Let me talk a little bit about how your work looks to many experimental psychologists — even today, many experimental psychologists consider your work very theoretical. A recent cognitive psychology text (Lachman, Lachman, & Butterfield, 1979) refers to "global modeling" in the following terms:

. . . their colleagues have mixed feelings about the global modelers. On the one hand, most . . . experimental information processing psychologists can see that they're asking the right questions. On the other hand, there is some objection to the movement away from the traditional experimentation. . . . The global modelers are similar to linguists in their willingness to use rational argument and they're similar to artificial intelligence specialists in their willingness to be pragmatic for the purpose of implementing parts of their models on computers. To at least some information processing psychologists and perhaps to many, these are character flaws. (p. 437)

I don't imagine you consider those to be a character flaws. How would you respond to that?

A: My usual response is to give people a lecture on how science is done in other sciences. You know, if people looked around a little more at geology, astrophysics, and a few other places, and didn't think that Newton's three laws of motion summed up all of science, they'd relax a little bit about methodology. One uses all sorts of devices to acquire theories. We look to computer programs as a source of hints for understanding psychology.

List processing is a great example of this. As I say, it was originally invented mostly as a response to some very practical programming needs. But it turned out that in order to meet those needs, you had to meet some conditions that *any* information-processing system that thinks has to meet.

And once having gotten this approach, it gave us a lot of clues as to how the human system works.

I mentioned geology because experimental psychologists could never be geologists — they don't believe in just looking at the world and looking at it hard! But that's the way we found out about glaciers and mountain raising and all those good things. That wasn't done by controlled experiments. That was done just by very careful observation of the details of nature.

And that's what we do with our work in protocol analysis, for example. We actually get some human beings to behave, and then we take their behavior seriously, because that's the phenomenon we want to explain. Those are data. And all of these old wives' tales about introspection and its woes just become irrelevant when you understand what to do with those data.

Q: From a common sense viewpoint it certainly seems reasonable to say that if you want to find out about people, *talk to them*! Experimental psychologists, however, have been very wary of doing that because of the absence of some agreed-upon theoretical representation for human language. How do you represent what people do when they talk to you? How do you represent meanings? Do you represent the speech signal? And so on. There are very great self-doubts, I think, among experimental psychologists about using that information. How would you justify your use of ordinary language?

A: In the same way I'd justify using any information. You can raise the same questions about finger pushes on keys. You know, How do you encode this? Do you encode the amount of pressure applied? Not usually done. All that's usually done is to encode which key is pressed. That already involves a theoretical position, already involves injecting some theory into your analysis of the data. And of course you do that in analyzing protocols as well as with anything else. It's no different than the physicist who has to have a physical theory of the instrumentation. Exactly the same thing.

Q: The difference is, I suppose, that within physics, there is good agreement regarding the meaning of the data.

A: Well, there's never good agreement on the frontiers, because at the frontiers there's always a hazy line between which part of what you're interpreting is really data and which part is a misinterpretation of your instrumentation. That's true in any experimental frontier, and it's true here. It's a real bootstrapping operation.

Q: Thus "the facts" themselves are ambiguous, or at least uninterpretable without some theory.

A: Only a geologist can squeeze a fact from a rock. A rock isn't a fact. A geologist looks at it and he scratches it and he makes all sorts of guesses. A lot of his observations are qualitative. What test do you perform on something to call it sandstone? Most geologists of my acquaintance just *look* at it. How subjective can you be?

Q: Of course, they can agree with each other when they look at it.

A: Yeah well, people who've looked at protocols can also agree. The disagreement is not among people who look at protocols; the disagreement is between them and people who don't look at protocols. A little like the prelates who were debating with Galileo, and they didn't want to look through his telescope because — I don't know what, maybe they were afraid of what they would see. I don't know of much disagreement in protocol analysis when you take actual protocols and analyze them. You can get very high reliability.

Q: So as we said before, to many mathematical computer scientists you are quite experimental, whereas to most experimental psychologists, your work is highly theoretical.

A: Well, it's always good if you've got people on both sides of you; then you know you're somewhere on course.

Q: What permitted you to take this position early on in the game, when everybody else within psychology was constrained by the rules of the behavioristic paradigm? What permitted you to do things that other people couldn't do?

A: I guess one very obvious thing was I was never trained in that paradigm. I never had a formal course in psychology. So I didn't know what you weren't supposed to do. I knew about behaviorism, I'd read about such things — not with great belief, but I knew it existed. But I was exposed to a number of other traditions in biology and in the social sciences, where people were very much more relaxed about the variety of things they took as data and the variety of ways in which they looked at it. The name of the game was to explain the phenomena.

Second, it isn't as though experimental psychology has had a rich collection of theoretical concepts adequate to describing complex behavior. There was a terrible poverty here. And if you compare the poverty of the formalisms of S–R psychology, where you do an S, an arrow, and an R and call that a theory, the comparison of that with the kinds of theoretical tools you have in logic or in mathematical economics made psychology look like a very backward nation. And since I had access to those other tools, I couldn't see why I shouldn't be using them in the problems that I had.

I think this is where computers really came into the act — the idea that symbolic processing could be described in formal terms. This idea fascinated me long before there were any computers around.

Q: The formal devices that you invented are not that different from those used by people like Clark Hull, for example. But your work has clearly worked out in a way in that Hull's never did. What do you think is the difference?

A: Hull's theoretical tools were very impoverished. He couldn't talk about the content of a symbol. He had "S" for stimulus, and he could give a subscript to it, so it was "stimulus one" and "stimulus two." He had no way of talking about the content of the symbol. He had nothing corresponding to the branch operation. He had nothing corresponding to the directed association. Just very impoverished formulas.

Q: The lesson that most experimental psychologists drew from the failure of Hull's theory is that we didn't have enough facts, and we should go back to the laboratory to get more data. And indeed Skinner (1957) has argued that one shouldn't build theories at all. But you went in the opposite direction — you became *more* theoretical rather than less.

A: Yeah, we saw a way of doing it — and that's the other important half of it. It's all very well to talk about virtue, but another thing is to *be* virtuous. And you have to ask: What makes it possible to be more theoretical in the appropriate way? Until some formalisms came along that we could apply to the problem, we were just preaching virtue.

Q: Do you think that mathematical formalisms would have been enough by themselves without the use of the computer?

A: Well, they got us a certain distance along the way. I ran a "controlled experiment" on that myself: I tried to do these things before computers and after computers. Before the computer we had a metaphor drawn from logic, whereby we could equate decision making with drawing conclusions from premises. But until the computer came along and allowed us to deal with the semantics of the situation and allowed us really to represent memories and to access information, these ideas still remained very vague.

Q: When would you say the main change took place in the views of scientific psychologists? George Miller suggests — facetiously, I think — that the shift took place on September 12, 1956, because there was a conference at that time where you and Allen Newell presented a paper on a system for discovering proofs of logic theorems; Green and Swets presented a paper on signal detection theory; and George Miller presented a paper on the magic number 7, plus or minus 2.

A: At that conference, Chomsky also gave one of his first presentations of the three theories of grammar. And there was the publication of the Bruner, Goodnow, and Austin (1956) book. All these ideas were enormously influential later on.

These events all took place in that year. Nineteen fifty-six was obviously the key year in terms of these things all coming to a jell. There were a lot of things that happened before 1956, but if one wants to have a starting point, then it's as good a place as any.

I'll give you a little bit of my own experience. I first got into contact with "precomputer" computers about 1938, when I was still in the municipal measurement business and was editing the statistical portions of a municipal yearbook. It all had to be done by hand, and I thought that this was a hell of a way to do it. I heard there was some sort of machine over at the University of Chicago bookstore. I found an old IBM calculating punch there, and I learned how to wire up the thing and converted the work to a machine operation. That alerted me to the notion that computation might be done by machine, and from then on I was sensitive to what was going on in that area.

Later on, I got to the West Coast and was involved in a big empirical field study in which we had more data than we knew what to do with. So I made use of the IBM Service Bureau out there. By that time they had wire plug-boards. I don't know if you've ever seen a plug-board machine. You essentially programmed it by wiring a plug-board. So, I got introduced to that. And then when the first real computers appeared, right after the war ended, I was fascinated. I had no idea it had anything to do with my work, but one can't limit one's interest to that. So I tried to follow what was going on.

In 1950, at an Econometric Society meeting in Cambridge, we had some discussion on the extent to which you could use the computer as a metaphor for the mind. A few were very skeptical. I was less skeptical because I saw that hierarchical structures in computers ought to have something to do with hierarchical structures in thinking processes. So, I was watching these things for a variety of reasons that had only a little bit to do with human problem solving. And by 1954, the IBM 701 was out, and I learned to program that. Then Al Newell and I went out to the RAND corporation, where they had a big air defense simulation, and Al had figured out a way of using a computer to generate maps that could be used on a simulated radar screen. That was my first introduction to the idea that you could use a computer for something other than producing numbers.

And all that began to interact with my general fascination with human thinking. In '54, Al and I went out to observe an air exercise out at March Air Force base, and on the way out we began talking about using the computer to simulate human thinking. Al got another injection when Selfrich and Dinneen came out there with their first programmed pattern recognizer (Dinneen, 1955). That's when Al really decided he'd better go to work.

Q: The idea that computers are *general* symbolic processors is fascinating. I think it is one of the really important points that's still not well understood in psychology.

A: Oh yeah, most people who don't deal with computers still don't understand this. Some computer scientists still don't understand it!

Q: You've said that in psychology, there are many things you can observe without easily quantifying them, and these may be quite objective in their own way. But in many psychologists' minds, being able to assign a number to something is still the *sine qua non* of science.

A: The *sine qua non* of science is to get interested in some set of phenomena and try to explain them. First you get some theories that explain the phenomena and then some evidence that the theories are right. I think it's ridiculous to think that that is limited to quantitative things. If you believe that, you have to rule out most natural science, outside of a few limited areas of physics.

Q: I suppose the question is, How do you get precision if you can't assign numbers?

A: I don't think there's any problem with getting real precision in a computer program. If you don't have precision, it doesn't run, does it? It does what it does in a very precise way. There's nothing I can think of more formal than a computer program for describing what a complex behaving system does.

Q: Every beginning psychology student is taught that in any respectable experiment you need an experimental group and a control group. Then if you find a statistically significant difference between the two you can claim to be verifying an hypothesis. The statistical test gives a quantitative measure of the probability of the truth of your hypothesis.

A: Well, it doesn't, of course. Part of the trouble is the abuse of the statistical procedures being used. With a few exceptions there are no standard statistical procedures for deciding whether *models fit data*. I could give you a long lecture on that. The idea is not original with me; you'll find a whole literature on this subject, which is steadily ignored by most writers of statistical textbooks for psychologists. I think that's one of the problems. Psychologists try to apply statistical tests as though a model were a null hypothesis. There are some fundamental things wrong with that.

Q: Many experimentalists seem ill at ease with global theories because they seem arbitrary, like a story somebody might tell — what if somebody else comes along with an entirely different story? It's not clear how you would show that one global theory is better than another.

A: The time to start worrying about that is when you have *two* global theories that explain the same facts. I don't know any alternative theories to EPAM (a model of short-term memory; see Simon, 1979, pp. 95–124), for example, that explain the facts that EPAM explains. Just name it!

Q: I imagine that you could set up some set of propositions that would explain the same facts.

A: Well, do it. And when somebody's done it, it'll be time to choose between them. Psychology is the only science I know of that is so possessed, so preoccupied with the notion of choosing between theories, when in the past it hasn't even had a single theory! Geologists don't behave this way, physicists don't behave this way. They feel gratified when they get *one* theory. Then when some other one comes along that will explain the same phenomenon, they begin to worry about testing the difference. But that doesn't happen very often.

Q: So you think theoretical adequacy — the ability to explain the phenomena in any way at all — is the important thing to look for.

A: Right. The important thing about Special Relativity wasn't that it resolved the paradox of the Michelson–Morley experiment. Einstein hardly knew about those experiments before. So it wasn't a choice between the Newtonian and Einsteinian theory. The problem was that there were electromagnetic phenomena that simply wouldn't fit *at all* with *any* theory known. Einstein discovered a theory that fit them. I don't know that any statistical test was ever applied to decide whether that was the right theory or not.

Q: Then you feel that you have an adequate theory of certain psychological phenomena — but it is hard to convince people that your theory is indeed adequate?

A: It's not so hard, they're coming over, coming over very fast now. Not enough of them know enough of the formalism yet. They're getting it in a kind of Bowdlerized form in these English language versions of the theory, so it'll be another generation before they get sufficiently mathematized to take it straight out of the bottle.

Q: In other words, as more people become familiar with computers and computational formalisms, then they should understand what you've been doing.

A: The ones who really read *Human Problem Solving* (1972) are much better off than the ones who merely read introductions to expository accounts.

Q: What constitutes persuasive evidence in science, and particularly in psychology? What do you think convinces people?

A: Big qualitative phenomena that are loud and clear, that you can talk about without statistical significance tests. The chess experiments are a good example. There are some very clear, powerful phenomena there that make more friends for this view of chunking, perception, and memory than anything else. So a good loud qualitative phenomenon and a plausible explanation are good enough.

Q: In a curious way, your viewpoint is not that different from Skinner's. That is to say, he would argue that statistical tests are useless, that you have to find dramatic phenomena. And furthermore he would argue that the real phenomena in psychology are to be found in the environment, rather than within the organism. Isn't that how you feel as well?

A: I think our positions are very close together. What I think Skinner leaves out are the very important characteristics of the organism that condition the way it has to deal with the environment. Skinner's theory is impoverished with respect to his description of the organism, and it doesn't have such constructions as a limited short-term memory or an associative long-term memory that has to be indexed in a particular way. But that's all the difference that I see.

Q: That's interesting. Skinner wrote an article a few years ago called "Why I Am Not a Cognitive Psychologist" (1977). He says:

The cognitive metaphor is based on behavior in the real world. We associate things by putting them together, store memoranda and retrieve them for later use, . . . [and] we describe contingencies of reinforcements in rules. These are the actions of real persons. It is only in the fanciful world of an inner person that they become mental processes. (p. 9)

Is he right that we have a metaphor that we simply take from actions in the physical world?

A: Certainly not. Oh, I don't know where we get the ideas originally, but the problem of psychology is to explain how the box that sits on your neck can do the things it does. And that's what an information-processing theory does explain. The fact is that you can find analogous processes in the physical world — I've been using the encyclopedia metaphor here all afternoon — the fact that an encyclopedia is indexed doesn't mean that my brain isn't. The principles of indexing might be different in the two cases.

Q: What I think is really central is the question of inferring unobservable phenomena — you can't see rules in other people's heads, and here Skinner uses the famous joke by Molière about . . .

A: About the opium?

Q: Yes, right. The medieval professor is trying to explain why opium makes you sleepy, and he claims that it is because of a "dormitive virtue" in the opium. He infers the explanatory construct that explains the phenomenon, without having any direct evidence about the inferred construct. And Skinner says that this kind of circular reasoning is all we do when we infer the existence of rules in people's heads.

A: From the fact that opium makes me sleep, I would certainly infer that there's some chemical properties of opium which, if I understood them, and understood the physiology of the brain, would tell me how this happened. And I guess people are beginning to understand now that there are certain parts of the brain that have an affiliation for opiates. I don't know the facts on that, but I see articles that seem to be talking that way in biological journals. And that will be the explanation of opium.

The biologists didn't give up and say, Well, all we need to know is that people go to sleep. They precisely went about finding out what the internal mechanism is that put them to sleep. That doesn't mean just naming it a "dormitive faculty." Physics would be in a very bad state if the only entities that were allowed in physics are the things we see with our eyes. No more quarks, no more atoms, no more molecules, no more electrons. I find it hard to debate that position of Skinner's because it seems to me so extraordinary.

Q: And by "theoretical explanation" you mean referring behavior to something that is not behavior.

A: Ultimately, yes. Explaining in terms of more primitive mechanisms than the behavior itself, a more parsimonious account than the behavior itself.

Q: It's curious in that respect that one of the strong arguments that behaviorists have used against theories is the argument from parsimony.

A: When you talk about parsimony of a theory, you have to ask not only how many words it takes to state the theory, but how much the theory explains. And I don't know very many things that Skinnerian doctrine explains, except that under favorable circumstances, if you reinforce an animal's behavior it might continue. And a few little facts about how the schedule of those reinforcements affects the pattern of behavior, for pigeons at least. But I don't see anything in Skinner that says anything about *shaping*—which is the real learning phenomenon. He says it exists and how you do it, but there's no formal theory of it.

Q: Why not?

A: Because I don't think you can build a formal theory with your hands tied behind your back by the limitation that you can't go inside the head.

Q: Skinner has had impressive success in persuading people of his viewpoint. How would you account for that success?

A: Well, I would account for it in considerable part by the attraction that simplicity and certainty have for a large number of people. You find this same phenomenon in economics with Milton Friedman. If you come along with a simple formula that when recited appropriately, will deal with almost any situation you're in, maybe you won't ask too hard whether the formula really deals with the situation.

Q: So you think that sheer simplicity is attractive.

A: Yeah, simplicity with a kind of broad applicability. I'll try to define what I mean by applicability there. There is nothing you could say about the world that Milton Friedman can't translate into a little discourse on neoclassical economics. And Fred Skinner can do the same thing with any behavioral phenomenon. He can turn it into something with contingencies and reinforcements.

Q: It seems to me that until now you have only looked at conscious, deliberate problem solving.

A: If you look at any of the models that we built, there's nothing in the model that represents the boundary between conscious and unconscious. That's a defect of the models. It also means that the models do not assume that all of this is going on in the conscious mind. In order to even talk about consciousness, you have to add mechanisms that are not present in any of those models, self-referential mechanisms. This involves the representation of your own processes you have access to.

Q: Why is it, do you think, that your work did not catch on sooner?

A: Some people understood what we were doing very early. George Miller, for example, understood what we did on the information-processing end of things, but I never understood why he didn't have the courage of his convictions on the computer side. I never understood it. He was one of the organizers of the 1958 RAND summer seminar, and probably the main author of *Plans and the Structure of Behavior* (Miller, Galanter, & Pribram, 1960).

Q: Was he aware of the computational approach at that time?

A: Oh, he sure was. At that summer institute he wrote a little parser for sentences.

Q: Have you talked to him about this?

A: Yeah, many times in many ways, and I just can't characterize his reactions. He somehow or other never 100% believed it was for real.

Q: His role in the paradigm shift is very interesting. He is perceived by many people to be the person who was just far enough ahead of the field to lead other people in that direction, but not so far as to be considered an outsider to the field.

A: That's right, that certainly has been his role. I couldn't understand it. It's a great mystery. I've known George for many many years, and I just find myself in wonder about this.

Well you know, partly this is my own reaction: I couldn't have stayed away from it. It just seemed to me that this was the most exciting thing happening in science. And he was one of the guys who helped bring about the shift. The paper on the "magic number seven" (1956) — you know at that time he was right in the forefront, he wasn't an intermediary, but in the forefront.

Q: What impact have you seen the cognitive shift have on other people in the field?

A: I guess the biggest impression I've taken away from this, and from other experiences that I've had, is that there just aren't very many adventurers in the world. They just aren't there. You know, science is a gambling game. If you play it for big stakes, you have to take big gambles. There just aren't very many people, including scientists, who feel very comfortable doing that. I thought in 1956 there would be a gold rush of people clamoring to get into this, even graduate students. But it was only five years ago when things like the DENDRAL mass spectograph program at Stanford (done by Lederberg and Feigenbaum) began to make Artificial Intelligence (AI) a little bit respectable, that graduate students in large numbers began to come to AI. For complicated reasons, this work got a good reception and changed attitudes about how iffy AI was, and that had an immediate impact on graduate students.

Q: Graduate students seem to be very careful, very perceptive.

A: Almost as careful as their professors.

Q: One of the remarkable questions in the history of behaviorism is why it is so tenacious, so that very many people who call themselves experimental psychologists are still . . .

A: Are still behaving that way.

Q: Do you have any thoughts on that?

A: Not really, except that once a paradigm gets entrenched in a field, people learn it and they practice it until there's some crushing reason for doing something else. And they pass it on to their graduate students, so that there is a great built-in inertia in the system. I've watched the same thing in other fields. Economics is another great one. How any grown-up, bright human being can go on satisfied with neoclassical theory is kind of hard to understand. Well, it has these nice formal properties, and it gives you some things you know how to do, particularly with respect to experimental methodologies. Economists learn how to do statistical regressions on economic data and things of that sort. They don't learn how to do interviews in a business firm. That's much more difficult for an economist to learn to do. Similarly, in psychology, I think it is much easier to accept the mental baggage of information-processing psychology than it is to take a protocol and analyze it. I think in many ways the behaviorists were successful because they provided a few experimental methodologies that people could learn in graduate school and keep on doing afterward.

Q: You're one of the few psychologists to have received a Nobel Prize.

A: Yes. There are of course the ethologists, such as Tinbergen and Lorenz. I'm not sure if they consider themselves psychologists. They got the biology prize, and von Békésy also, and Pavlov if we go back in history a little. Pavlov, of course, did not get it for conditioning, but for his work on the digestive system. Mine is for my work on the economics of the firm.

Q: You've told me that you consider all of your work to be part of problem-solving psychology. Do you think the Nobel committee was aware of this, and recognized the psychological aspect of your work?

A: Well, again, I can't read the minds of the committee, but I know them, and they are economists who do the things economists do. The things they know about my work are largely in economics. As a matter of fact, I'd feel uncomfortable about the prize if I thought it had been given to me for the psychological work, which obviously would have had to be a joint prize with Allen Newell. But trying to be as objective as one can be about these things, I think the work I've done that has had a direct impact on economics could explain their choice reasonably well. I suppose my general notoriety doesn't hurt. But I was a real early card-carrying member of the Econometric Society, and a Fellow of the Econometric Society at the time I did the work for which they cited me.

Q: You would say that there's a great continuity in all of the work that you've done, and indeed that there's an impressive continuity across "artificial systems" as you call them (Simon, 1969/1981), which includes living systems. Would you say, then, that in spite of your Nobel Prize, this continuity is still not recognized very widely?

A: I certainly would agree with that. I think that the new "cognitive science" slogan is a long step in that direction.

Q: "Cognitive science," you mean, as being the interdisciplinary area that has grown up in recent years between psychologists, Artificial Intelligence people, linguists, philosophers, and so on.

A: Yes, that's the whole point of the journal *Cognitive Science,* and the whole point of the Sloan Foundation effort to fund activities in cognitive science.

Q: And would you say that psychology in general is moving in the direction that you've pioneered with Allen Newell?

A: Well, I've got to believe that, because I believe that in the long run, reality determines which way science is going to go. Because we know how the world is in reality, it's got to come this way. And I'm prepared to be very patient about it.

Donald A. Norman:
Cognitive Science and the Future of Psychology

Donald A. Norman (b. 1935) has made notable empirical contributions to the study of cognition, especially on the topics of short-term memory and selective attention. He has also devoted a major effort to global theoretical models, even though such models have been more difficult to publish in the psychology journals (*e.g.*, Norman & Rumelhart, 1975). In addition, his textbooks on cognition are quite well known, and have been translated into several foreign languages (Norman, 1967/1976; Lindsay & Norman, 1977). And finally, Donald Norman has shown considerable leadership in the founding group of "cognitive science," both in the journal and in the society of that name. For instance, his article "Twelve Issues in Cognitive Science" (1981) sketches out an ambitious program for cognitive science in the investigation of such classically thorny psychological issues as consciousness and emotion.

Like the other "Nucleators" presented in this chapter, Norman began his career outside of conventional psychology. After receiving his BS in engineering from MIT, he attended graduate school at the University of Pennsylvania (where some of the early computers had been developed), specializing in electrical and computer engineering. Several physicists and mathematicians were developing a Mathematical Psychology program at Penn at that time, and, intrigued by what seemed to be the most powerful computer around — the human brain — Norman decided to switch to psychology. After receiving his doctorate at Penn in 1962, Norman spent some time at the Harvard Center for Cognitive Studies, where George Miller and Jerome Bruner were having great influence on the direction of early cognitive work. Since then he has served on the faculty of the University of California, San Diego, as director of its Cognitive Science Laboratory and member of the Center for Human Information Processing.

The present interview differs somewhat from the others in this volume, because Professor Norman requested a new interview, some years after having given a conventional one, to emphasize his optimism and excitement about the newest developments in cognitive science. I was most pleased to give him this opportunity.

Interview with Donald A. Norman

Q: How do you feel that psychology has changed recently?

A: Well, today I'm an optimist. I have a good feeling about the way the field has developed in the recent years, and the way it might develop in the future. When I started off, I had to justify the study of the mind, the study of information-processing mechanisms.

Q: That was about 20 years ago?

A: In the early 1960s. The word "mind" was not allowed. The study of information processing didn't really exist — not in psychology. Over the years, human information processing and cognitive psychology have become the dominant themes in psychology. "Mind" is a respectable word today, and the study of consciousness is a respectable study. Today we're talking even in broader terms: not just of cognitive psychology, or even of a cognitive science, but bringing in other disciplines — finally relating what happens in the brain to what happens to the total organism, to what happens with interactions among people, among ourselves and society and culture and the environment; looking at the way the nervous system shapes our behavior. It's an exciting era, and I think that now is a good time to talk about it, because new developments in cognitive science are just beginning: cognitive psychology has become a mature discipline. It's so mature, in fact, that some people feel that its days are over — that information-processing psychology is no longer the appropriate view — that cognitive psychology is suspect, and that it will be replaced with new paradigms. But to me, the new paradigms are well within the same spirit. We simply are seeing an emergence of new views of the human. And that's good, that's proper. Even though they may look like internal bickerings and arguments from close up, from a distance they're all moving in the same direction.

Q: So you feel very positive toward the field right now.

A: Yes, on the whole, I think we're developing very well. I think that the congruence of fields, the combination of cognitive psychology, linguistics, cognitive anthropology, sociology, the neurosciences, and especially neuropsychology, philosophy, and Artificial Intelligence are all positive. At the moment there really isn't a good synthesis of all these fields. What we have, rather, are small groups of people from two or three of these disciplines working together. That has meant an influx of ideas from many different viewpoints, an influx that has just begun. There haven't been any spectacular developments yet. I suspect that within 5 to 10 years there may be.

Q: Why do you think that this interaction between all these fields is possible today and was not possible 20 years ago or 40 years ago?

A: Well, I think it was possible 80 years ago, less possible 60 years ago, and then it disappeared. A lot of that has to do with the history of American psychology, the development of behaviorism, the development of a way of thought in psychology that really discouraged the analysis of internal mechanisms. And this was true not only in psychology, but in other disciplines as well. The information sciences didn't exist. We knew very little of the concepts of information and communication. Those sciences and the appropriate mathematics didn't exist. The study of linguistics was primarily — the study of individual languages. Linguists were looking at languages and trying to write dictionaries and grammars. The study of anthropology viewed the human in a very peculiar light, a very degrading light, actually, for the societies that were being studied. Most of the disciplines, I feel, were very narrow in their outlook.

What has happened since the 1950s or '60s has been the emergence of a new science of information processing. Now, I think that there are a large number of common origins for this. In the neurosciences, people were concerned with the mechanisms by which the body regulates its own behavior. In engineering there has been the development of servomechanisms, the development of computational devices — most of them analogue — and then the first inklings of a digital computer. The concepts of digital computation have been around for a long time, 100 years or longer. The notion of information flow has been around, but it was slowly being refined. The work of Shannon was clearly a critical impetus (*e.g.*, Shannon & Weaver, 1949). Around the end of the 1950s there were a group of people from the neurosciences, from mathematics, from engineering, who shared common backgrounds and were trying to develop a common view about the importance of the processing of information. In fact, in the late 1950s there was a spate of conferences on what today we would call Artificial Intelligence, which in those days tended to be called other things. There was Her Majesty's Conference on the Mechanisms of Thought; there were the Macy conferences (see Heims, 1975); Norbert Wiener was a major figure in the development of cybernetics, the attempt to apply mathematical methods to the understanding of human behavior (Wiener, 1961). What we would today call cognitive psychologists played a role, although this didn't fit within the discipline of psychology in the United States. I think that was a turning point in the late 1950s. I feel that Artificial Intelligence, as a discipline, was developed out of those early conferences, and I think that the first inklings of change in psychology came about then as well.

Contemporary psychology has been characterized by some as being dominated by the computer metaphor, as just following the developments in computer science. I think that's false. I think that, in fact, we grew out of a common origin. The people who developed information-processing psychology grew up in the same spirit and at the same time as the people who developed Artificial Intelligence. So when McCarthy, Simon, Newell, and Minsky were developing their ideas in computer science, so, too, were people like Miller, and people like me, much younger, coming from the engineering tradition. I learned first from people like Shannon and Wiener, then took a course with Chomsky. Then I began developing my own ideas about computers, because that's what I was doing in those days, building computers. I learned of the work of Simon and Newell at Carnegie–Mellon and then slowly developed my own notions of how the human information-processing system might be studied. I think that this was the common groundswell of the field. It was the *Zeitgeist* of the times; no one field grew out of the other.

In fact, you could argue that computer science grew out of psychology. A naïve psychology of sorts, but Von Neumann, when he talked of the computer (1958), clearly had in mind the mechanism by which people solved problems; the standard computer design of today—the Von Neumann computer—was intended to copy the human processing system.

Q: The idea of information seems to be critical: What is the study of information processing, and how is it different from studying just behavior or just the brain?

A: If you look just at behavior, then you miss all of the internal processes that take place. If you look just at the brain, you learn something about the kinds of mechanisms that exist and the neural pathways; but in order to understand what is happening, you must know about the informational *signals* that are being transmitted over those pathways and what happens to them. Formally, information is that abstract entity that allows one to distinguish among alternatives. And the information is defined to have a minimum unit—the bit—that distinguishes between just two alternatives. That formal definition has not been too useful in psychology, but if you examine that definition you'll see that it requires that there be a lot of other things present. If a signal is to discriminate between two alternatives, that means you must have set out those two alternatives in the beginning. It means that it must be possible to generate a signal in some medium that is transmitted over distance. There must therefore be some means of generating the signal and transmitting it, some means of receiving it, some means of interpreting the signal. In order to interpret a signal, the receiver must know beforehand what the alternatives are, and then it must determine which one of those alternatives is signified by the signal. "Information," then, involves transmission of signals, their encoding to specify some particular set of alternatives, and then the reception and decoding of these signals, which means the attempt to understand which of the alternatives might have been meant. Now, in communication theory, there is little problem with all this, because beforehand everybody gets together and agrees on what the alternative states are going to mean. When you talk about the human organism, however, the problems are not the same, because we can only *infer* what the other person might have had in mind when communicating with us by speaking to us or writing to us or signalling us. Even within the brain, it is not clear that the formal requirements of information theory are met. But nonetheless, I think it provides a basic paradigm. We can then move from the paradigm to manipulate it for our own purposes, to understand the brain better. The basic notion of information processing, I think, is that of abstract signals that are transmitted from person to person, from the culture to the person, within the person, within the brain, that are interpreted by and within the brain.

Q: And so, in a sense, information is independent of the physical medium that is used to transmit the signals?

A: In the formal definition, yes. Within the human, not necessarily so. There's a debate about that just barely beginning that promises to be very important. In the early days of the study of human information processing, we were looking at mechanisms of mind, and we divided the human into various classes of mechanisms. We said that there was clearly sensation, perception, memory, language, thought, skills. A set of different kinds of processes. We started off by analyzing the kinds of phenomena that humans exhibited, and then we looked at the kinds of processing mechanisms we thought could underlie those phenomena. Then we moved from the study of the individual mechanisms to an emphasis on the problem of representation. This really meant, therefore, that we were dominated by studies of memory and language and thought. This led, eventually, to the problems of representing ideas in memory, the development of semantic networks, the notion of propositional representation, of analogical representation, and ultimately to the development of the concept of a schema. A schema is an overall, large-scale organizing concept within the memory that is used to guide processing.

Q: What's the importance of schemata? I am genuinely puzzled about what schemata do for cognitive psychologists. It just seems to be another data structure.

A: There are several different ways of viewing the schema. The concept of the schema is very important because it says that the memory structures are organized into small units of information—that new structures can be built only by analogy to old structures or by addition to old structures. It says that we don't just experience something and build up a whole new memory representation. The concept of schema is not well defined. It has been greatly criticized as being fuzzy and sloppy, and it *is* both fuzzy and sloppy. But I think this is because it's in an early stage of development. The concept is very important because, as I said, it argues for a certain kind of structure of the knowledge within memory that is heavily based on experience; it says that once you start developing a particular set of knowledge structures, you're committed to them for the rest of your life, essentially. They will color your interpretation of everything, and these interpretations will be very difficult to change. Possible, but difficult.

This morning I was talking with Dave McNeill, who wrote a book on language, action, and thought (McNeill, 1979), which revives the Whorfian hypothesis. Essentially the Whorfian hypothesis says that different peoples in different cultures come to view the world differently, and their mental structures for the world are different.

Q: By "view of the world," you mean the way they experience the world?

A: I mean the way people experience the world, and what is important in the world for people in our culture may be quite different from what is important for people in some other culture, even if the environment were the same. Their language and their thoughts would reflect that. It's not that thought follows linguistic structure; it's that the culture determines the *mental structures*, and both thought and language reflect the mental structures. The notion of schemas fits this analysis very well. In fact, schemas tend automatically to lead to this idea. The way you originally organize your data structures will determine your future organization.

But so far the development of cognitive concepts has excluded a number of things. It's excluded feelings, it's excluded emotions, it's excluded images and other analogical representations. Psychologists are just now beginning to look at the mechanisms controlling action—how we actually do things. Even the first few studies have led us to realize that skilled actions are done automatically, without attentional resources. That fact forces us for the first time, I think, to confront the fact of consciousness. The problem of consciousness, as you well know, is not a new problem, and it has been brought up before, but never well. Only a few people have written about consciousness. The word is appearing more and more frequently in the literature, but seldom with much content. I think that as we start looking at performance and the way we actually do our tasks, we are going to be faced with coming to grips with consciousness, because there seems to be a distinct difference in the way in which we perform unskilled acts under conscious control and the way we perform skilled acts with apparently no conscious control whatsoever — oftentimes with no conscious awareness of doing the act. There's no way to study that without getting into the details of what it *means* to have conscious control. That's only one aspect of consciousness.

One other area that's being revived is the study of learning, which is, today, coming from research in memory. Once upon a time the study of learning dominated psychology — psychology *was*, in a sense, the study of learning and motivation.

But in those days it was a global characterization of the organism. Today it's an attempt to understand what goes on inside the mind, what it is that is changing with learning. I feel that learning may be the most difficult concept, because understanding learning will also involve the understanding of consciousness. I believe that consciousness is essential for certain kinds of learning.

Q: You feel that consciousness is necessary for some kinds of learning but not others?

A: Well, as you know, David Rumelhart and I have distinguished several classes of learning. We call them accretion, restructuring, and tuning (Rumelhart & Norman, 1978). Accretion is just the accumulation of new information where schemas already exist; you are simply acquiring new information that can fit within existing schemas. "Tuning" refers to the situation where the schemas exist but they're inefficient; with repeated practice they become specialized or "tuned" to the particular task at hand. "Restructuring" is done least often, but it is most important — that's where you essentially learn a whole new way of viewing the world. Here the proper schema does *not* yet exist. You must create new schemas; usually by analogy from schemas from other areas. I believe that tuning does not require consciousness. Restructuring does. And I don't know about accretion.

In the past we've tended to view the mind as a relatively homogeneous medium. There was learning, yes, there was memory, yes, language, and thought. The whole image was of a general memory where all knowledge resided, and a general processing mechanism that took care of language or thought, took care of this, took care of that. We're now changing that. We're realizing that the knowledge people have about one domain doesn't seem to transfer well to other domains. We can have people who reason flawlessly, apparently effortlessly, with great depth and sophistication about one domain, and when they move to a new domain, they're like children. They make the most elementary reasoning errors. Professors of logic, who are very sophisticated in the use of implication, can make the most elementary errors when they come to other domains. We're also beginning to believe there are specialized brain mechanisms which handle various things that we do, and that hasn't yet sunk home. We still don't know if this means that there's a single memory or whether there are separate memories. Is there a separate memory for faces that's different from a memory for words, or different from a memory for emotions, or a memory for events? We don't know, we really don't know.

Jerry Fodor has written a book on what he calls "the modularity hypothesis." He argues the extreme view: specialized mechanisms for everything (Fodor, 1983). I suspect that this will become a big debate in the next decade, with extreme opponents on either side. And as is the nature of such debates, the answer will be in the middle. I think there is much more specialization than we previously believed; but I suspect that the specialization is not as strong as Fodor, at the moment, seems to be advocating.

We are now learning more neurological information. We haven't paid much attention to neuropsychology, the effects of brain damage, the way the nervous system may be organized, and about the constraints the nervous system puts on the organism. And again, as you know, when you start looking at the effects of brain damage you find patients who have perfect memory except they can't remember faces anymore. Or people will seem to know most words quite well, but they won't be able to handle function words, just as though there *were* a separate memory for function words such as "the," "of," "which," and the like. That seems strange on the face of it, until you realize that function words don't have meanings in the same way that other words do. They seem to be processing pointers. So the word "the" is a pointer for how to process the noun that is going to follow. Maybe that involves a separate mechanism that can be damaged separately.

Q: Have you just gone from psychology to neurophysiology?

A: No. I've expanded from cognitive psychology to cognitive science. That's what I've done. It means that the information that we look at from brain damage is of critical importance. This happens to coincide with increasing sophistication on the part of those who look at neurological structures and brain-damaged patients. The neighboring sciences are all interacting in a positive way.

There are new views of memory as well. If you look at the brain and consider the way it seems to be interconnected, you soon develop completely new computational devices. The new book by David Rumelhart and Jay McClelland (in press) is what I have in mind, or the earlier book by Hinton and Anderson (1981).

Q: One of the things that comes up for me is the old mind–body problem. If you look at the introspectionists and the behaviorists, it really seems that they were fundamentally concerned with that. The behaviorists certainly were taking a physicalistic view that "everything is body." The introspectionists seem to be somewhere in the middle, and now we are going to be talking about consciousness again. The question is, is consciousness real? Does that raise the same old philosophical questions again?

A: I think it does, but I leave that for the philosopher. I prefer to do my science. Jerry Fodor is very good at explaining what I'm doing. I don't find the mind–body problem to be a difficult one, however. If you grow up in the era of information processing, you have realized that the symbols that one uses for information are physical symbols. This analogy is relevant to the mind–body problem. The mind is this abstraction that results from all of the physical processes. I don't believe that there is anything mysterious about the physical processes; my attempt is to understand those physical processes.

Q: But in informational terms.

A: I would like to be able to relate them to the phenomena. Dreyfus (1979) has argued strongly that the phenomenal experiences are the important things, and that we in fact cannot capture those phenomena in these information-processing concepts. I think he's wrong and right. When I'm performing intensely at some skill, say playing table tennis, I feel that the world closes in on me; I feel that I'm sort of "one" with my paddle. I don't compute where the ball is; I simply move, and I hit the ball, and it goes across the net, and I'm ready for the return. The phenomenal experiences are very compelling. We can't explain them. But I feel that the behavior can all be explained in information-processing terms. And eventually I would hope to be able to include the role of consciousness in the control of my actions and the role of attention in focusing on what is happening. Now the leap from that point to explaining the internal, subjective feelings is a big one, and I don't know how to do that. And I'll leave that for others. Maybe that is, in fact, the philosophical issue.

Q: Well, would you hope for some kind of convergence between the objective data and the experiences that people go through?

A: I think that we will show that whenever you have this subjective feeling, we have these physical events going on. But I feel that to explain the phenomenal experiences, we're going to have to go to a different level of description. We don't describe the operation of electronic circuits by recourse to fundamental physics. We don't describe how a bridge is constructed and the strength of beams by recourse to fundamental physics. In a similar way, I don't think that we need to describe mental operations by recourse to the fundamental biochemistry. And the phenomenal experiences may also require their own level, which cannot be described, maybe even at the psychological level.

Q: No new approach to emotion and feeling has yet come out of the cognitive revolution. Is there any current work in which cognitive science people are looking at feelings and emotions in an interesting way?

A: There have been a number of attempts, a number of conferences and books. Zajonc has argued that emotions require no information processing, that they are immediate, and direct. I think that he and I differ only in our definition of information processing. For me, for a particular sight to have an emotional impact, it has to be interpreted, and that interpretation requires information processing. Subjectively though, it is very fast, immediate, and direct. I'd like to be able to understand that subjective emotion, and the role that emotions play in processing. They seem to involve a different processing structure, probably chemically based, probably from different sources, than our conventional communication. Emotions are continually with us.

Roy D'Andrade (1981) wrote an article in *Cognitive Science* on the role of emotion in the development of culture. One view of emotions is that they're a remnant of our earlier age, and that they're out of place in today's modern human. D'Andrade makes just the opposite argument. He says that lower animals have fewer emotions, and as you go higher up on the scale you find more and more emotions. He feels that humans have emotions because they're necessary for our lives, necessary to interpret the world. It's a very interesting approach. I don't know yet how to interpret it.

But it's also the case that if you look at the brain, you look at the body. Most of the body is body! The brain is a very small part of us, and I suspect that the intellectual part of the brain is only a small part of the brain, and the rest has to do with regulation, with reproduction, with survival — factors that we have been ignoring as psychologists, probably to our discredit. We oftentimes think of the intellectual function as serviced by the regulatory function. It may be the other way around: Maybe the regulatory function is what's primary, and perhaps the intellectual function grew up in order to regulate ourselves better. That's quite a different view of the person, and it would put emotions in a much more primary role.

Q: Does it seem to some extent that we're recapitulating the points that Freud made around the turn of the century?

A: I think we often move in cycles, but one would hope it's more of a spiral than a cycle. Each time we circle around we're further up. Freud has been rediscovered. I think Freud proposed very sophisticated, intelligent mechanisms. That may be a surprise for people outside experimental psychology to hear, because Freud has had such wide influence in our culture. He's had almost no influence in experimental psychology. In fact, it is a surprise to hear positive things about Freud said within psychology, and they're being said by many people, not just me. Marvin Minsky, I have discovered, is a fan of Freud's. He's particularly interested in the interpretation of dreams, and the role of dreams. I think Freud was a very important figure and will become more important.

Q: It's interesting, along those lines, that so far in cognitive psychology we don't deal with "irrational" kinds of processes, such as dream processes or drowsy thought. Is Minsky trying to understand those kinds of things?

A: Well, maybe. As you know, Minsky is not a psychologist; he's interested in his own pursuits regarding the way that processing might go on. The irrational is very hard to handle, so it's not just that we're afraid to tackle it. We don't have the tools yet. Hilgard has been trying to look at hypnosis for quite a while (*e.g.*, 1971) and I think he has given us many interesting insights, but we still don't have the proper tools to understand hypnosis.

Q: Along similar lines, if you look at early behaviorism as a sort of "casting out" from psychology of all the commonsense terms that we have for talking about people, then you can view cognitive psychology as a way of bringing most of those terms back into psychology. But we haven't dealt with *all* of the commonsense terms, and one that we haven't dealt with yet is "self." Are there any inklings that cognitive scientists might start to deal with that sort of thing?

A: I haven't seen them. The notion of "self" is interesting. I don't think we're ready yet. I think we may need to understand more about the role of consciousness, the role of processing structures, and "self" seems intimately linked with the notion of consciousness and of awareness.

Q: In contemporary psychology there are quite a few behaviorists who are doing work that, within their own terms, seems to be very fruitful. Is there any movement in the direction of unification of psychological research? For example, are cognitive scientists looking at conditioning as a phenomenon that needs to be explained?

A: Well, that's interesting. I haven't seen the signs of reconciliation of these points of view yet. I do think, though, that as we start to look at automatic behavior, we're starting to look at exactly the sort of behavior that the behaviorists have described so well and have good tools for. It may very well be that automatic behavior is essentially behavioristic behavior, in which we are controlled primarily by the environment. "Cognitive" behavior is perhaps the less skilled behavior. Cognitive behavior is important for learning or for dangerous situations or acquiring ill-learned concepts. Now, to say that something is automatic and behavioristic, however, is still not saying that there isn't a lot going on that we need to understand. But it may be much more like the kinds of things that are looked at in behavioristic psychology. Most of what we do is automatic; language is usually automatic. Language, the most cognitive of our activities! We don't think and plan the words that we speak; we're usually unaware of them. Sometimes I'm so much unaware of planning my speech that when I hear myself say something, I'll stop and think about it and say, "Hey, that's very interesting. Why did I say that?" So there's one area where we might see reconciliation.

Q: What about operant conditioning as a sort of motivational technique?

A: I haven't seen operant techniques come in. I would think that operant psychology, though, is much more relevant to what we're talking about than classical conditioning. I was recently speculating with two senior, well-known psychologists, whose names I will not reveal. And they were saying, "I wonder what it would be like to be frozen for a hundred years, and then to wake up and be able to pick up an introductory text in psychology, to see what concepts they had. Would those texts mention conditioning?" And these two were speculating that no, conditioning would be absent from the text 100 years from now. It would be seen as much less important than it has been in current psychology. The other side of that, I might point out, is that some people believe that conditioning, both classical and operant, is in fact an example of the kind of learning that requires consciousness. It requires awareness to link the action that you do and the result that occurs. So it may be, in fact, transformed into an essentially cognitive operation.

Q: The word "purpose" hasn't cropped up very much in this conversation. But that was one of the things that, in a sense, operant conditioning was designed to avoid.

A: I think that people are purposeful organisms, that we do things for goals. Some of the new work in operant literature is very suggestive of this—that the animal is attempting to accomplish some goal, and the means are not important. One other reason for the gulf between the operant literature and the cognitive literature is that operant psychologists have relied so heavily on the use of animals, most often the rat or the pigeon. That makes it very difficult for cognitivists. Operant experiments become quite complex, with many different stages; and many different technical aspects are necessary to get the animals to perform. Those things leave me very confused. I always have great difficulty when I try to translate the results of an operant experiment into cognitive terms. How would this work in the world, when there *aren't* all these conditions? Their experiments are amazingly complex! So, there's a difference imposed by the technology, not just by the theoretical insights.

Q: In view of the fact that we're "spiralling" back today to the same ideas that William James was talking about in 1890, suppose you were talking to William James today—how would you explain to him what the difference is between what he was doing and what we seem to be doing?

A: William James is one of my favorite authors. I love to read him; I learn from him. But I suspect we couldn't communicate very well. I suspect that our languages are different. The notion of information processing, which is so central to our ideas, would be completely foreign to him. He would have to develop a whole new set of concepts. I think it's much easier for us to read James and reinterpret it in our terms, than it would be for James to understand what we say and interpret it in his terms. Though I think we'd be in good company on the analysis of the critical phenomena for psychology to understand; we could talk and enjoy each other.

Q: William James could not understand us as well as we could understand him: Is the current point of view more encompassing?

A: Well, perhaps. But I might also remind you of what I said earlier about the differences in cultures. I may very well be misunderstanding James. I may simply be imposing my own views onto what James has written, and he might disapprove strongly of my reading of his works.

A case in point: Donald Broadbent wrote what we consider to be one of the major works in cognitive psychology (Broadbent, 1958). We consider that to be a landmark in the development of information-processing psychology. He developed some of the notions of short-term memory. He gave us the selective-attention experiments. But he considers that book to be widely misinterpreted. Cognitive psychology was not his message, and in fact if you look at the book again, you discover that he uses those terms only in the first chapter. And the rest of the book has to do with the effects of stress on people's behavior (see also Broadbent, 1971). Donald Broadbent is a behaviorist and has been most upset by the strong cognitive interpretation given to his views. I personally think he should be pleased. But it goes to show that when we claim to have good insight into a person or a book, it does not necessarily mean that we have interpreted things the way they were intended.

8

Toward an Integrated Psychology: A Summary and Critique

Nature has no departments. — ALFRED NORTH WHITEHEAD

At first glance, the world of psychology resembles a vast, fragmented mosaic. Just looking at the most scientifically well-established parts of psychology, we have a number of disciplines, each with its own empirical techniques, communicating only rarely with one another. Psychophysics, operant psychology, information-processing psychology, perceptual psychology, developmental psychology, social psychology, cognitive science, psychophysiology, mathematical psychology, psychometrics, comparative psychology, clinical psychology, and all the various subareas within each of these specializations — they seem to represent a number of separate fiefdoms, with little sense of a shared psychological foundation. There is agreement among the various ministates about the importance of empirical evidence, but unlike the mature sciences, there appears to be little agreement among psychologists about the fundamental problems to be solved, or even about the language in which to express the fundamental questions. It is no wonder that most laypersons have only a confused and sketchy notion of the psychological world.

This book has presented evidence for a major shift of metatheory in scientific psychology. The meaning of that shift, we have argued, is the freeing of the theoretical imagination. That is, the cognitive metatheory is open to theoretical constructs that are not themselves immediately observable, but which may be used because of their explanatory force. What is missing today in psychology is a unifying theory: It is only theory that gives a sense of unity to physics, chemistry, and the other mature sciences. If the major thesis of this book is correct, we may be moving today toward the first shared theory for psychological science.

In this chapter we will briefly review the evidence presented in this book, and then cast a speculative look at the future.

What have we learned? For a cognitive psychologist, the interviews in this book present a small treasury of insights into the most explicit and formal kind of cognition in which people engage — namely, the practice of science. Science is evidently much richer and more swayed by elements of the human comedy than current cognitive models suggest. The psychologists interviewed here have touched on hundreds of issues. We can only comment on a few.

The Behaviorists: Radical, Neo, and Clinical

Scientific revolutions, like political ones, are neither simple nor one-sided. Like any idealistic human enterprise, the history of a scientific revolution is apt to be liberally sprinkled with irony, enough to go around for all sides. Both the behavioral and cognitive revolutions amply illustrate the point.

Behaviorism came on the scene in 1913, a home-grown American psychology as rash and boastful as America at the turn of the century, and it radically altered the self-imposed mission of scientific psychology. In a sense, behaviorism constituted a populist revolt against the foreign-trained psychological elite. Instead of examining the human mind, carefully, systematically, and with no thought of satisfying more than intellectual curiosity, John Watson proclaimed that scientific psychology could change the world. Once the true scientific method was applied to human beings, it would inevitably work to revolutionize and perfect our lives by controlling our environment. Most subsequent behaviorists were a good deal less sanguine than Watson, but the strain of utopian idealism has carried through to this day, primarily in the writings of B. F. Skinner.

The enormous influence of behaviorism between 1913 and 1960 was supported by more than utopian optimism. Given the physicalistic view of science taught by the philosophers, behaviorism became the only reasonable way for scientific psychology to proceed. The world was clearly physical, and claims about the world that lacked obvious physical reference were held to be meaningless. Although neurophysiology was one legitimate physical way to describe human beings, it did not address those immediate and pressing questions that seemed to demand some sort of psychological answers. But if psychology was to be a science, it required a physical domain of its own, and the observable behavior of intact organisms seemed the only logical choice. Many psychologists may have felt uncomfortable with the resulting obligation to reject the concepts of human consciousness, goals, thoughts, and feelings, but even to the skeptics, the logic of the philosophical argument must have seemed unassailable. To be modern and rational, one had to be a scientist; to be relevant to human concerns, one had to be a psychologist; to be modern, rational, *and* relevant to human beings, one had no choice but to be a behaviorist. Idealistic youngsters became behaviorists in this way (*e.g.*, Skinner, 1978; Krasner, 1978). Because behaviorism demanded great self-discipline in the use of scientific language in order to do respectable scientific psychology, they sacrificed the psychology of everyday life. As one consequence, psychologists were compelled to lead a double life: Everyday living still required a psychological language replete with mentalisms, but respectable scientific discourse required one to repudiate it. Everything was to be reduced to observable, physical stimuli and responses.

Given these severe restrictions, behaviorists accomplished marvels in restating the psychology of common sense in stimulus–response terms. Perhaps the most brilliant was Skinner, who make it possible to talk about goal-directed action without any reference to goals. Indeed, it often comes as a surprise to students of psychology to learn that "the field of the operant is the field of purpose"—that operant conditioning is a behavioristic way of studying the purposefulness of action, which any child in our culture learns to understand in the first few years of life. It may be futile to speculate whether operant psychology might have succeeded without such linguistic transformations. The fact is that the technology of operant conditioning proved useful in psychology and other biological sciences: Animals of almost any species can be trained to do nearly anything a researcher might like. And some valuable scientific discoveries have been made: notably, schedules of reinforcement, biofeedback control of autonomic functions, and ways of controlling specific psychopathologies, such as phobias.

Our interviews in Chapter 3 present three kinds of contemporary behaviorists. The radical wing is well represented by B. F. Skinner and Howard Rachlin; Irving Maltzman and Howard Kendler present the neobehaviorism of Hull and Spence; and the very vigorous movement in behavior therapy is given voice in the interview with Alan O. Ross. These individuals present a reasonable picture of contemporary behaviorism in a world increasingly dominated by the cognitive perspective. They also present a variety of coping strategies with the cognitive challenge. Skinner and Rachlin would appear to accuse cognitive psychologists of unscientific, perhaps even "religious" tendencies, and continue to argue that every legitimate topic in psychology can be handled adequately by an operant behaviorism. Maltzman maintains strongly that cognitive psychology, insofar as it is at all legitimate, is nothing new. Kendler is inclined as well to see continuities rather than revolutionary change. And Ross views his clinical behaviorism as essentially an application of findings from basic research in psychology, so that the metatheoretical arguments do not affect his work directly.

It seems likely that a minority of psychologists will continue to be behaviorists. This is probably healthy for the future of psychology. Behaviorists will continue viable research programs, and their presence may serve as a useful reminder to other psychologists of the virtues of theoretical self-discipline and empirical rigor.

Perhaps the main lasting contribution of behaviorism has been its overwhelming emphasis on experimentally verifiable fact, which still dominates scientific psychology. It is still far easier to publish an experimental finding with minimal theory than a theoretical argument expressed in a genuine theoretical language. There is a great deal of disagreement over these priorities; but like it or not, the fact is that psychologists at present have only experimental proof-procedures. As genuine theoretical languages for psychology, based on computer languages, come into wider use, it is possible that theoretical contributions may come to be appreciated more, as they have been in the more developed sciences.

The Cognitive Shift

As suggested, then, although a number of behaviorists continue to work productively, they are a distinct minority. More and more, the cognitive metatheory is consolidating its hold on the psychological community. Areas that were strongholds of behavioral thought, such as animal psychology and behavior therapy, are currently in a state of flux. As we look back to our interviews about the origins of the cognitive perspective, what can we conclude?

Cognitive Psychology and Common Sense

In Molière's late-Medieval farce *The Bourgeois Gentleman*, a newly wealthy bourgeois hires a scholar to make him as sophisticated as he is rich. Among other absurdities, the scholar proposes to teach the bourgeois the difference between prose and poetry, defining prose as the kind of language that we speak all of our lives. This strikes the bourgeois as re-markable — "You mean that I've been speaking *prose* all of my life?" he asks with pride. This is a question that cognitive psychologists might well ask themselves, because it seems that we have been doing cognitive psychology all of our lives. And indeed we have: Commonsense psy-chology *is* a kind of cognitive psychology, in that we naturally infer unobservable things about ourselves and other people. We do not see directly that someone is upset; we observe a certain tone of voice, posture, and facial expression. Yet we can often tell very accurately when someone is upset, making use of shared cultural knowledge that is truthful and testable, and helpful in getting along in the world. Indeed, when it comes to our commonsense understanding of ourselves and others, we live in a largely theoretical world. Given that we are surviving rather well in this world, our commonsense theories about ourselves and other people probably have quite a bit of truth in them. And so it is not surprising that ever since the cognitive revolution, psychologists have been redis-covering common sense.

Common sense psychology has no professional advocates. But if they existed, one might forgive them a bit of gentle laughter at the expense of 20th-century scientific psychology. After all, experimental psychologists early in the century rejected all of everyday psychology with great fan-fare, only to rediscover it, in a somewhat more subdued mood, 50 years later. In the intervening years, what, if anything, has been gained?

First, psychologists have developed consensual proof-procedures, methods by which any member of the scientific community can present evidence to be checked by others. In principle, this kind of evidence must be acknowl-edged as true by any rational person who understands it. Much of this we owe to the behaviorists, who insisted on public proof-procedures. Iron-clad canons of evidence may be even more important to psychology than to any other science, because humans are so prone to wishful thinking in psychological matters. The more we invest in some point of view, the more likely it is to sway our interpretation of reality; and most people are deeply invested in some particular view of the human condition.

Second, and of great importance for the future, psychologists appear to be ac-quiring a true theoretical language, one that can naturally represent the elements of psychological reality. In recent years we have been able to represent the perceptual world of sound and sight more adequately than ever before, and also the major components of language and meaning. The new theoretical languages even support working models of psychopathologies, such as neurosis and paranoid psychosis (Boden, 1977). Although much remains to be done to develop methods for testing these theories empirically, work of this sort represents a major leap forward in theoretical sophistication over anything done before.

Third, there is a new maturity in scientific psychology that makes it unnecessary to reject common sense, and relieves psychologists of the need to slavishly imitate other sciences. If behaviorism can be viewed as the adolescence of psychology — with its need to define an identity separate from its predecessors, its absolute insistence on the trappings of physical science, and its rejection of inherited wisdom — cognitive work signals perhaps a stage of early maturity. Rather than rejecting common sense, today we are rather impressed by it, and indeed sometimes awed by its complexities. Rather than making an absolute separation between psychology and philosophy or neurophysiology, many cognitive scientists are intrigued by the possibilities of working with scholars in these disciplines, to our mutual benefit (Norman, 1981). And rather than importing the logic of the physical sciences, a good deal of modern research is constrained by an inner logic all its own.

Was Scientific Psychology in Crisis before the Cognitive Shift?

In this book we have avoided using Kuhn's terminology for scientific revolutions, especially the controversial word "paradigm," for fear of being caught up in irrelevant and distracting issues. Nevertheless we can ask questions that stem from Kuhn's analysis. For instance, I suggest that the behavioristic and cognitive revolutions turned on metatheoretical issues rather than specifically psychological issues. (To be sure, a viable metatheory must have a promising research program associated with it, one that seems likely to lead to adequate psychological theory.) Further, we can ask along with Kuhn, Are scientific revolutions caused by a period of crisis in the discipline, a time when the community appears to run into paradoxical events that cannot be explained in its current frame of reference?

Certainly the shift from "introspectionism" to behaviorism could have been motivated by an apparent paradox. William James, who wrote the great American textbook prior to behaviorism (1890), insisted absolutely on the *primacy* of consciousness in psychology. And yet, James attempted to provide *physical* explanations of the mind–brain connection — of perception and action in the physical world. Holding both of these beliefs, James was inevitably forced to deal with the mind-body paradox, for how could consciousness be primary if it was somehow *caused* by physical events? James's position was paradoxical and provided a shaky foundation on which to build the new science. Watson's behavioristic solution to the mind–body puzzle was radical, but at least coherent: If we assume that all reference to consciousness can be expunged from psychology, then we can indeed build on a consistent physicalistic basis.

Thus behaviorism in its early years gave coherence to the enterprise of psychology at the cost of limiting its domain. Starting in the early 1930s, Clark Hull developed a research program to unify the missing parts — notably, the fact that behavior is evidently purposeful — by proposing to reduce such phenomena to potentially observable, physical, internal stimuli and responses. This physicalistic reduction was necessary to make his higher-level constructs scientifically respectable, or so it seemed. In our interview with George Mandler, he refers to the Yale of Hull as the "home of the Holy Grail," and neobehaviorists such as Irving Maltzman and Howard Kendler continue to regard their training with Kenneth Spence at Iowa as the most exciting intellectual period of their careers. But about 1950 the Hull–Spence program failed by its own rigorous criteria, and the confusion and despair that resulted was comparable to the hopes it had raised before. So we can answer our basic question by suggesting that, yes, the cognitive shift in psychology *was* preceded by a period of crisis in the received approach.

During the 1950s the alternatives must have seemed bleak, as witness the directions taken by the more than 75 Spence PhD students. The radical behaviorism of Skinner was still going strong, because its atheoretical position was not affected by the failure of Hullian theory. But it had nothing to say about the kinds of general questions Hull tried to answer. Physiological psychology was promising, but it seemed to lead to a kind of neurological reductionism that denied the need for psychology. Other research programs seemed weak and unpromising by the very tough methodological standards advocated by the neobehaviorists. Finally, some Hull–Spence students chose to work on applied problems, a direction that led some of them toward the new behavior therapy (Kalish, 1981).

In retrospect, a cognitive psychologist might say that Hull's problem was not his attempt to develop theory, but his use of a weak theory to explain extraordinarily complex phenomena. It is doubtful whether any neobehaviorists felt this way. They had seen the failure of the most highly theoretical attempt to do psychology, and they continued to view large-scale theory work with deep suspicion.

Thus a Kuhnian analysis of the origins of the cognitive shift seems very much on target. It may be forever impossible to prove without a doubt that the crisis in Hullian theory helped to make psychologists receptive to a cognitive approach, given the difficulty of proving anything about history conclusively. But it certainly seems plausible.

The Adapters

The Adapters (Chapter 5) are those behaviorists who changed with the revolution to a more cognitive perspective — in this book, Marvin Levine, James J. Jenkins, and George Mandler. Of the three, Levine occupies an interesting intermediate position, in that he sees little conflict and many continuities between the behavioral and cognitive positions. Levine's personal development in psychology has more continuity than the personal history of Jenkins, for example. Hence Levine views the cognitive shift in an evolutionary way, while Jenkins perceives revolutionary changes.

Jenkins's history reflects some of the major conflicts of the '50s and '60s. Trained in industrial psychology, Jenkins became fascinated with the problem of language early in his career. His first move was to perform an extremely thorough test of the "mediational model" of language learning, a model that postulated invisible stimuli and responses along the lines of Hull and Osgood. In spite of early promising results, the program to prove mediation theory failed, driving Jenkins in the direction of Chomskyan linguistics as a source of alternative ideas. Again, the early results of a Chomskyan program of psycholinguistic research were encouraging, until Chomsky himself "pulled the rug out from under the program" by altering his theoretical position (Chomsky, 1965). Once more, Jenkins was forced to reexamine his assumptions. Most recently he has been attracted to a Gibsonian approach to psychology (see also the interviews with Neisser and Weimer). (Thus the interview with Jenkins could equally well have gone into Chapter 6, "The Persuaders.")

Mandler's experience was different from both Jenkins's and Levine's. He was not affected by Chomsky's work to the same extent that Jenkins was, being influenced more by Gestalt conceptions of the organizational properties of memory. (In addition, he has carried on a parallel research program on emotion that combines influences from psychoanalytic thinking and social psychology.) Mandler views behaviorism as a kind of scientific purge, a "housecleaning" process to remove unsupported theoretical concepts from the scientific language. Conversely, he considers the cognitive revolution to be "the great liberation of the '60s" — a time when one no longer needed to apologize for using theoretical constructs. But he also raises the possibility of another purge in the future.

Was the cognitive shift evolutionary or revolutionary? Is Levine right about the continuities between behaviorism and cognitive psychology, or are Jenkins and Mandler correct about the discontinuities? The answer is, of course, that both perceptions are correct. It appears that our perception of similarities and differences between ourselves and other people is very much a function of our own history, and perhaps of our need to differentiate ourselves from others. In a large scientific community, no one has a privileged position from which to view large sociological movements. Instead, we make inferences about the community based on a rather limited amount of local information. If we look very closely at the cognitive shift, we can probably find many continuities. But many small differences can add up to a few great differences, and those on opposite ends of a continuum are likely to emphasize such great differences. There is little question about the differences between Jenkins and Mandler on the one hand, and Skinner and Rachlin on the other. But Levine (a cognitive psychologist) is very similar indeed to Kendler (a neobehaviorist). Revolution or evolution? The answer must be: "both."

The Persuaders: The Role of Nonconformists within the Community

Just as it is unwise to make hard-and-fast distinctions between all cognitive and all behavioral psychologists, it is also important to acknowledge commonalities between our three groups of cognitive psychologists, the "Adapters," "Persuaders," and "Nucleators." Nevertheless, our four Persuaders (Chapter 6) stand out as nonconformists in the psychological community, though sometimes in subtle ways. Ulric Neisser states his own nonconformist tendencies very clearly when he notes his feeling of being "uncomfortable in the mainstream." Ironically, his *Cognitive Psychology* (1967) defined and named the new "mainstream" point of view in psychology. *Cognitive Psychology* appeared at exactly the right time, saying exactly the right things. Thus the book had very little persuasion to do, because its readers had already persuaded themselves by the time they read it.

Neisser's more recent books are more nonconformist. In *Cognition and Reality* (1976) he criticized the new cognitive viewpoint for being out of touch with the reality of everyday life. This position has not been universally accepted in cognitive psychology, though the need for more "ecologically valid" approaches is widely acknowledged. Thus Neisser has worked himself out of the "uncomfortable mainstream" into a position as a useful critic of current psychology.

The nonconformity of Ernest R. Hilgard is a great deal more subtle. His basic outlook developed in the years before behaviorism came to dominate American psychology, under the influence of what may be called "broadminded functionalism." During the behavioristic era one might have thought Hilgard to be the quintessential behaviorist because of his classic text *Conditioning and Learning* (Hilgard & Marquis, 1940), which was required reading for all graduate students in behavioristic psychology departments. In fact, in concluding their book, Hilgard and Marquis decided that the behavioristic program of reducing all learning to stimulus–response conditioning was not going to work. Hilgard's subsequent book, *Theories of Learning* (1948), expanded on the flaws of behavioral theories, but proposed no major alternative. And a few years later, Hilgard began his long-term research program into hypnosis, a phenomenon that clearly defies many of the simpler ideas about human functioning. In sum, Hilgard was never a behaviorist, but for some time his work was very central to behavioristic thinking. In a curious way he is an "establishmentarian nonconformist".

The nonconformity of our next two Persuaders is very evident. Neither Weimer nor Wapner have published experimental work, though both are remarkably thoughtful psychologists. Wapner is a good example of a "scientific isolate," one of many in the history of science, and we have argued that the existence of such isolates is important to the development of science in the same way that biological diversity is important to the adaptability of a species. When scientific communities are confronted with a basic paradox, some isolated scientist may come to the fore with a fully developed alternative point of view. In just this way Einstein was a complete outsider in the physics community until 1905, when he published the first of a series of papers showing how one could resolve several paradoxes emerging from Newtonian physics. In all likelihood scientific isolates exist at all times, but they become known only if the scientific community runs into trouble in its established course.

All of the Persuaders must face a trade-off between developing their ideas in depth and their ability to communicate with others. The more they go their separate ways, the more difficult it will be to persuade others to adopt their ideas. In this trade-off it would seem that Hilgard has chosen to communicate the most: next, perhaps Neisser, Weimer, and, finally, Wapner. On the other hand, if one can disregard the need to communicate, one may be able to develop a point of view in much greater depth than otherwise. It may be that a nonconforming scientist is forced to choose between developing a profoundly different perspective and being badly understood, or being understood and adopting a less profound point of view.

The Nucleators

The Nucleators presented in Chapter 7 are very much like the Persuaders, except for the fact that they developed quite independently of official psychology. In physics, a "nucleator" is a particle that serves as the nucleus of a new cluster of particles, the way snowflakes will form around tiny dust-motes in the atmosphere. There is a strong streak of nonconformity in these individuals as well. Chomsky points out in his interview that he may not have the academic credentials to be a linguist, in spite of the fact that he is certainly the best-known linguist in this century! Simon is a very unusual economist (his best-known work in economics involves decision making in the firm, an unusual topic for an economist), an unusual computer scientist (he treats computers empirically rather than mathematically), and an unusual psychologist (he is much more theoretically inclined than most psychologists). The psychology community was compelled to expand its domain in order to incorporate the work of Nucleators such as Simon and Chomsky, and to a lesser extent that of Fodor and Norman. But this process of expansion takes a long time. All four individuals in this chapter experienced some degree of rejection of their work by the psychological community. Probably they are still only partially understood by mainstream psychologists.

It is interesting to speculate what might have happened if the early Chomsky or Simon had tried to "make it" in the psychological community of the '50s and '60s. Most likely they would have failed to find a niche. Even Fodor and Norman, who published experiments in the experimental psychology literature, might have had difficulty had the community not taken a more theoretical direction.

Some Conclusions about Scientific Psychology

What lessons can we draw from all this? Can we gain some deeper understanding of psychology, or of science in general? Based on the interviews and historical chapters in this book, there are some trends and themes that seem especially noteworthy.

Science as an Ecosystem

In Chapter 1 we suggested several useful metaphors for approaching the cognitive shift in psychology, among them the notion that the scientific community functions like a biological ecosystem. Each scientist or small group of scientists must find its own niche, which is defined not just by material resources, but by intellectual resources as well. New niches are created when some promising new resource is opened up (by the invention of a new research tool, a new theoretical insight, *etc.*). By the same token, a research domain may become overexploited and exhausted. This metaphor has proved useful in this book in making sense of the actions and thoughts of psychologists in many different situations. It may well be worth exploring in much more detail.

Diversity in Science

After reading the 17 interviews in this book, one is left with a strong impression that the psychological community is marked more by diversity than consensus. This is true even within each major framework: behaviorists such as Kendler and Skinner disagree deeply on many points, as do cognitive psychologists such as Simon and Jenkins, or Chomsky and Norman. For any pair of interviews in this book, one can imagine numerous issues on which the interviewees might disagree. Areas of agreement exist of course, but even these are more like "family resemblances" than they are a reflection of fundamental axioms shared by everyone in the community.

This diversity of opinion may happen more often in "adolescent" sciences such as psychology than in older disciplines. But diversity of opinion may be fundamentally important even in the developed sciences. We may tend to overestimate the degree of consensus in science: To be sure, there is considerable consensus, but it is mostly about a relatively small number of facts and assumptions that have managed to withstand a very contentious process of critical examination. Indeed, the existence of disagreement and diversity of views does not *contradict* the fact of consensus — it is precisely this diversity which leads to a consensus about those ideas, and findings that manage to stand against critical attack. All significant facts and concepts must endure a trial by fire. Only the surviving ones are likely to command broad consent.

This is not to say that there are no rules in science. Even children discover very quickly that we must stick to some rules to play a game, or else it will be impossible to know who won or lost. In the case of science, those rules are ultimately the empirical proof-procedures, which meet the test of reality as far as we can know it. But of course even proof-procedures change in science, as we can see so graphically in the cognitive revolution: If our thesis about the *metatheoretical* nature of the cognitive shift is correct, the main contention between behaviorists and cognitive psychologists has been about the rules of the game.

If *diversity* is indeed as important as consensus in science, it would lend support to the idea of the scientific community as an ecosystem (Chapter 1). Imagine a semantic space with as many dimensions as there are reasonable and fruitful orientation issues in the discipline. There is only a limited number of promising combinations of these issues, and they define the desirable "niches" in the semantic ecosystem. Each niche must be sufficiently different from the others to enable the scientist to claim it as his or her own. There is no payoff for doing research that exactly duplicates the work of others. But there is great incentive for being identifiably different from others. Indeed, following this logic, a scientific community could suffer sometimes from too much consensus, so that individual niches become cramped and sterile.

Another attractive image might present the scientific community as a collection of Leibnitzian monads, perfect glass spheres dancing through a semantic space, occasionally touching other spheres, exchanging messages, shoring up boundaries, and moving on. It is as if each scientist defines a set of issues that differentiate him or her from the others, and together these boundary issues constitute a point of view. Because no one can know the future, many of these issues may ultimately turn out to be irrelevant or wrongly posed. But they permit one to hold a rhetorical position, one that is well defended against all predictable avenues of attack. One of the virtues of such a secure point of view is to create simplicity in the midst of great complexity—empirical, theoretical, and even philosophical complexity. This in turn permits one to focus on certain isolated empirical questions that seem to provide promising avenues of research. The *cost* of a truly secure and well-defended position is that it may blind us to the virtues of other (apparently incompatible) positions—reality may pass us by and we may simply not notice.

Although mixing metaphors may be poor literary style, it provides a vocabulary rich and imaginative enough to help us characterize the nature of the scientific ecosystem—a bit like a jungle, a bit like a debating society, a bit like the Leibnitzian monadology—a society of perfect luminous spheres, now touching, now repelling each other. Some mix of such images may give us a first approximation of the reality.

Are There "Recessive" as Well as "Dominant" Paradigms?

The cognitive metatheory is nothing new. Commonsense psychology routinely makes inferences about people's ideas, feelings, and attitudes. And clinical theories such as psychodynamics are clearly cognitive in the metatheoretical sense. Thus, the cognitive metatheory has existed for a long time, even when behaviorism dominated psychology. One might speak of cognitive ideas during this time as having been "recessive." Presumably such recessive ideas continue to exist even when they are not popular because various Persuaders and Nucleators continue to hold on to unpopular ideas. Similarly, one may argue that psychological physicalism existed long before John Watson published his famous paper on behaviorism in 1913 (see Chapter 2). Is this sort of "recessive" framework unique in the history of psychology, or does it occur elsewhere in the history of science?

Conceivably "recessive" theoretical ideas exist even in the more developed sciences. One can point to numerous cases in which ideas were disbelieved for centuries, leading a shadowy existence until they became part of a new, dominant framework. The heliocentric theory of planetary motion was certainly anticipated by the Greeks, and the seeds of evolutionary theory can be found in the Greeks as well. Newton's great competitor Leibnitz had severe doubts about Newton's concepts of absolute space, doubts that were justified a few centuries later with the advent of Einsteinian physics. Certainly not all ideas in science are anticipated centuries before: But it is not uncommon to find "recessive" theoretical ideas continuing to exist even when they are excluded by the dominant framework. A complete conception of science must be able to account for the continued existence of such unpopular ideas.

The Persistence of the Mind–Body Problem

In a story so full of ironies, perhaps the most marvelous one concerns the philosophical mind–body problem. Nineteenth-century psychologists were philosophically sophisticated, and agonized over the paradoxes of mind and body, but the 20th century seemed to have the answer once and for all. To be scientific was to be physical, and because the whole universe was the proper domain for science, a scientific psychologist had to be a physicalist. Everything had to be reducible to physical events as a touchstone of respectability; and of course the conception of physical causality was not the sophisticated sort of causality associated with modern physics, but a kind of 19th-century, no-nonsense, billiard-ball causality. Respectable empirical scientists were duly suspicious of any preoccupation with philosophical questions; "Armchair speculation" was one of the milder epithets directed at such unscientific activity.

And yet when we look at the three historic phases of scientific psychology — 19th-century psychology of consciousness, behaviorism, and cognitive psychology — it seems all too clear that the mind–body problem is at the bottom of them all. Wilhelm Wundt believed that physical and mental laws were incommensurable, though he denied being a dualist. His kind of "functional dualism" was acutely conscious of its philosophical underpinnings. John Watson and his followers were self-conscious physicalists, and indeed denied the existence of any mind–body problem at all. As for cognitive psychologists, who claim that mental states can be inferred on the basis of physical evidence — they currently avoid any stand on the ontological status of conscious contents. If cognitive psychologists were to think about the issue (which they do rarely), they would probably adopt the standard position called "dual-aspect monism" — the view that conscious experience and physical reality constitute two perspectives on a single world.

The mind–body problem may be the kind of foundation paradox that psychology can neither solve nor ignore for very long. Indeed, it may be inherent in any "cognitive system" — in any system that can represent some part of its world. Mathematicians are familiar with several foundation paradoxes of this kind, and the fact that philosophers have not been able after two millenia to resolve numerous difficulties emanating from the mind–body problem suggests that it may never be fully resolved. Yet good scientific psychology may be possible without solving this foundation paradox, just as good physics is possible without solving the puzzles inherent in action at a distance, the Heisenberg Uncertainty Principle, or some of the more fantastic implications of quantum mechanics.

If all this is true, then we would expect the history of psychology to exhibit slow, pendular swings between different views of the mind–body paradox, because, even if it cannot be solved, different perspectives will reveal different aspects of human psychology. And this is, of course, exactly what the history does show. Indeed, the oldest kind of psychology may not be Western psychology at all, but the sophisticated philosophical praxis inherent in Vedic and Taoist writings of 4,000 years ago. If we count this kind of "psychophilosophy" as a true, empirical psychology — armed with its own techniques and theories, having its own community of experts — then the pendulum has swung from a true mentalism in ancient psychology, to a hesitant quasimentalistic dualism in the psychology of Wundt and James, to a total physicalism in the behaviorism of Watson and the physiological reductionism of Pavlov. In fact, from this point of view, Watson and Pavlov become *world-historic* figures — they represent the very extreme physicalistic swing of the mind–body pendulum, which even now may be ponderously moving back in the direction of greater mentalism.

This is in fact the accusation made by Skinner (see the interview). Skinner does not distinguish between cognitive psychology and introspectionism, arguing that any taint of unobservable explanatory entities leads back to the unscientific sin of mentalism. The accusation is probably incorrect, because most cognitive psychologists believe *in principle* in physicalistic reductionism. But with the coming of the computer, the terms of the argument have begun to change: A computer can be analyzed physically in terms of its switching circuits, but it is perfectly all right to refer to its operation at a higher systems-level in terms of goals, decisions, and representations. Indeed, a purely physical analysis of the computer would completely miss its informational aspect: Information inherently presupposes reference ("intentionality," in philosophical terms), including reference to possible but nonexistent states of the world. "Information" is something that is preserved under any number of transformations in the physical medium used to encode it. As a signal is transmitted from a magnetic disk to a bubble memory, to an electrical signal flowing in a copper wire, to a radio signal, to a hole in a paper tape, or to a stream of electrons activating the phosphor on a viewing screen, the information remains constant. So perhaps Skinner is right after all in suspecting that our current ventures in cognition may lead in some distant future to a true mentalism. Perhaps the new theoretical precision in the cognitive sciences may permit us to clarify the mind–body problem more than ever before, so that we can distinguish those cases where it can lead us into difficulty from others, where it may be merely a necessary aspect of cognition.

Serious scholars have suggested that mind–body problems emerge even in physics, especially with the notion of information. Information plays a fundamental role in physics as the inverse of entropy, and the physical facts also suggest that information is biologically central. Living systems can be considered to be local exceptions to the general rule of entropy. Further, the genetic code of all living things is carried by the information-bearing molecules DNA and RNA. Thus information is a core conception in physics and biology, and we have already reviewed arguments for considering information fundamental in psychology as well (Chapter 4). Mind–body problems also emerge in connection with relativity, the Heisenberg Uncertainty Principle, and even standard notions such as "potential energy." All these useful physical constructs require a representation of alternatives that go beyond current reality, representations that often seem critically dependent on the observer. Two well-known scholars, a psychologist and a physicist, have suggested that information should be considered a fundamental quantity, much like mass and energy, but governed by very different laws (*e.g.*, Bakan, 1980; Szilard, 1929/1964). Information is a foundation concept in cognitive science, and it will be interesting to see if this train of thought will help to revive interest among cognitive scientists in a new, rigorously scientific analysis of the mind–body issue, involving fundamental physical and psychological insights. Such a development, if it ever takes place, is not likely to happen soon. But it is certainly not beyond the bounds of possibility.

Psychology as a Bridge between the Two Cultures

In the second half of the 20th century, we have grown up in a world divided by competing perspectives, especially the perspectives of the "two cultures" (Snow, 1959). The world of physical science is increasingly well understood objectively. It has its own wonder and beauty, but it seems to have no place for human values. The world of the humanities is full of color, complexity, and human value, but it is increasingly considered to be out of touch with hard scientific reality. Psychology exists as a natural bridge between the two cultures, but for most of this century, scientific psychology has turned its face only toward the physical sciences. The very real concerns shared by psychology and the humanities have been largely ignored. Thus psychology has abdicated its natural role as an integrative force between the sciences and humanities.

It is possible that with its new-found maturity, psychology will begin increasingly to adopt this bridging role. Scientific psychologists must have a commitment to hard evidence, but at the same time they are interested primarily in the content of the humanities: human knowledge, consciousness, feelings, imagination. It may yet be possible to build a coherent scientific worldview in which human values follow not from the laws of religion, but from the nature of humanity.

The Neglect of Psychodynamic Thought

There is still one glaring exception to this growing maturity of scientific psychology, and that is the continued neglect of psychodynamic thought. Psychodynamic psychologies have developed largely independently of academic experimental psychology, even though many experimental psychologists of all persuasions have long had a private fascination with psychodynamic ideas (see Chapter 2 and the interviews with Mandler, Neisser, and Hilgard). In that psychodynamics postulates unobservable conflicts between unobservable emotions, it is clearly cognitive. Yet the cognitive shift has thus far produced only glimmerings of interest in the very rich theoretical treasure of psychodynamic thought (see Erdelyi &

Goldberg, 1979, Erdelyi, 1985). But some of the major barriers are down; there are now no metatheoretical obstacles to an adequate scientific evaluation of psychodynamic concepts.

Psychodynamic thought is often equated with psychoanalytic orthodoxy, certainly an understandable historical association. But it may be harmful to carry the custom of identifying psychodynamics with psychoanalysis too far. First, there is such a thing as "commonsense psychodynamics," the kind we all use when we say that someone is in conflict over a decision, or is blaming another person for his own faults. This commonsense psychodynamics predates the beginnings of psychoanalysis by millenia. Further, confusing all psychodynamic thought with psychoanalytic orthodoxy often leads to an all-or-none approach to this fascinating and vital area of human psychology, as if believing in ego-defense mechanisms, for example, forces us necessarily to believe in the Oedipus complex, the death instinct, or other, more problematic products of Freud's genius. A truly scientific approach to psychodynamics should probably focus first on intermediate-level constructs that can be tested most easily, such as the defense mechanisms. Finally, psychodynamic ideas are often confused with the *practice* of psychoanalytic therapy, as if psychodynamic theory necessarily leads to traditional psychoanalysis as the therapy of choice for all emotional problems. Clinical researchers in recent years have made a convincing case for very specific, "superficial," problem-oriented therapy to relieve human psychological misery. Nevertheless, there is much to be learned from the older ideas, even if they do not immediately lead to practical therapeutic results.

Thus, none of the usual confusions of psychodynamics with orthodox psychoanalysis, with the Oedipus complex or death instinct, or with the practice of psychotherapy is really necessary. It is essential to make a distinction between psychodynamics as a treasury of important psychological ideas, many of which deserve serious testing, and these other confounds. Psychodynamic thought, broadly conceived, has probably provided the richest and most humanly relevant vein of psychological theorizing in this century. Experimental psychologists even today seem to ignore this important intellectual influence, not on the basis of its own faults or merits, but essentially because of a sociological taboo. This is surely the single greatest neglected topic in contemporary scientific psychology. Probably at some time in the near future these ideas will be reexamined, using the very good empirical and theoretical tools that are available to contemporary experimental psychologists (*e.g.*, Erdelyi, 1985; Fisher & Greenberg, 1977; Baars, 1985).

Some observers have suggested that the bias against psychodynamic thinking reflects the kind of people who choose to become experimental psychologists. Psychodynamics is, after all, the domain of emotion, and it is sometimes suggested that experimental psychologists do not examine psychodynamic thought because they do not wish to examine their own emotions. This criticism may be discounted when it is made by psychoanalysts, because it seems self-serving. But sometimes we hear a similar criticism from more disinterested sources. In *The Psychology of Science* (1966) Abraham Maslow attacked "various behaviorisms," arguing that

More than any other scientists we psychologists have to contend with the astonishing fact of resistance to the truth. More than any other kind of knowledge we fear knowledge of ourselves. . . . And the closer our probings approach to our personal core, the more resistance there will be. . . .

One must sometimes talk to one's graduate students in the social and psychological sciences as if they were going off to war. One must speak of bravery, of morals and ethics, of strategy and tactics. The psychological or social scientist must *fight* to bring truth about the hot subjects. (pp. 16–17)

Furthermore,

Science . . . can be a defense. It can be primarily a safety philosophy, a security system, a complicated way of avoiding anxiety and upsetting problems. In the extreme instance it can be a way of avoiding life, a kind of self-cloistering. It can become — in the hands of some people, at least — a social institution with primarily defensive, conserving functions, ordering and stabilizing rather than discovering and renewing. (p. 33)

Similarly, Erdelyi and Goldberg (1979) hint broadly that modern cognitive psychologists have repressed repression: "What is to be made of this blanket silence?" they ask. "Is it really a reflection of bias against psychoanalytic notions in general and, through guilt by association, against psychodynamics in particular? Or is there perhaps some simpler and more reasonable explanation?" (pp. 356–357). In fairness it should be pointed out that the notion of repression presents difficult problems of experimental measurement, though probably not insuperable ones (*e.g.*, Baars, 1985). Further, until very recently, cognitive psychologists have studiously avoided not just problems of the unconscious, but problems presented by consciousness as well (see Baars, 1983a, in press).

But it may be true that scientific psychology attracts individuals who need to distance themselves in some way from the human reality that we know through common sense psychology. Certainly the wholesale rejection of common sense by experimentalists during the behavioristic period suggests something of this sort. In the older sciences the attempt has been not so much to *reject* common sense as to *transcend* it. But in psychology, until rather recently, scientists openly took satisfaction in the degree to which their ideas violated common sense.

The Study of Consciousness Has Ethical Implications

In recent years cognitive psychologists have started to address the issue of consciousness again in a serious way (*e.g.*, Baars, in press; Underwood, 1982; Mandler, 1975). There is a growing consensus about the information-processing properties of consciousness, although there is still a good deal of theoretical uncertainty in interpreting these properties.

But a new acceptance of consciousness may change our view of the world in certain fundamental ways. For example, contemporary researchers tend to use animals as expendable materials, no different from paper supplies or laboratory equipment that may be discarded after use. If we ever learn to see animals as conscious beings, capable of suffering much like ourselves, this facile disregard for their lives may well begin to change. During the behavioristic era it was almost a point of honor to consider animals (and humans, too) as nothing more than physical objects. Cognitive psychologists have not yet changed this attitude very much, though they see animal nervous systems as amazingly complex and sophisticated information processors, as complex as human brains in those particular capacities for which an animal is biologically specialized. It is difficult to see how that view can coexist with the cavalier disregard for animals that we find so surprisingly often (Singer, 1975). Animals are routinely "sacrificed" once they have learned a task, because the next experiment will require animals uncontaminated with previous conditioning.

None of this is meant to suggest that animal experimenters are deliberately cruel, but rather that they are often committed to a philosophical perspective that has no place for the idea that animals can experience suffering like ourselves. Facts, and our beliefs about facts, can have powerful implications for our values.

One may wonder whether the computational analogy favored by cognitive psychologists will have a dehumanizing effect as well. If we view people as information processors, does that mean that we can treat them like computers? Many people have expressed concern about this possibility (*e.g.*, Weizenbaum, 1976). Curiously enough, the effect so far has been to humanize rather than dehumanize our scientific conception of human beings. Compared with the older perspective in psychology, cognitive psychology sees people not as passive, but as active; not as physical in any simple sense, but as information-dependent; not as agglomerations of simple S–R links, but as awesomely complex organisms, representing and integrating their world in a holistic fashion; not as fundamentally superstitious, swayed by irrational emotions and duped by religious illusions, but as reality-oriented and indeed reality-creating creatures. The cognitive view of the organism may well shake our conception of ourselves, whether rightly or not, but so far, compared with the previous way of looking at people, the new perspective has increased rather than decreased human self-respect (e.g., Boden, 1977). Nevertheless, our generation has learned to look at science, too, with a degree of skepticism; and as the tools of cognitive science become more and more powerful, it will be increasingly important for cognitive scientists to make a serious effort to ensure that their knowledge will not be abused. At this point there is no sign that this realization has yet begun to strike home.

Toward an Integrated Psychology

What will psychology be like in 20 or 50 years? We can only speculate, but there are interesting signs that we may be moving toward a first theoretical integration. With all the reservations that are appropriate in the chancy business of predicting the future course of a science, here are my predictions:

1. The coming theoretical integration will probably be based on some sort of information-processing foundation. Indeed, the notions of "representation" and "information processing" are likely to be so obvious to the coming generations of students — having grown up with computers — that they will not be able to understand what all the controversy in the first century of psychology was about.

2. In a matter of decades we will have a dominant theory of human mental processes.

3. The new theoretical framework will deal with both conscious and unconscious processes as foundation concepts.

4. With the rapid advances in neurophysiological measurement techniques, which allow on-line monitoring of neural and psychological processes as they occur, there will likely be an integration between psychological and neurophysiological theory as well. Since most neuroscientists seem comfortable with information-processing language, this should pose no fundamental obstacle. The difference between neuroscience and psychology will begin to resemble the difference between "hardware" and "software" in computer science.

5. Behavioristic research programs will become increasingly theoretical. They may continue to employ a different vocabulary for some

time, but ultimately, as they develop more computer simulations of behavioral data, they will begin to postulate theoretical constructs just as current cognitive researchers are doing. Behavioral researchers may begin to tie their constructs more closely to neuroscientific observations.

6. As language psychologists become more confident of their semantic models, other fields that are based in good part upon language — clinical psychology, the study of motivation, problem solving, social interaction, education, and the like — will develop a strong theoretical basis, closely connected to the underlying mental processes.

7. In motivational psychology, there will be an integration of a wide range of ideas originating in current social and personality research, operant conditioning, and psychodynamics. These currently warring communities will find what unifies them to be more significant than whatever has separated them.

8. Applied and clinical psychology will continue to be a mix of behavioral, motivational, self-exploratory, cognitive, and neurochemical approaches. The first four of these will be effectively indistinguishable from one another, except on a purely pragmatic basis. Neurochemical treatment will be increasingly guided by a genuine understanding of individual neurochemistry, rather than the haphazard empirical approach that is used today.

9. There will be significant attempts to bridge the gap between "the real world" and "the laboratory," aided by new observational and mathematical techniques. There will be an increasing flow of information in both directions. The use of computers to monitor outcomes, within ethical boundaries, will become so common that there will be no clear dividing line between pure and applied investigation.

10. Intelligent computer-based software will be increasingly used to perform fundamental psychological research.

11. One of the major ethical issues will be to define appropriate boundaries between individual and societal access to psychological information about individuals. Computer-based systems will be used to defend individuals from undue probing, as well as to do whatever probing seems acceptable.

The Consequences of Success in Scientific Psychology

In the last half of the 20th century, we have learned that science is often a double-edged sword. Nuclear physics is one of the intellectual jewels of our century, but it has also created the most destructive weapon of the century. Psychologists have not experienced the ambiguities of scientific success as much as their colleagues in the natural sciences; there are some advantages to practicing a young and uncertain science. But the possibility of misusing psychological knowledge clearly exists, especially if we view psychology essentially as *a means for manipulating others*.

There is another way of looking at psychology, and that is as *a source of insight* into human beings, *including* ourselves. In this light the very wish to manipulate others may become something to examine. "Psychology as an opportunity for insight" leads to a more optimistic way of viewing the uses of psychology—we might imagine a tyrant, who wants to "predict and control" masses of people, turning instead to examine his own needs for manipulation, and finding other ways to satisfy those needs. A fantasy? Perhaps. But the history of science shows again and again that the consequences of science are fundamentally unpredictable. Is it too much to hope that the future of psychology may yet have some happy surprises in store?

References

Allport, F. H. *Theories of perception and the concept of structure.* New York: Wiley, 1955.

Allport, G. W. (Ed.). *Psychoanalysis as seen by analyzed psychologists, a symposium.* Washington, DC: American Psychological Association, 1953.

Anderson, J. R. *Cognitive psychology and its implications.* San Francisco: Freeman, 1980.

Anderson, J. R., & Bower, G. H. *Human associative memory.* Washington, DC: Winston, 1973.

Andreski, S. *Social sciences as sorcery.* New York: St. Martin's Press, 1972.

Ashby, F. G., & Townsend, J. T. Decomposing the reaction time distribution: Pure insertion and selective influence revisited. *Journal of Mathematical Psychology,* 1980, *21,* 93–123.

Atkinson, R. C., & Shiffrin, R. M. Human memory: A proposed system and its control processes. In K. Spence & J. Spence (Eds.), *The psychology of learning and motivation* (Vol. 2). New York: Academic Press, 1968.

Ayer, A. J. *Language, truth and logic.* New York: Dover Publications, 1946.

Baars, B. J. "Cognitive" vs. "conscious": Letter to the editor. *American Psychologists,* 1981, *36*(2), 223–224.

Baars, B. J. Conscious contents provide the nervous system with coherent, global information. In R. Davidson, G. Schwartz, & D. Shapiro (Eds.), *Consciousness and self-regulation* (Vol. 3). New York: Plenum, 1983a.

Baars, B. J. *Willlam James as the unintentional progenitor of behaviorism.* Paper presented at the Eastern Psychological Association, May 1983b.

Baars, B. J. Can involuntary slips of the tongue reveal a state of mind? — with an addendum on the problem of conscious control of action. In T. S. Shlechter & A. Toglia (Eds.), *New directions in cognitive science.* New York: Plenum, 1985.

Baars, B. J. *A cognitive theory of consciousness.* London: Cambridge University Press, in press.

Bakan, D. On the effect of mind on matter. In R. W. Rieber (Ed.), *Body and mind: Past, present and future.* New York: Academic Press, 1980.

Bandura, A. *Principles of behavior modification.* New York: Holt, Rinehart & Winston, 1969.

Bateson, G. *Mind and nature: A necessary unity.* New York: Bantam Books, 1979.

Baver, R. A. *The New Man in Soviet psychology.* Cambridge, MA: Harvard University Press, 1959.

Beck, A. T., Rush, A. J., Shaw, B. F., & Emery, G. *Cognitive therapy of depression.* New York: Guilford Press, 1979.

Bergmann, G., & Spence, K. W. Operationism and theory construction. *Psychological Review,* 1941, *48,* 1–14.

Bergson, H. *Creative evolution* (A. Mitchell, Trans.). New York: Holt, Rinehart & Winston, 1926. (First published, 1907.)

419

Berlyne, D. E. *Conflict, arousal, and curiosity*. New York: McGraw-Hill, 1960.

Bernstein, N. *The coordination and regulation of movement*. New York: Pergamon Press, 1967.

Bettelheim, B. *Freud and man's soul*. New York: Knopf, 1983.

Bever, T. G., Fodor, J. A., & Garrett, M. A formal limitation of associationism. In T. R. Dixon & D. L. Horton (Eds.), *Verbal behavior and general behavior theory*. New York: Prentice-Hall, 1968.

Blumenthal, A. L. *Language and psychology: Historical aspects of psycholinguistics*. New York: Wiley, 1970.

Blumenthal, A. L. A reappraisal of Wilhelm Wundt. *American Psychologist*, 1975, *30*, 1081–1088.

Blumenthal, A. L. *The process of cognition*. New York: Publisher, 1977a.

Blumenthal, A. L. Wilhelm Wundt and early American psychology: A clash of cultures. *Annals of the New York Academy of Sciences*, 1977b, *291*, 13–20.

Blumenthal, A. L. Wilhelm Wundt, the founding father we never knew. *Contemporary Psychology*, 1979, *24*(7), 547–550.

Blumenthal, A. L. Wilhelm Wundt—problems of interpretation. In W. G. Bringman & R. D. Tweney (Eds.), *Wundt studies*. Toronto: Hogrefe, 1980.

Boden, M. *Artificial intelligence and natural man*. New York: Basic Books, 1977.

Boring, E. G. *A history of experimental psychology* (2nd ed.). New York: Appleton-Century-Crofts, 1950. (First published, 1929.)

Boring, E. G., & Lindzey, G. (Eds.). *A history of psychology in autobiography*. New York: Appleton-Century-Crofts, 1967.

Bousfield, W. A. The occurrence of clustering in the recall of randomly arranged associates. *Journal of General Psychology*, 1953, *49*, 229–240.

Bower, G. H., & Trabasso, T. R. Reversals prior to solution in concept identification. *Journal of Experimental Psychology*, 1963, *66*, 409–418.

Bransford, J. D. *Human cognition, learning, understanding, and remembering*. CA: Wadsworth, 1979.

Bransford, J. D., & Franks, J. J. The abstraction of linguistic ideas. *Cognitive Psychology*, 1971, *2*, 331–350.

Bransford, J. D., & Franks, J. J. The abstraction of linguistic ideas: A review. *Cognition*, 1972, *1*, 221–249.

Brentano, F. *Psychology from an empirical standpoint* (A. C. Rancurello & D. B. Terrell, Trans.). London: Routledge & Kegan Paul, 1973. (First published, 1874.)

Bridgman, P. W. *The logic of modern physics*. New York: Macmillan, 1927.

Briskman, L. B. Is a Kuhnian analysis applicable to psychology? *Science Studies*, 1972, *2*, 87–97.

Broadbent, D. E. *Perception and communication*. New York: Pergamon Press, 1958.

Broadbent, D. E. *Decision and stress*. New York: Academic Press, 1971.

Bruner, J. S. Jerome S. Bruner. In C. Murchison (Ed.), *A history of psychology in autobiography*. Worcester, MA: Clark University Press, 1936.

Bruner, J. S. *In search of mind: Essays in autobiography*. New York: Harper & Row, 1984.

Bruner, J. S., Goodnow, J. J., & Austin, G. A. *A study of thinking*. New York: Wiley, 1956.

Bruner, J. S., & Postman, L. Emotional selectivity in perception and reaction. *Journal of Personality*, 1947, *16*, 69–77.

Brunswik, E. Points of view. In P. L. Harriman (Ed.), *Encyclopedia of psychology*. New York: Philosophical Library, 1946.

Burtt, E. A. *The metaphysical foundations of modern physical science*. New York: Doubleday, 1954.

Buss, A. R. The structure of psychological revolutions. *Journal of Behavioral Sciences*, 1978, *14*, 57–64.

Cannon, W. *The wisdom of the body.* New York: Norton, 1932.

Chase, W. E., & Simon, H. A. The mind's eye in chess. In W. Chase (Ed.), *Visual information processing.* New York: Academic Press, 1973.

Cherry, E. C. Some experiments on the recognition of speech with one and with two ears. *Journal of the Acoustical Society of America,* 1953, *25,* 975–979.

Chew, S. L., Larkey, L. S., Soli, S. D., Blount, J., & Jenkins, J. J. The abstraction of musical ideas. *Memory and Cognition,* 1982, *10,* 413–423.

Chomsky, N. Three models for the description of language. *IRE Transactions on Information Theory,* September 1956, *IT-2*(3), 113–124.

Chomsky, N. *Syntactic structures.* The Hague, The Netherlands: Mouton, 1957.

Chomsky, N. Review of Skinner's *Verbal behavior. Language,* 1959, *35,* 26–58.

Chomsky, N. *Aspects of the theory of syntax.* Cambridge, MA: MIT Press, 1965.

Chomsky, N. *Cartesian linguistics.* New York: Harper & Row, 1966.

Chomsky, N. *American power and the new mandarins.* New York: Pantheon, 1969.

Chomsky, N. *Language and mind.* New York: Harcourt Brace Jovanovich, 1972.

Chomsky, N. *The logical structure of linguistic theories.* New York: Plenum Press, 1975.

Chomsky, N. *Lectures on government and binding: The Pisa lectures.* Dordrecht, The Netherlands: Foris Publications, 1982.

Chomsky, N., & Halle, M. *The sound pattern of English.* Englewood Cliffs, NJ: Prentice-Hall, 1972.

Chomsky, N. & Miller, G. A. Finite-state languages. *Information and Control,* 1958, *1,* 91–112.

Clark, H. H., & Clark, E. V. *Psychology and language: An introduction to psycholinguistics.* New York: Harcourt Brace Jovanovich, 1977.

Cofer, C. N. (Ed.). *Verbal learning and verbal behavior.* New York: McGraw-Hill, 1961.

Cofer, C. N., & Musgrave, B. S. (Eds.) *Verbal behavior and learning: Problems and processes.* New York: McGraw-Hill, 1963.

Cohen, D. *J. B. Watson, the founder of behaviorism: A biography.* Boston: Routledge & Kegan Paul, 1979.

Cooper, L. A., & Shepard, R. N. Chronometric studies of the rotation of mental images. In W. G. Chase (Ed.), *Visual information processing.* New York: Academic Press, 1973.

D'Andrade, R. G. The cultural part of cognition. *Cognitive Science,* 1981, *5,* 179–195.

Danziger, K. The positivist repudiation of Wundt. *Journal of the History of the Behavioral Sciences,* 1979, *15,* 205–226.

Deese, J. Meaning and change of meaning. *American Psychologist,* 1967, *22,* 641–651.

Deese, J. *Psychology as science and art.* New York: Harcourt Brace Jovanovich, 1972.

de Groot, A. D. *Thought and choice in chess.* Amsterdam: Mouton, 1965.

Dember, W. Motivation and the cognitive revolution. *American Psychologist,* 1974, *29,* 161–168.

Dewey, J. The reflex arc concept in psychology. *Psychological Review,* 1896, *3,* 357–370.

Dinneen, G. P. Programming pattern recognition in modern computers. *Proceedings of the 1955 Western Joint Computer Conference.*

Dixon, T. R., & Horton, D. L. (Eds.). *Verbal behavior and general behavior theory.* Englewood Cliffs, NJ: Prentice-Hall, 1968.

Dollard, J., & Miller, N. E. *Personality and psychotherapy: An analysis in terms of learning, thinking and culture.* New York: McGraw-Hill, 1950.

Donders, F. C. Die Schnelligkeit psychischer Processe. *Archiv für Anatomie und Physiologie,* 1868, 657–681.

Dreyfus, H. L. *What computers can't do: A critique of artificial reason* (2nd ed.). New York: Harper & Row, 1979.

Duncker, K. On problem solving. *Psychological Monographs,* 1945, *58*(270).

Ellenberger, H. *The discovery of the unconscious: The history and evolution of dynamic psychiatry.* New York: Basic Books, 1970.

Ellis, A. *Reason and emotion in psychotherapy.* New York: Lyle Stuart, 1962.

Erdelyi, M. H. A new look at the New Look: Perceptual defense and vigilance. *Psychological Review,* 1974, *81,* 1–25.

Erdelyi, M. H. *Psychoanalysis: The cognitive psychology of Sigmund Freud.* San Francisco: Freeman, 1985.

Erdelyi, M. H., & Goldberg, B. Let's not sweep repression under the rug: Toward a cognitive psychology of repression. In J. F. Kihlstrom & F. J. Evans (Eds.), *Functional disorders of memory.* Hillsdale, NJ: Erlbaum, 1979.

Ericsson, K. A., & Simon, H. A. Verbal reports as data. *Psychological Review,* 1980, *87,* 215–251.

Esper, E. A. *A history of psychology.* Philadelphia: Saunders, 1964.

Esper, E. A. Max Meyer: The making of a scientific isolate. *Journal of the History of the Behavioral Sciences,* 1966, *2*(4), 341–356.

Esper, E. A. Max Meyer in America. *Journal of the History of the Behavioral Sciences,* 1967, *3*(2), 107–131.

Esper, E. A. *Mentalism and objectivism in linguistics.* New York: American Elsevier, 1968.

Estes, W. *Handbook of learning and cognitive processes.* Hillsdale, NJ: Halstead Press, Division of Wiley, 1975.

Eysenck, H. J. The effects of psychotherapy. In *Behavior therapy and the neuroses.* London: Pitman Medical Publishing, 1960.

Feigenbaum, E. A., & Feldman, J. (Eds.). *Computers and thought.* New York: McGraw-Hill, 1963.

Fermi, L. *Illustrious immigrants: The intellectual migration from Europe, 1930–1941.* Chicago: University of Chicago Press, 1971.

Feyerabend, P. *Against method: Outline of anarchistic theory of knowledge.* London: NLB, 1975.

Fisher, S., & Greenberg, R. P. *Scientific credibility of Freud's theories and therapy.* New York: Basic Books, 1977.

Fisher, S., & Greenberg, R. P. *Scientific evolution of Freud's theories and therapy.* New York: Basic Books, 1978.

Fodor, J. A. Could meaning be an r_m? *Journal of Verbal Learning and Verbal Behavior,* 1965, *4,* 73–81.

Fodor, J. A. *Psychological explanation: An introduction to the philosophy of psychology.* New York: Random House, 1968.

Fodor, J. A. *The language of thought.* New York: Thomas Crowell, 1975.

Fodor, J. A. The mind–body problem. *Scientific American,* January 1981, *244*(1).

Fodor, J. A. *The modularity of mind.* Cambridge, MA: MIT Press, 1983.

Fodor, J. A., Bever, T. G., & Garrett, M. *The psychology of language.* New York: McGraw-Hill, 1974.

Fodor, J. A., & Garrett, M. Some syntactic determinants of sentential complexity. *Perception and Psychophysics,* 1967, *2,* 289–296.

Fodor, J. A., Garrett, M. F., & Bever, T. G. Some syntactic determinants of sentential complexity. II: Verb structure. *Perception and Psychophysics,* 1968, *3,* 453–461.

Fodor, J. A., Jenkins, J. J., & Saporta, S. Psycholinguistics and communication theory. In F. E. X. Dance (Ed.), *Human communication theory.* New York: Holt, Rinehart & Winston, 1967.

Franks, J. J., & Bransford, J. D. Abstraction of visual patterns. *Journal of Experimental Psychology,* 1971, *90,* 65–74.

Freud, S. The interpretation of dreams. *Standard Edition,* 1953, *3.* London: Hogarth Press. (First published, 1900.)

Freud, S. *Introductory lectures on psychoanalysis.* New York: Norton, 1970. (First published, 1920.)

Freud, S. *An outline of psychoanalysis.* New York: Norton, 1940.

Freud, S. Postscript to the question of lay analysis. *Standard Edition*, 1961, *20*, 1–74. London: Hogarth Press. (First published, 1927.)

Frick, F. C., & Miller, G. A. A statistical description of operant conditioning. *American Journal of Psychology*, 1951, *64*, 20–36.

Frijda, N. H., & de Groot, A D. *Otto Selz: His contribution to psychology.* The Hague, Paris, & New York: Mouton.

Garfield, S. Psychotherapy: A 40-year appraisal. *American Psychologist*, 1981, *36*(2), 179–183.

Garner, W. R. *Uncertainty and structure as psychological concepts.* New York: Wiley, 1962.

Ghiselin, B. (Ed.). *The creative process.* New York: New American Library, 1952.

Gibson, E. *Principles of perceptual learning and development.* New York: Appleton-Century-Crofts, 1969.

Gibson, J. J. *The senses considered as perceptual systems.* Boston: Houghton Mifflin, 1966.

Gibson, J. J. *The ecological approach to visual perception.* Boston: Houghton Mifflin, 1979.

Gleitman, H., Nachmias, J., & Neisser, U. The S-R reinforcement theory of extinction. *Psychological Review*, 1954, *61*, 23–33.

Gray, J. A., & Wedderburn, A. A. Grouping strategies with simultaneous stimuli. *Quarterly Journal of Experimental Psychology*, 1960, *12*, 180–184.

Greenspoon, J. *The effect of verbal and non-verbal stimuli on the frequency of numbers of two verbal response classes.* Unpublished doctoral dissertation, Indiana University, 1951.

Gregory, R. L. *Eye and brain: The psychology of seeing.* New York: McGraw-Hill, 1966.

Gregory, R. L. *The intelligent eye.* New York: McGraw-Hill, 1970.

Griffin, D. R. *The question of animal awareness.* New York: Rockefeller University Press, 1976.

Guthrie, E. R. *The psychology of learning.* New York: Harper & Row, 1935.

Hadamard, J. *The psychology of invention in the mathematical field.* Princeton, NJ: Princeton University Press, 1945.

Harlow, H. F., & Suomi, S. J. Nature of love — simplified. *American Psychologist*, 1970, *25*, 161–168.

Hayek, F. A. *The counter-revolution of science.* Glencoe, IL: Free Press, 1952.

Hayek, F. A. *New studies in philosophy, politics, economics, and the history of ideas.* Chicago: University of Chicago Press, 1978.

Healy, W., Bronner, A. F., & Bowers, A. M. *The structure and meaning of psychoanalysis.* New York: Knopf, 1929.

Hebb, D. O. *The organization of behavior.* New York: Wiley, 1949.

Heidbreder, E. *Seven psychologies.* New York: Appleton-Century-Crofts, 1933.

Heims, S. Encounter of behavioral sciences with new machine-organism analogies in the 1940s. *Journal of the History of the Behavioral Sciences*, 1975, *5*(2), 368–373.

Helmholtz, H. von *Treatise on physiological optics* (3 vols. in English translation; J. P. C. Southall, Trans.). New York: Dover, 1962.

Herbart, J. F. Psychology as a science, newly founded upon experience, metaphysics and mathematics. In T. Shipley (Ed.), *Classics in psychology.* New York: Philosophical Library, 1961.

Hilgard, E. R. *Theories of learning.* New York: Appleton-Century-Crofts, 1948.

Hilgard, E. R. *Personality and hypnosis: A study of imaginative involvement.* Chicago: University of Chicago Press, 1970. (2nd ed., 1979.)

Hilgard, E. R. Hypnotic phenomena: The struggle for scientific acceptance. *American Scientist*, 1971, *59*(5), 567–577.

Hilgard, E. R. Autobiography of Ernest R. Hilgard. In G. Lindzey (Ed.), *A history of psychology in autobiography* (Vol. 6). Englewood Cliffs, NJ: Prentice-Hall, 1974.

Hilgard, E. R. Neodissociation theory of multiple cognitive control systems. In G. E. Schwartz & D. Shapiro (Eds.), *Consciousness and self-regulation* (Vol. 1). New York: Plenum, 1976.

Hilgard, E. R. *Divided consciousness: Multiple controls in human thought and action.* New York: Wiley, 1977.

Hilgard, E. R. Consciousness and control: Lessons from hypnosis. *Australian Journal of Clinical and Experimental Hypnosis*, 1979, *7*(2), 103–115.

Hilgard, E. R. Consciousness in contemporary psychology. *Annual Review of Psychology*, 1980a, *31*, 1–26.

Hilgard, E. R. The trilogy of mind: Cognition, affection, and conation. *Journal of the History of the Behavioral Sciences*, 1980b, *16*(2), 107–117.

Hilgard, E. R. *Psychology in America: A historical summary.* New York: Harcourt Brace Iovanovich, 1986.

Hilgard, E. R., & Marquis, D. G. *Conditioning and learning.* New York: Appleton-Century-Crofts, 1940.

Hilgard, J. R. *Personality and hypnosis: A study of imaginative involvement.* Chicago: University of Chicago Press, 1970.

Hinton, G., & Anderson, J. *Parallel models of associative memory.* Englewood, NJ: Erlbaum, 1981.

Hirst, W., Spelke, E., Reaves, C., Caharack, G., & Neisser, V. Dividing attention without alternation or automaticity. *Journal of Experimental Psychology*, 1980, *109*(1), 98–117.

Hochberg, E. Effects of the Gestalt revolution: The Cornell symposium on perception. *Psychological Review*, 1957, *64*, 73–383.

Hofstadter, R. *Anti-intellectualism in American life.* New York: Random House, 1963.

Horton, D. L., & Kjeldergaard, P. M. An experimental analysis of associative factors in mediated generalization. *Psychological Monographs*, 1961, *75*, No. 11.

Hovland, C. I., Janis, I. L., & Kelley, H. H. *Communication and persuasion: Psychological studies of opinion change.* New Haven, CT: Yale University Press, 1959.

Hull, C. L. The concept of the habit-family hierarchy and maze learning: Part 1. *Psychological Review*, 1934, *34*, 33–54.

Hull, C. L. Mind, mechanism, and adaptive behavior. *Psychological Review*, 1937, *44*, 1–32.

Hull, C. L. *Principles of behavior.* New York: Appleton-Century-Crofts, 1943.

Hull, C. L. *A behavior system: An introduction to behavior theory concerning the individual organism.* New Haven, CT: Yale University Press, 1952.

Hull, C. L., Hovland, C. I., Ross, R. T., Perkins, D. T., & Fitch, F. G. *Mathematico-deductive theory of rote learning: A study in scientific methodology.* New Haven, CT: Yale University Press, 1940.

Hulse, S. H., Fowler, H., & Honig, W. K. (Eds.). *Cognitive psychology in animal behavior.* Hillsdale, NJ: Erlbaum, 1978.

Hume, D. An inquiry concerning human understanding. In A. Flew (Ed.), *David Hume: On human nature and understanding.* New York: Collier, 1962. (First published, 1777.)

Hunter, W. S. The delayed reaction in animals and children. *Animal Behavior Monographs*, 1913, *2*, 21–30.

James, W. *Principles of psychology.* Cambridge, MA: Harvard University Press, 1983. (First published, 1890.)

Jammer, M. *The concept of force: A story in the foundations of dynamics.* Cambridge, MA: Harvard University Press, 1957.

Jenkins, J. J. Mediated associations: Paradigms and situations. In C. N. Cofer & B. S. Musgrave (Eds.), *Verbal behavior and learning: Problems and processes.* New York: McGraw-Hill, 1963.

Jenkins, J. J. Comments on pseudomediation. *Psychonomic Science*, 1965, *2*, 97–98.

Jenkins, J. J. *The role of experimentation in psycholinguistics*. Paper presented at the Meeting of the American Psychological Association, 1966.

Jenkins, J. J. Remember that old theory of memory? Well, forget it! *American Psychologist*, 1974, *29*(11), 785–795.

Jenkins, J. J., & Foss, D. J. An experimental analysis of pseudomediation. *Psychonomic Science*, 1965, *2*, 99–100.

Jenkins, J. J., & Palermo, D. S. Mediation processes and the acquisition of linguistic structure. In U. Bellugi & R. W. Brown (Eds.), The acquisition of language. *Monographs of the Society for Research in Child Development*, 1964, *3*, 158–160.

Jenkins, J. J., & Paterson, D. G. *Studies in individual differences*. New York: Appleton-Century-Crofts, 1961.

Jenkins, J. J., & Russell, W. Associative clustering during recall. *Journal of Abnormal Social Psychology*, 1952, *47*, 818–821.

Jones, E. *The life and work of Sigmund Freud* (Vol. 1). New York: Basic Books, 1953.

Joynson, R. B. The breakdown of modern psychology. *Bulletin of the British Psychological Society*, 1970, *23*, 261–9.

Jung, C. G. *Studies in word-association* (M. D. Eder, Trans.). London: Heinemann, 1918.

Kalish, H. I. *From behavioral science to behavior modification*. New York: McGraw-Hill, 1981.

Katona, G. *Organizing and memorizing: Studies in the psychology of learning and teaching*. New York: Columbia University Press, 1940.

Kazdin, A. E. *History of behavior modification: Experimental foundations of contemporary research*. Baltimore: University Park Press, 1978.

Keller, F. S., & Schoenfeld, W. N. *Principles of psychology: A systematic text in the science of behavior*. New York: Appleton-Century-Crofts, 1950.

Kendler, H. H. What is learning? — A theoretical blind alley. *Psychological Review*, 1952, *59*, 269–277.

Kendler, H. H. Kenneth W. Spence. *Psychological Review*, 1967, *74*, 335–341.

Kendler, H. H. Environmental and cognitive control of behavior. *American Psychologist*, 1971, *26*(11), 962–973.

Kendler, H. H. The making of a neobehaviorist. In T. S. Krawiec (Ed.), *The psychologists*. New York: Oxford University Press, 1974.

Kendler, H. H. *Psychology: A science in conflict*. New York: Oxford University Press, 1981.

Kendler, H. H. *Behaviorism and psychology: An uneasy alliance*. In S. Koch & D. Leary (Eds.), *A century of psychology as science*. New York: McGraw-Hill, 1985.

Kendler, H. H., & Kendler, T. Vertical and horizontal processes in problem solving. *Psychological Review*, 1962, *69*(1), 1–16.

Kendler, H. H., & Kendler, T. From discrimination learning to cognitive development: A neobehaviorist odyssey. In W. K. Estes (Eds.), *Handbook of learning and cognitive processes*. Hillsdale, NJ: Erlbaum, 1975.

Kendler, H. H., & Spence, J. Tenets of neobehaviorism. In H. Kendler & J. Spence (Eds.), *Essays in neobehaviorism: A memorial volume to Kenneth W. Spence*. New York: Appleton-Century-Crofts, 1971.

Kimble, G. A. *Hilgard and Marquis' conditioning and learning* (2nd ed.). New York: Appleton-Century-Crofts, 1954.

Koch, S. Clark L. Hull. In W. K. Estes *et al.*, *Modern learning theory*. New York: Appleton-Century-Crofts, 1954.

Koch, S. Behavior as "intrinsically" regulated: Work notes towards a pre-thory of phenomena called "motivational." In M. R. Jones (Ed.), *Nebraska Symposium on Motivation*. Lincoln, NE: University of Nebraska Press, 1956.

Koch, S. *Psychology: The study of a science*. New York: McGraw-Hill, 1959.

Koch, S. Psychological science versus the science–humanism antinomy: Intimations of a significant science of man. *American Psychologist*, 1961, *16*, 629–639.

Koch, S. More verbal behavior from Dr. Skinner. *Contemporary Psychology*, 1976, *21*(7), 453–457.

Koestler, A. *The ghost in the machine*. Chicago: H. Regnery, 1967.

Köhler, W. Gestalt psychology today. *American Psychologist*, 1959, *14*, 727–734.

Krantz, D., Hall, R., & Allen, D. William McDougall and the problem of purpose. *Journal of the History of Behavioral Sciences*, 1969, *5*, 25–38.

Krasner, L. Studies of the conditioning of verbal behavior. *Psychological Bulletin*, 1958, *55*, 148–170.

Krasner, L. The therapist as a social reinforcement machine. In H. H. Strupp & L. Luborsky (Eds.), *Research in psychotherapy* (Vol. 2). Washington, DC: American Psychological Association, 1962.

Krasner, L. *25 years of clinical psychology*. Paper presented at New York State Psychological Association, NYC, April 13, 1973.

Krasner, L. On the death of behavior modification: Some comments from a mourner. *American Psychologist*, 1976, *31*(5), 387–388.

Krasner, L. The future and the past in the behaviorism–humanism dialogue. *American Psychologist*, 1978, *33*(9), 799–804.

Krechevsky, I. "Hypotheses" in rats. *Psychological Review*, 1932, *39*, 516–532.

Kuhn, T. S. *The structure of scientific revolutions* (Vol. 2, No. 2). Chicago: University of Chicago Press, 1962. (2nd ed., 1970.)

Kuhn, T. S. Reflection on my critics. In I. Lakatoš & A. Musgrave (Eds.), *Criticism and the growth of knowledge*. London: Cambridge University Press, 1970.

Lachman, R., Lachman, J. L., & Butterfield, E. C. *Cognitive psychology and information processing: An introduction*. Hillsdale, NJ: Erlbaum, 1979.

Lakatoš, I. Falsification and the methodology of scientific research programmes. In I. Lakatoš & A. Musgrave (Eds.), *Criticism and the growth of knowledge*. London: Cambridge University Press, 1970.

Lakatoš, I., & Musgrave, A. (Eds.). *Criticism and the growth of knowledge*. London: Cambridge University Press, 1970.

Lakoff, G., & Johnson, M. *Metaphors we live by*. Chicago: University of Chicago Press, 1980.

Lang, P. J., & Lazovik, A. D. Experimental desensitization of a phobia. *Journal of Abnormal and Social Psychology*, 1963, *66*, 519–525.

Larson, C., & Sullivan, J. Watson's relation to Titchener. *Journal of the History of the Behavioral Sciences*, 1965, *1*, 338–354.

Lashley, K. S. *Brain mechanisms and intelligence*. Chicago: University of Chicago Press, 1929.

Lashley, K. S. Basic neural mechanism in behavior. *Psychological Review*, 1930, *37*, 1–24.

Lashley, K. S. The problem of serial order in behavior. In L. A. Jeffress (Ed.), *Cerebral mechanisms in behavior*. New York: Wiley, 1951.

Lazarus, A. A. *Behavior therapy and beyond*. New York: McGraw-Hill, 1971.

Lees, R. P. Review of "Syntactic Structures" by Noam Chomsky. *Language*, 1957, *33*, 375–408.

Lepley, U. M. A theory of serial learning and forgetting based upon conditioned reflex principles. *Psychological Review*, 1932, *39*, 279–288.

Levine, M. A model of hypothesis behavior in discrimination learning set. *Psychological Review*, 1959, *66*, 353–366.

Levine, M. Hypothesis behavior by humans during discrimination learning. *Journal of Experimental Psychology*, 1966, *71*(3), 331–338.

Levine, M. Hunting for hypotheses. In M. H. Siegel & H. P. Ziegler (Eds.), *Psychological research: The inside story*. New York: Harper & Row, 1976.

Levine, M. Principles of spatial problem solving. *Journal of Experimental Psychology: General*, 1982, *111*(2), 157–175.

Levine, M., & Fingerman, P. Nonlearning: The completeness of blindness. *Journal of Experimental Psychology*, 1974, *102*(4), 720–721.

Levine, M., & Phillips, S. Probing for hypotheses with adults and children: Blank trials and introtacts. *Journal of Experimental Psychology*, 1975, *104*(4), 327–254.

Lindsay, P. H., & Norman, D. A. *Human information processing: An introduction to psychology*. New York: Academic Press, 1977.

Luchins, A. S. Mechanization in problem solving: The effect of "Einstellung." *Psychological Monographs*, 1942, *54*(6), 1–95.

Lynn, R. *Attention, arousal, and the orientation reaction*. New York: Pergamon, 1966.

MacCorquodale, K. On Chomsky's review of Skinner's Verbal Behavior. *Journal of Experimental Analysis of Behavior*, 1970, *13*, 83–99.

MacKay, D. G. Aspects of the theory of comprehension, memory, and attention. *Quarterly Journal of Experimental Psychology*, 1973, *25*, 22–40.

MacKay, D. M. *Information, mechanism, and meaning*. Cambridge, MA: MIT Press, 1969.

Mackenzie, B. D. Behaviorism and positivism. *Journal of the History of the Behavioral Sciences*, 1972, *8*, 221–231.

Mahoney, M., & Arnkoff, D. Cognitive and self-control therapies. In S. L. Garfield & A. E. Bergin (Eds.), *Handbook of psychotherapy and behavior change* (2nd ed.). New York: Wiley, 1978.

Maltzman, I. R. Theoretical conceptions of semantic conditioning and generalization. In T. R. Dixon & D. L. Horton (Eds.), *Verbal behavior and general behavior theory*. Englewood Cliffs, NJ: Prentice-Hall, 1968.

Maltzman, I. R., & Cole, M. (Eds.). *A handbook of contemporary Soviet psychology*. New York: Basic Books, 1969.

Mandler, G. From association to structure. *Psychological Review*, 1962, *69*(5), 415–427.

Mandler, G. Parent and child in the development of the Oedipus complex. *Journal of Nervous and Mental Disease*, 1963, *136*(3), 227–235.

Mandler, G. *Memory research reconsidered: A critical view of traditional methods and distinctions*. Center for Human Information Processing, University of California, San Diego, 1976.

Mandler, G. The generation of emotion: A psychological theory. In R. Plutchik & H. Kellerman (Eds.), *Emotion: Theory, research, and experience* (Vol. 1: *Theories of emotion*). New York: Academic Press, 1980.

Mandler, G. *Mind and body*. New York: Norton, 1984.

Mandler, G. *Cognitive psychology: An essay in cognitive science*. Hillsdale, NJ: Erlbaum, 1985.

Mandler, G., & Kessen, W. *The language of psychology*. New York: Wiley, 1959.

Mandler, J. M., & Mandler, G. The diaspora of experimental psychology: The Gestaltists and others. *Perspectives in American History*, 1968, *2*, 371–419.

Marr, D. *Vision: A computational investigation into the human representation of visual information*. San Francisco, W. H. Freeman, 1982.

Marr, D., & Nishihara, H. K. Visual information processing: Artificial intelligence and the sensorium of sight. *Technology Review*, 1978, *81*(1), 28–49.

Maslow, A. H. *Toward a psychology of being*. New York: Van Nostrand, 1962.

Maslow, A. H. *The psychology of science*. South Bend, IN: Gateway Editions, 1966.

Masserman, J. H. *Behavior and neurosis: An experimental psycho-analytic approach to psychological principles*. Chicago: University of Chicago Press, 1943.

Masterman, M. The nature of a paradigm. In I. Lakatoš & A. Musgrave (Eds.), *Criticism and the growth of knowledge*. London: Cambridge University Press, 1970.

McCulloch, W. S., & Pitts, W. A. A logical calculus of the ideas immanent in nervous activity. *Bulletin of Mathematical Biophysics*, 1943, *5*, 115.

McDougall, W. *Outline of psychology*. New York: Scribner's, 1923.

McGeoch, J. A. *Psychology of human learning.* New York: Longmans, Greene, 1942.

McNeil, D. *The conceptual basis of language.* Hillsdale, NJ: Erlbaum, 1979.

Meese, C. E. K. Scientific thought and social reconstruction. *Sigma Xi Quarterly*, 1934, *22*, 13–24.

Meichenbaum, D. H., & Goodman, J. Training impulsive children to talk to themselves: A means of developing self-control. *Journal of Abnormal Psychology*, 1971, *77*, 115–126.

Miller, G. A. *Language and communication.* New York: McGraw-Hill, 1951.

Miller, G. A. Human memory and the storage of information. *IRE Transactions on Information Theory*, 1956, *IT-2*(3), 128–137.

Miller, G. A. The magical number seven, plus or minus two: Some limits on our capacity for processing information. *Psychological Review*, 1956, *63*, 81–97.

Miller, G. A. *Psychology: The science of mental life.* Harmondsworth, Middlesex, England: Penguin Books, 1962.

Miller, G. A. *Mathematics and psychology.* New York: Wiley, 1964.

Miller, G. A. Toward a third metaphor for psycholinguistics. In W. Weimer & D. Palermo (Eds.), *Cognition and the symbolic processes.* Hillsdale, NJ: Erlbaum, 1974.

Miller, G. A. *Spontaneous apprentices: Children and language.* New York: Seabury, 1977.

Miller, G. A. *A very personal history.* Talk to Cognitive Science Workshop, MIT Cognitive Science Group, June 1, 1979.

Miller, G. A., & Chomsky, N. A. Finitary models of language users. In R. D. Luce, R. R. Bush, & E. Galanter (Eds.), *Handbook of mathematical psychology* (Vol. 2). New York: Wiley, 1963.

Miller, G. A., & Frick, F. C. Statistical behavioristics and sequence of responses. *Psychological Review*, 1949, *56*, 311–324.

Miller, G. A., Galanter, E., & Pribram, K. H. *Plans and the structure of behavior.* New York: Holt, Rinehart & Winston, 1960.

Miller, G. A., & Johnson-Laird, P. N. *Language and perception.* Cambridge, MA: Belknap Press, 1976.

Minsky, M. *Semantic information processing.* Cambridge, MA: MIT Press, 1968.

Moruzzi, G. A., & Magoun, H. W. Brain stem reticular formation and activation of the EEG. *Electroencephalogy and Clinical Neurophysiology*, 1949, *1*, 455–473.

Mowrer, O. H. *Learning theory and personality dynamics.* New York: Ronald Press, 1950.

Murray, S. Gatekeepers and the Chomskian revolution. *Journal of the History of the Behavioral Sciences*, 1980, *16*, 73–88.

Natsoulas, T. Consciousness. *American Psychologist*, 1978a, *33*(10), 906–914.

Natsoulas, T. Residual subjectivity. *American Psychologist*, 1978b, *33*(3), 269–283.

Neisser, U. An experimental distinction between perceptual process and verbal response. *Journal of Experimental Psychology*, 1954, *47*, 399–402.

Neisser, U. Decision-time without reaction-time: Experiments in visual scanning. *American Journal of Psychology*, 1963a, *76*, 376–385.

Neisser, U. The imitation of man by machine. *Science*, 1963b, *139*, 193–197.

Neisser, U. *Cognitive psychology.* New York: Appleton-Century-Crofts, 1967.

Neisser, U. *Cognition and reality.* San Francisco: W. H. Freeman, 1976.

Neisser, U. Is psychology ready for consciousness? Review of Hilgard's *Divided consciousness. Contemporary Psychology*, 1979, *24*(2), 99–100.

Neisser, U. *Memory observed: remembering in natural contexts.* San Francisco: W. H. Freeman, 1982.

Newell, A. The knowledge level. *AI Magazine*, 1981, *2*(2), 1–20.

Newell, A., Shaw, J. C., & Simon, H. A. Elements of a theory of human problem solving. *Psychological Review*, 1958a, *65*, 151–166.

Newell, A., Shaw, J. C., & Simon, H. A. Chess-playing programs and the problem of complexity. *IBM Journal of Research and Development*, 1958b, *2*, 320–335.

Newell, A., Shaw, J. C., & Simon, H. A. Report on a general problem-solving program for a computer. In *Information processing: Proceedings of the International Conference on Information Processing*. Paris: UNESCO, 1960.

Newell, A., & Simon, H. A. The Logic Theory Machine: A complex information processing system. *IRE Transactions on Information Theory*, 1956, *IT-2*(3), 61–79.

Newell, A., & Simon, H. A. General Problem Solver, a program that stimulates human thought. In E. A. Feigenbaum & J. Feldman (Eds.), *Computers and thought*. New York: McGraw-Hill, 1963.

Newell, A., & Simon, H. A. *Human problem-solving*. Englewood Cliffs, NJ: Prentice-Hall, 1972.

Norman, D. A. *Memory and attention: An introduction to human information processing* (2nd ed.). New York: Wiley, 1976. (1st ed., 1967.)

Norman, D. A. Twelve issues in cognitive science. In D. A. Norman (Ed.), *Perspectives on cognitive science*. Norwood, NJ: Ablex, 1981.

Norman, D. A., & Rumelhart, D. E. *Explorations in cognition*. San Francisco: W. H. Freeman, 1975.

Olds, J. A preliminary mapping of electrical reinforcing effects in the rat brain. *Journal of Comparative and Physiological Psychology*, 1956a, *49*, 281–285.

Olds, J. Pleasure centers in the brain. *Scientific American*, 1956b, *195*, 105–116.

Olds, J. Self-stimulation of the brain. *Science*, 1958, *127*, 315–323

Olds, J. Hypothalamic substrates of reward. *Physiological Review*, 1962, *42*, 554–604.

Olds, J., & Milner, P. Positive reinforcement produced by electrical stimulation of septal area and other regions of the rat brain. *Journal of Comparative Physiological Psychology*, 1954, *47*, 419–427.

Osgood, C. E. *Method and theory in experimental psychology*. New York: Oxford University Press, 1953.

Osgood, C. E. Meaning cannot be an r_m? *Journal of Verbal Learning and Verbal Behavior*, 1966, *5*, 402–407.

Osgood, C. E. A dinosaur caper: Psycholinguistics past, present, and future. *Annals of the New York Academy of Sciences*, 1975, *263*, 16–26.

Osgood, C. E., Suci, C. J., & Tannenbaum, P. H. *The measurement of meaning*. Urbana, IL: University of Illinois Press, 1957.

Paivio, A. *Imagery and verbal processes*. New York: Holt, Rinehart & Winston, 1971.

Palermo, D. Is a scientific revolution taking place in psychology? *Scientific Studies*, 1971, *1*, 135–155.

Pavlov, I. P. *Conditioned reflexes* (G. V. Anrep, Trans.). London: Oxford University Press, 1927. (Reprinted, New York: Dover, 1960.)

Peterson, L. R., & Peterson, M. J. Short-term retention of individual verbal items. *Journal of Experimental Psychology*, 1959, *58*, 193–198.

Platt, J. Strong inference. *Science*, 1964, *146*(3642), 347–353.

Plutchik, R. Operationism as methodology. *Behavioral Science*, 1968, *8*, 234–241.

Poincaré, H. *Science and hypothesis* (G. B. Halsted, Trans.). New York: The Science Press, 1913.

Polanyi, M. *Personal knowledge*. New York: Harper & Row, 1958.

Polanyi, M. *The tacit dimension*. Garden City, NY: Doubleday, 1966.

Posner, M. I. *Cognition: An introduction*. Glenview, IL: Scott, Foresman, 1973.

Posner, M. I. *Chronometric explorations of mind*. Hillsdale, NJ: Erlbaum, 1978.

Posner, M. I., & Keele, S. W. On the genesis of abstract ideas. *Journal of Experimental Psychology*, 1968, *77*, 353–363.

Posner, M. I., & Schulman, G. Cognitive science. In E. Hearst (Ed.), *The first century of experimental psychology*. Hillsdale, NJ: Erlbaum, 1979.

Posner, M. I., & Warren, R. E. Traces, concepts and conscious constructions. In A.

W. Melton & E. Martin (Eds.), *Coding processes in human memory*. Washington, DC: Winston, 1972.

Postal, P. M. Underlying and superficial linguistic structure. *Harvard Educational Review*, 1964, *34*, 246-266.

Postman, L. Organization and interference. *Psychological Review*, 1971, *78*, 290-302.

Postman, L., & Brown, D. The perceptual consequences of success and failure. *Journal of Abnormal and Social Psychology*, 1952, *47*, 13-221.

Postman, L., Bruner, J. S., & McGinnies, E. Personal values as selective factors in perception. *Journal of Abnormal and Social Psychology*, 1948, *43*, 142-153.

Pribram, K. *Language of the brain*. Englewood Cliffs, NJ: Prentice-Hall, 1971.

Putnam, H. *Mind, language, and reality: Philosophical papers* (Vol. 2). London: Cambridge University Press, 1975.

Rachlin, H. Scaling subjective velocity, distance, and duration. *Perception and Psychophysics*, 1966, *1*, 77-82.

Rachlin, H. *Introduction to modern behaviorism*. San Francisco: W. H. Freeman, 1970.

Rachlin, H. Self-control. *Behaviorism*, 1974, *2*, 94-107.

Rachlin, H. Reinforcing and punishing thoughts. *Behavior Therapy*, 1977a, *8*, 659-665.

Rachlin, H. Reinforcing and punishing thoughts: A rejoinder to Ellis and Mahoney. *Behavior Therapy*, 1977b, *8*, 678-681.

Rachlin, H. A review of M. J. Mahoney's *Cognition and behavior modification*. *Journal of Applied Behavior Analysis*, 1977, *10*, 369-374.

Rachlin, H. Who cares if the chimpanzee has a theory of mind? *Behavioral and Brain Sciences*, 1978, *1*, 593-594.

Rachlin, H. Skinner and the philosophers: Review of P. Harzem and T. R. Miles (Eds.), *Conceptual issues in operant psychology*. *Contemporary Psychology*, 1979, *24*(3), 184-185.

Rachlin, H. Economics and behavioral psychology. In J. Staddon (Ed.), *Adaptation to constraint: The biology, economics, and psychology of individual behavior*. New York: Academic Press, 1980.

Rachlin, H. Absolute and relative consumption space. In D. Bernstein (Eds.), *Nebraska Symposium on Motivation*. Lincoln, NE: University of Nebraska Press, 1981.

Rachlin, H., Kagel, J., & Battalio, R. Substitutability in time allocation. *Psychological Review*, 1980, *87*(4), 355-374.

Rachlin, H., Kagel, J., Battalio, R., & Green, L. Maximization in behavioral psychology. *Behavioral and Brain Sciences*, 1981, *3*, 371-418.

Razran, G. The observable unconscious and inferable conscious in current Soviet psychophysiology: Interoceptive conditioning, semantic conditioning, and the orienting reflex. *Psychological Review*, 1961, *68*, 81-147.

Razran, G. Russian physiologists' psychology and American experimental psychology: A historical and a systematic collation and a look into the future. *Psychological Bulletin*, 1965, *63*, 42-64.

Reichenbach, H. *Experience and prediction*. Chicago: University of Chicago Press. 1938.

Reitman, W. *Cognition and thought: An information-processing approach*. New York: Wiley, 1965.

Restle, F. The selection of strategies in cue learning. *Psychological Review*, 1962, *69*, 329-343.

Rieber, R. W. *Body and mind: Past, present, and future*. New York: Academic Press, 1980.

Roback, A. A. *History of American psychology*. New York: Collier Books, 1964.

Rogers, C. R. *On becoming a person*. Boston: Houghton-Mifflin, 1970.

Rosch, E. Cognitive representation of semantic categories. *Journal of Experimental Psychology: General*, 1975, *104*(3), 192-233.

Rosch, E., & Lloyd, B. *Cognition and categorization*. Hillsdale, NJ: Erlbaum, 1978.

Rosenblueth, A., Wiener, N., & Bigelow, J. Behavior, purpose, and teleology. *Philosophy of Science*, 1943, *10*, 18–24.

Ross, A. O. *The practice of clinical child psychology*. New York: Grune & Stratton, 1959.

Ross, A. O. *The exceptional child in the family*. New York: Grune & Stratton, 1964.

Ross, A. O. *Psychological disorders of children: A behavioral approach to theory, research, and therapy*. New York: McGraw-Hill, 1974.

Ross, A. O. *Psychological aspects of learning disabilities and reading disorders*. New York: McGraw-Hill, 1976.

Rumelhart, D. E., & McClelland, J. *Parallel distributed processing: Studies in the microstructure of cognition*. Cambridge, MA: Bradford Books, in press.

Rumelhart, D. E., & Norman, D. A. Accretion, tuning, and restructuring: Three models of learning. In J. W. Cotton & R. Klatzky (Eds.), *Semantic factors in cognition*. Hillsdale, NJ: Erlbaum, 1978.

Russell, B., & Whitehead, A. N. *Principia mathematica* (Vol. 1). London: Cambridge University Press, 1910.

Ryle, G. *The concept of mind*. London: Cambridge University Press, 1949.

Salzinger, K. Pleasing linguists: A parable. *Journal of Verbal Learning and Verbal Behavior*, 1970, *9*, 725–727.

Salzinger, K. Inside the black box, with apologies to Pandora: A review of Ulric Neisser's *Cognitive psychology*. *Journal of the Experimental Analysis of Behavior*, 1973, *19*, 369–378.

Samelson, F. History, origin myth and ideology: "Discovery" of social psychology. *Journal for the Theory of Social Behavior*, 1974, *4*, 217–231.

Savage, C. W. Introspectionist and behaviorist interpretations of ratio scales of perceptual magnitudes. *Psychological Monographs: General and Applied*, 1966, *80*(19), Whole No. 627.

Schachter, S., & Singer, J. Cognitive, social, and physiological determinants of emotional state. *Psychological Review*, 1962, *69*(5), 379–399.

Schafer, R. *A new language of psychoanalysis*. New Haven, CT: Yale University Press, 1976.

Schank, R. C., & Colby, K. M. (Eds.). *Computer models of thought and language*. San Francisco: W. H. Freeman, 1973.

Schuell, H., Jenkins, J. J., & Jimenez-Pabon, E. *Aphasia in adults: Diagnosis, prognosis, and treatment*. New York: Harper & Row, 1964.

Sears, R. R. *Survey of objective studies of psychoanalytic concepts*. New York: Social Science Research Council, Bulletin 51, 1943.

Selfridge, O. G., & Neisser, U. Pattern recognition by machine. *Scientific American*, 1960, *203*, 60–68.

Selz, O. *Über die Gesetze des geordneten Denkverlaufs. Eine experimentelle Untersuchung*. Erster Teil, Stuttgart: Spemann, 1981.

Shakow, D., & Rapaport, D. The influence of Freud on American psychology. *Psychological Issues*, 1963, *4*(1), Monograph 13, Whole issue.

Shallice, T. Dual functions of consciousness. *Psychological Review*, 1972, *79*(5), 383–393.

Shallice, T. The Dominant Action System: An information-processing approach to consciousness. In K. S. Pope & J. L. Singer (Eds.), *The stream of consciousness: Scientific investigations into the flow of experience*. New York: Plenum, 1978.

Shannon, C. E., & Weaver, W. *The mathematical theory of communication*. Urbana, IL: University of Illinois Press, 1949.

Shapiro, A. K. A contribution to the history of placebo effect. *Behavioral Science*, 1960, *5*, 109–135.

Shaw, R., & McIntyre, M. Algoristic foundations for cognitive psychology. In W. B. Weimer & D. S. Palermo (Eds.), *Cognition and the symbolic processes*. Hillsdale, NJ: Erlbaum, 1974.

Shaw, R. E., & Wilson, B. E. Conceptual knowledge: How we know what we know. In D. Klahr (Ed.), *Cognition and instruction*. Hillsdale, NJ: Erlbaum, 1976.

Simon, H. A. *Administrative behavior*. New York: Macmillan, 1947.

Simon, H. A. *Models of thought*. New Haven, CT: Yale University Press, 1979.

Simon, H. A. *The sciences of the artificial*. Cambridge, MA: MIT Press, 1981. (First published, 1969.)

Singer, P. *Animal liberation*. New York: Avon Books, 1975.

Skinner, B. F. *The behavior of organisms*. New York: Appleton-Century-Crofts, 1938.

Skinner, B. F. Review of Hull's *Principles of behavior*. *American Journal of Psychology*, 1944, *57*, 276–281.

Skinner, B. F. *Walden two*. New York: Macmillan, 1948.

Skinner, B. F. Are theories of learning necessary? *Psychological Review*, 1950, *57*, 193–216.

Skinner, B. F. *Science and human behavior*. New York: Macmillan, 1953.

Skinner, B. F. *Verbal behavior*. New York: Appleton-Century-Crofts, 1957.

Skinner, B. F. John Broadus Watson, behaviorist. *Science*, 1959, *129*, 197–198.

Skinner, B. F. A lecture on "having" a poem. In *Cumulative record*. New York: Appleton-Century-Crofts, 1961, 345–354.

Skinner, B. F. Behaviorism at fifty. *Science*, 1963, *140*, 951–958.

Skinner, B. F. Some responses to the stimulus "Pavlov." *Conditional Reflex*, 1966, *1*, 74–78.

Skinner, B. F. B. F. Skinner. In E. G. Boring & G. Lindzey (Eds.), *A history of psychology in autobiography* (Vol. 5). New York: Appleton-Century-Crofts, 1967.

Skinner, B. F. *Beyond freedom and dignity*. New York: Knopf, 1971.

Skinner, B. F. *Cumulative record: A collection of papers* (3rd ed.). New York: Appleton-Century-Crofts, 1972.

Skinner, B. F. *About behaviorism*. New York: Random House, 1974.

Skinner, B. F. *Particulars of my life*. New York: Knopf, 1976.

Skinner, B. F. Why I am not a cognitive psychologist. *Behaviorism*, 1977, *5*(2), 1–11.

Skinner, B. F. *The shaping of a behaviorist*. New York: Knopf, 1979.

Skinner, B. F. *A matter of consequences*. New York: Knopf, 1983.

Skinner, B. F., Solomon, H. C., & Lindsley, O. R. Studies in behavior therapy. Metropolitan State Hospital, Waltham, MA, Status Report 1, November, 1953.

Smith, M. L., & Glass, G. V. Meta-analysis of psychotherapy outcome studies. *American Psychologist*, 1977, *132*, 752–760.

Snow, C. P. *The two cultures and the scientific revolution*. London: Cambridge University Press, 1959.

Snygg, D., & Coombs, A. W. *Individual behavior*. New York: Harper & Row, 1949.

Sokolov, E. N. *Perception and the orienting reflex*. New York: Macmillan, 1963.

Spearman, C. The proof and measurement of association between two things. *American Journal of Psychology*, 1940a, *15*, 72–101.

Spearman, C. "General intelligence," objectively determined and measured. *American Journal of Psychology*, 1940b, *15*, 201–292.

Spence, K. W. Cognitive versus stimulus–response theories of learning. *Psychological Review*, 1950, *57*, 159–172.

Sperling, G. The information available in brief visual presentations. *Psychological Monographs*, 1960, *74*(11), Whole No. 498.

Sternberg, S. High-speed scanning in human memory. *Science*, 1966, *153*, 652–654.

Sternberg, S. The discovery of processing stages: Extension of Donder's method. In W. G. Koster (Ed.), *Attention and performance II*. Amsterdam: North-Holland, 1969. (Reprinted from *Acta Psychologica*, 1969, *30*, 276–315.)

Stevens, K. N. Toward a model for speech recognition. *Journal of the Acoustic Society of America*, 1960, *32*, 47–55.

Stevens, S. S. The operational definition of psychological concepts. *Psychological Review*, 1935, *42*, 517–527.

Stevens, S. S. Operations or words? *Psychological Monographs: General and Applied*, 1966, *80*, 33–38.

Stich, S. S. *From folk psychology to cognitive science: The case against belief.* Cambridge, MA: MIT Press, 1983.

Strange, W., Jenkins, J. J., & Johnson, T. Dynamic specification of coarticulated words. *Journal of the Acoustical Society of America*, 1984, *74*, 695–705.

Strange, W., Keeney, T., Kessel, F. S., & Jenkins, J. J. Abstraction over time of prototypes from distortions of random dot patterns. *Journal of Experimental Psychology*, 1970, *83*, 508–510.

Suppes, P. Stimulus–response theory of finite automata. *Journal of Mathematical Psychology*, 1969, *6*, 327–355.

Swets, J. A., & Birdsall, T. G. The human use of information. III: Decision-making in signal detection and recognition situations involving multiple alternatives. *IRE Transactions on Information Theory*, 1956, *IT-2*(3).

Szilard, L. On the decrease in entropy in a thermodynamic system by the intervention of intelligent beings (A. Rapoport & M. Knoller, Trans.). *Behavioral Science*, 1964, *9*, 301–310. (First published, 1929, in German.)

Thorndike, E. L. *Human learning.* New York: Appleton-Century-Crofts, 1931.

Titchener, E. On "Psychology as the behaviorist views it." *Proceedings of the American Philosophical Society*, 1914, *53*, 1–17.

Tolman, E. C. A behaviorist's definition of consciousness. *Psychological Review*, 1927, *34*(6), 433–439.

Tolman, E. C. *Purposive behavior in animals and men.* New York: Appleton-Century-Crofts, 1932.

Tolman, E. C. Cognitive maps in rats and men. *Psychological Review*, 1948, *55*, 189–208.

Troland, L. T. *The fundamentals of human motivation.* New York: Van Nostrand, 1928.

Tulving, E. Episodic and semantic memory. In E. Tulving & W. Donaldson (Eds.), *Organization and memory.* New York: Academic Press, 1972.

Turing, A. M. Computing machinery and intelligence. *Mind*, 1950, *LIX*(236).

Ullmann, L. P., & Krasner, L. *A psychological approach to abnormal behavior.* Englewood Cliffs, NJ: Prentice-Hall, 1969, (2nd ed., 1975.)

Underwood, G. *Aspects of consciousness* (Vol. 3). London: Academic Press, 1982.

Von Foerster, H. Biologic. In E. E. Bernard & M. R. Care (Eds.), *Biological prototypes and synthetic systems* (Vol. 1). New York: Plenum Press, 1962.

Von Neumann, J. *The computer and the brain.* New Haven, CT: Yale University Press, 1958.

Wachtel, P. Z. *Psychoanalysis and behavioral therapy.* New York: Basic Books, 1977.

Warren, N. Is a scientific revolution taking place in psychology? Doubts and reservations. *Science Studies*, 1971, *1*, 407–413.

Warren, R. M., & Warren, R. *Helmholtz on perception, its physiology and development.* New York: Wiley, 1968.

Washburn, M. F. *The animal mind.* New York: Macmillan, 1908.

Watson, J. B. Psychology as the behaviorist views it. *Psychological Review*, 1913, *20*, 158–177.

Watson, J. B. *Psychology from the standpoint of a behaviorist.* Philadelphia: Lippincott, 1919.

Watson, J. B. *Behaviorism.* New York: Norton, 1925.

Watson, J. B. *Behaviorism.* (rev. ed.). New York: Harper's, 1930.

Watson, J. B. John B. Watson. In C. Murchison (Ed.), *A history of psychology in autobiography* (Vol. 3). Worcester, MA: Clark University Press, 1936.

Watson, J. B., & Raynor, R. *Psychological care of infant and child.* New York: Norton, 1928.

Watson, R., & Merrifield, M. Characteristics of individuals eminent in psychology in temporal perspective. *Journal of the History of the Behavioral Sciences*, 1973, *9*, 339–359.

Weimer, W. B. Psycholinguistics and Plato's paradoxes of the *Meno*. *American Psychologist*, 1973, *28*, 15–33.

Weimer, W. B. A conceptual framework for cognitive psychology: Motor theories of the mind. In R. Shaw & J. D. Bransford (Eds.), *Perceiving, acting, and knowing*. Hillsdale, NJ: Erlbaum, 1977a.

Weimer, W. B. Science as a rhetorical transaction: Toward a non-justificational conception of rhetoric. *Philosophy and Rhetoric*, 1977b, *10*(1), 1–29.

Weimer, W. B. *Notes on the methodology of scientific research*. Hillsdale, NJ: Erlbaum, 1979.

Weimer, W. B. Psychotherapy and philosophy of science: Examples of a two-way street in search of traffic. In M. J. Mahoney (Ed.), *Psychotherapy process*. New York: Plenum, 1980.

Weimer, W. B., & Palermo, D. S. Paradigms and normal science in psychology. *Science Studies*, 1973, *3*, 211–244.

Weimer, W. B., & Palermo, D. S. (Eds.). *Cognition and the symbolic processes*. Potomac, MD: Erlbaum, 1974.

Weizenbaum, J. *Computer power and human reason: From judgment to calculation*. San Francisco: W. H. Freeman, 1976.

Wertheimer, M. Relativity and Gestalt: A note on Albert Einstein and Max Wertheimer. *Journal of the History of the Behavioral Sciences*, 1965, *1*, 86–87.

Whyte, L. L. *The unconscious before Freud*. New York: Doubleday, 1962.

Wiener, N. *Cybernetics: On control and communication in the animal and the machine* (2nd ed.). Cambridge, MA: MIT Press, 1961.

Williams, M. D., & Hollan, J. D. The process of retrieval from very long-term memory. *Cognitive Science*, 1981, *5*(2), 87–120.

Winograd, T. Understanding natural language. *Cognitive Psychology*, 1972, *3*, 1–191.

Wolpe, J. Cognition and causation in human behavior and its therapy. *American Psychologist*, 1978, *33*(5), 437–446.

Wolpe, J. Behavior therapy vs. psychoanalysis: Therapeutic and social implications. *American Psychologist*, 1981, *36*(2), 159–164.

Woodworth, R. S. A revision of imageless thought. *Psychological Review*, 1915, *22*, 1–27.

Woodworth, R. S. *Experimental psychology*. New York: Holt, 1938.

Woodworth, R. S., & Schlosberg, H. *Experimental psychology* (rev. ed.). New York: Holt, Rinehart & Winston, 1954.

Wundt, W. *Lectures on human and animal psychology* (J. E. Creighton & E. B. Titchener, Trans.). London: Swan Sonnenschein, 1894. (Reprinted in D. N. Robinson (Ed.), *Significant contributions to the history of psychology, 1750–1920*. Washington, DC: University Publications of America, 1978.)

Wundt, W. *An introduction to psychology* (R. Pintner, Trans.). London: George Allen, 1912. (Reprinted by Arno Press, New York, 1973.)

Zadeh, L. A. (Ed.). *Fuzzy sets and their applications to cognitive and decision processes*. New York: Academic Press, 1975.

Zajonc, R. B. Feeling and thinking: Preferences need inferences. *American Psychologist*, 1980, *35*(2), 151–175.

Zilboorg, G. *A history of medical psychology*. New York: Norton, 1941.

Index

adaptation, 273

Adapters, in the cognitive shift, 197–269, 195, 402

additive factors method, 178

adequacy of behaviorism, 46

adequacy of cognitive theory, 159

adolescent quality of early psychology, 14, 15, 400, 406

ambiguities of scientific success, 416, 417

ambiguities of terms used, 5, 6, 158

ambiguity in the experience of events, 321

American cultural difficulties with psychoanalysis, 76

American psychology, 257

animal psychology, 242

animals, ethical treatment of, 83, 84, 414

anthropomorphism, 88

anticipatory goal responses (*see* fractional anticipatory goal responses)

anti-intellectualism, American, in behaviorism 44

antitheoretical trends in behaviorism, 62, 219, 265

antivitalism, 22

aphasia, 248

Artificial Intelligence, 94, 159, 167, 169, 173, 177, 180, 181, 184, 185, 307, 308, 338, 341, 348, 362, 379, 382, 386

associationism, 30, 49, 116, 120, 167, 198, 257, 264, 365

associations, 230, 258

atheoretical approaches, 162, 220

attention, 145, 170, 257

automata, finite, 342, 344

automata, mathematical theory of, 148, 153, 314, 339, 366

B

Bacon, Francis, 19

Bakan, David, 22

Bandura, Albert, 136

Bartlett, Frederick C., 54, 142, 259

Bateson, Gregory, 27, 28, 155

behavior modification (*see* behavior therapy)

behavior therapy, 67, 68, 74–80, 96, 118, 397

behaviorism, viii, 7 (*and see especially* Chapters 1–3, and 8)

Bergmann, Gustav, 100, 101, 115

Bernard, Claude, 22, 23, 28

Bernstein, N., 142

bit, 150

Boring, Edwin G., viii, 30, 52, 62, 73, 202, 204, 288

bottom-up flow of information, 169

Bower, Gordon, 261

Bransford, John, 169, 238, 243, 250, 304, 306, 314, 324

DATE DUE